BIOCHEMISTRY
FOR CLINICAL MEDICINE

BIOCHEMISTY FOR CLINICAL MEDICINE

Ira Thabrew
BSc PhD
Professor and Head
Department of Biochemistry and Clinical Chemistry
Faculty of Medicine
University of Kelaniya
Ragama
Sri-Lanka

Ruth M Ayling
PhD MRCP MRCPath
Consultant Chemical Pathologist
Department of Clinical Biochemistry
King's College Hospital
London
UK

with a contribution by

Claire Wicks
BSc SRD PhD
Post Doctoral Research Fellow
Alton Ochsner Medical Foundation
New Orleans
Lousiana
USA

© 2001

GREENWICH MEDICAL MEDIA LTD
137 Euston Road
London
NW1 2AA

ISBN 1 900151 081

First Published 2001

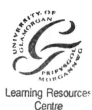
British Library Cataloguing in Publication Data

A Catalogue record for this book is available from the British Library

Typeset by Saxon Graphics Ltd, Derby

Printed in Spain by Grafos

CONTENTS

PREFACE

Developments in biochemistry have contributed immensely to the rate at which medical knowledge has expanded in recent years. In parallel with this expansion of biochemistry is the expansion in the number and variety of published textbooks of biochemistry and clinical biochemistry. However, our aim, in adding yet another to the bookshelf, is to produce a book containing both basic and clinical biochemistry in which we have tried to reduce the factual load to an essential core of knowledge that we consider relevant to students of medicine and other related disciplines.

The book is divided into two sections. Section 1 progresses from chapters providing an understanding of basic cell biology and concepts of membrane transport, cellular energetics, information storage, transmission and expression, to chapters describing the chemistry and metabolism of cellular biomolecules and clinical conditions that arise from disturbances in their metabolism. In section 2, a "systems" approach is used in the organisation of chapters presenting clinical biochemistry.

We thank Dr William Marshall for his support and encouragement during the preparation of this book and thank Geoff Nuttall and the editorial staff of GMM, especially Gavin Smith, for assistance with its publication.

Our aim has not been to produce a complete textbook of biochemistry but a book that will provide a basic knowledge of biochemistry enabling a fuller appreciation of clinical medicine.

Ira Thabrew
Ruth M Ayling
Sri-Lanka & London
September 2000

1

CELLS, ORGANELLES, AND TRANSPORT ACROSS MEMBRANES

Objectives

To understand:

- The types of living cells and the distinguishing characters of each type

- The organisation of cells within the body

- The structure and functional organization of a typical eukaryotic cell and disorders associated with defective cell organelles

- Human chromosomes and chromosomal disorders

- Transport of molecules and ions across cell membranes

Cells are the fundamental structural and functional units of the body. Two thirds of the body mass is cellular and the vast majority of biochemical reactions occur within cells. A knowledge of their structure and function, and organisation into tissues and organs is therefore essential for an understanding of the body and its operation.

TYPES OF LIVING CELLS

Living cells may be subdivided into two major groups based on the nature of the nucleus.

- **Prokaryotes** (e.g. bacteria) lack a well defined nucleus. They usually contain only one chromosome which consists of a single molecule of DNA densely coiled to form a nuclear zone.

- **Eukaryotes** (e.g. animals, plants, algae, fungi, and protozoa), have a well defined nucleus surrounded by a nuclear membrane.

Both eukaryotic and prokaryotic cells are bounded by a *plasma membrane* that separates the cell interior from the extracellular environment. In prokaryotes, however, this plasma membrane is usually surrounded by a rigid *cell wall*. A eukaryotic cell, besides containing a well defined nucleus and nuclear membrane, also has extensive intracellular membrane-bounded organelles and membrane systems, and many of their metabolic reactions are segregated within these intracellular compartments.

ORGANISATION OF CELLS WITHIN THE BODY

The average human body contains about 10^{15} cells.

There are many different types of cells, and within the body, groups of specialised cells are joined together to form *tissues* and *organs*, each of which performs specific tasks essential for the proper functioning of the body. Integration of functions between tissues is mediated by chemical signals (*hormones*) that are secreted by specialised glands (*endocrine glands*). Local chemical messengers that act as *autocrine* (acting on self), or *paracrine* (acting on near neighbours) factors also assist in the interaction and communication between certain specific cell types such as neurones and lymphocytes. In many tissues, communication between neighbouring cells occur through aqueous channels known as *gap junctions*. Each of these channels is formed by a hexagonal arrangement of 12 molecules of the transmembrane protein *connexin* High $[Ca^{2+}]$ and low pH in cells causes closure of these channels.

STRUCTURAL AND FUNCTIONAL ORGANISATION OF A TYPICAL EUKARYOTIC CELL

The structure of eukaryotic cells varies from organism to organism, and from tissue to tissue within an organism. Figure 1.1 shows a diagrammatic representation of a typical eukaryotic cell. The cell boundary is delineated by the *plasma membrane*. Between the plasma membrane and the *nucleus* is the *cytoplasm* composed of an aqueous phase known as the *cytosol*, within which are distributed several different *organelles* (*mitochondria, lysosomes, golgi complex, peroxisomes,* and *the endoplasmic reticular network*), each performing a specific function within the cell.

PLASMA MEMBRANE AND MEMBRANES SURROUNDING INTRACELLULAR ORGANELLES

Cell membranes are mainly assemblies of *lipid* and *protein* molecules held together by non-covalent interactions (Figure 1.2). Some of the proteins and lipids (exclusively those on the external side of the membrane) may be covalently linked to carbohydrate residues to form *glycoproteins* or *glycolipids* respectively. The proportions of protein:lipid vary widely from membrane to membrane. For example, the plasma membrane has a protein:lipid ratio of 1:4, while the inner mitochondrial membrane has a corresponding ratio of 3:2. Generally, a membrane with many functions (e.g. the inner mitochondrial membrane), has a high protein content; whereas a membrane with fewer

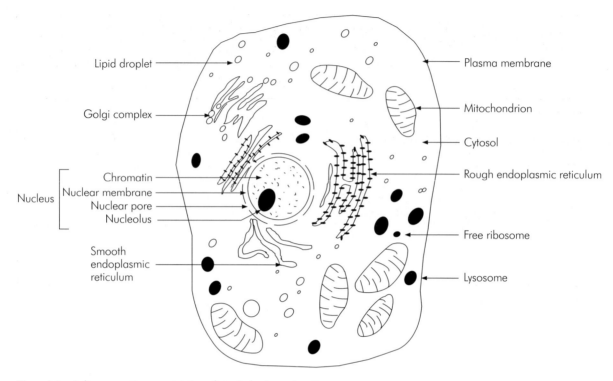

Figure 1.1 – A diagrammatic representation of a typical eukaryotic cell.

functions (e.g. myelin) has much less protein (protein: lipid ratio in myelin is 0:3). The specific properties of a particular membrane are usually due to the protein while more general characteristics such as electrical resistance and passive permeability are features of the lipid component.

Membrane lipids

The lipid molecules in membranes are usually arranged as a continuous bilayer (Figure 1.2). Molecules forming this bilayer are mainly *phospholipids*, together with small amounts of *cholesterol* and *glycolipids*. All these molecules are *amphipathic*, and possess a hydrophobic or non-polar end and a hydrophilic or polar end. In order to achieve the greatest stability, these molecules are arranged with the hydrophilic portions facing the exterior of each lipid layer, and the hydrophobic portions projecting towards the interior of the membrane. As shown in Table 1.1, the proportions of the different classes of lipids vary from membrane to membrane; they are, however, remarkably constant for a particular membrane type.

Lipids are not distributed uniformly in membranes. For example, in the plasma membrane, all the glycolipids and most of the phosphatidyl choline are in the extracellular side whereas phosphatidyl ethanolamine and phosphatidyl serine are predominantly in the cytoplasmic side. There is also evidence that under certain circumstances (e.g. in response to hormonal stimuli), molecules of a similar class of lipids cluster together within a particular part of a bilayer.

Membrane proteins

According to the currently accepted *lipid-protein mosaic model* of Sanger and Nicolson (Figure 1.2), membrane proteins may be *peripheral* (bound at the membrane surface) or *integral* (embedded partly or wholly in the lipid bilayer). Most membrane proteins are integral. Peripheral proteins are usually attached by electrostatic and hydrogen bonds to integral proteins, or to polar lipid head groups. Proteins may cluster together in specific areas of the membrane to form *multienzyme complexes*, or *respiratory complexes*. Different membranes also have characteristic protein compositions (Table 1.2).

The integral proteins that penetrate the lipid bilayer are exposed to both external and internal environments, and provide a means of communication across the bilayer that may be useful in the transport of metabolites, ions, and water or as in the plasma membrane, in

LIPID COMPOSITION (PERCENTAGE OF TOTAL LIPID) OF DIFFERENT MEMBRANES IN A HUMAN LIVER CELL			
Lipid	Plasma membrane	Endoplasmic reticulum	Mitochondrion
Cholesterol	20	5	3
Phosphatidyl choline	19	48	38
Phosphatidyl ethanolamine	12	19	29
Phosphatidyl serine	7	4	trace
Sphingomyelin	12	5	–
Cardiolipin	–	–	14
Glycolipids	trace	–	–

Table 1.1

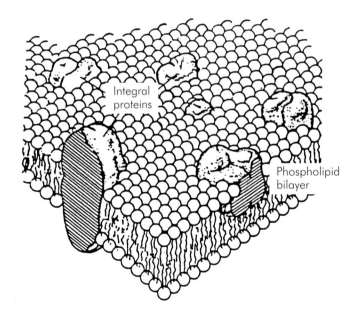

Integral proteins

Phospholipid bilayer

Figure 1.2 – The Singer-Nicholson fluid mosaic model of membrane structure. The model shows globular integral proteins (with stippled surfaces) randomly distributed in the plane of the phospholipid bilayer. (With kind permission from Luzio, J.P. and Thompson, R.J., Molecular Medical Biochemistry, Cambridge University Press, Cambridge, 1990, p99).

the transmission of signals in response to external stimuli provided by hormones, antibodies or other cells. The presence of specific energy dependent transport proteins enables membranes to be *selectively permeable* and allow only certain types of molecules to be transported into and out of cells and organelles, and also maintain ionic gradients between their internal and external environments.

THE CYTOSOL

The cytosol is the non-sedimentable, *soluble fraction of the cytoplasm* in which all the subcellular structures are suspended. It is also the site where many biochemical processes are localised. The major metabolic processes associated with the cytosol are:

• biosynthesis and catabolism of carbohydrates

SOME CHARACTERISTIC PROTEINS IN SELECTED MEMBRANES	
Membrane type	Characteristic protein
Plasma membrane	5'-Nucleotidase Na+/K+ ATPase
Endoplasmic reticulum	Glucose-6-phosphatase
Inner mitochondrial membrane	Succinate dehydrogenase Cytochrome oxidase
Golgi complex	Glycosyl transferase
Lysosomes	Acid phosphatase β-Glucuronidase

Table 1.2

- biosynthesis of fatty acids and steroids

- biosynthesis of purines and pyrimidines

Electron microscopy and immunofluorescence techniques have revealed the presence of a structural lattice in the cytosol that gives the cell its shape, and provides a basis for its movements. This lattice contains *microtubules* which traverse the cytoplasm, *microfilaments* that are adjacent to the plasma membrane and *intermediate filaments* that form a fine web within the cytoplasm. Each of these types is composed of a different type of contractile protein. The microfilaments (7 nm in diameter) contain mainly actin, and are involved in cell movements and clot retraction. Intermediate filaments (7–11 nm in diameter) contain keratin and several other proteins that contribute to the mechanical stability of the cell and internal structures. Microtubules (about 30 nm diameter) contain mainly α- and β-tubulins and participate in chromosome separation in mitosis and movement of cilia, and intracellular transport of vesicles and organelles.

Clinical disorders associated with cytoskeletal abnormalities

Cytoskeletal abnormalities have been implicated as being important determinants of certain disease states. For example, in *Immotile Cilia Syndrome*, the microtubules of the respiratory epithelial cilia interfere with the ability of such epithelium to clear inhaled bacteria which predisposes to lung infections. *Male sterility* may be caused by defects in microtubules in spermatozoa inhibiting their motility.

THE NUCLEUS

This is the largest intracellular organelle (about 4–6 μm in diameter), and is surrounded by a double-membraned envelope (Figure 1.1). It is present in all cells of the body except mature red blood cells. Most cell types contain a single nucleus, but muscle cells and some liver cells are multinucleate. The nuclear contents communicate with the cytosol through pores in the nuclear envelope. The nucleus contains *chromatin* which consists of *15% DNA, 10% RNA and 75% protein*. It acts as the main repository of cellular DNA, and is the site of DNA-directed processes including DNA replication and DNA-directed RNA biosynthesis. The DNA of human cells is organised into *chromosomes* and is usually associated with basic proteins called *histones*. Sperm contain another protein called *protamine* in place of histones.

Chromatin is usually amorphous except during cell division when the individual chromosomes become visible. Specialised areas in the nucleus, the *nucleoli* (one or more per nucleus) are the only morphologically distinct bodies within the nucleus at other times. They are rich in RNA and are the sites where ribosomal RNA is synthesised and temporarily stored before it is assembled into ribosomal precursors and transported out of the nucleus.

MITOCHONDRIA

Mitochondria are the major site of energy (ATP) production. Each mitochondrion (Figure 1.3) consists of four compartments.

A central *matrix* is surrounded by an *inner mitochondrial membrane* with which are associated cytochromes of the respiratory chain and the enzymes of oxidative phosphorylation (Chapter 2). This membrane is thrown into a number of folds or *cristae* which penetrate deeply into the matrix and serve to increase the surface area of the membrane. This membrane is also studded with small spherical particles that are attached by short stalks. The spherical particles contain the proteins involved in ATP synthesis. The inner membrane is impermeable to sucrose and most metabolites, and contains many specific and elaborate transport systems which help to move substances in and products out. Outside this membrane is the *outer mitochondrial membrane* which separates the mitochondrion from the rest of the cytoplasm. The space between the inner and outer membranes is sometimes referred to as the *sucrose permeable space*.

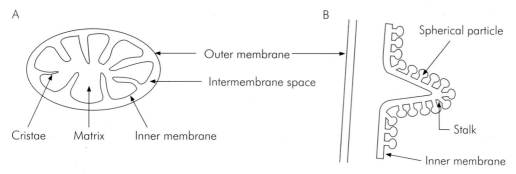

Figure 1.3 – A diagrammatic representation of (A) a mitochondrion (section), and (B) arrangement of the spherical particles on the inner mitochondrial membrane.

As shown in Table 1.3, each of the mitochondrial compartments has its characteristic complement of enzymes, and this subdivision is vital for the overall control of metabolism.

In addition to the enzymes listed, the matrix also contains mitochondrial DNA, ribosomes and other components necessary for the synthesis of some mitochondrial proteins. Mitochondrial DNA lacks histones and is not organised into chromosomes.

Clinical disorders associated with mitochondrial defects

Defects in the structure and function of mitochondria (mitochondrial cytopathies) underlie development of some *chronic neuromuscular diseases* with widely varying clinical expressions, but the exact biochemical mechanisms are not well understood.

Mitochondrial cytopathies associated with severe impairment of aerobic metabolism in organs such as the heart, kidney, liver and brain are likely to be incompatible with life. Less severe mitochondrial deficiencies may become clinically apparent at a level of cell activity at which the energy demand is not satisfied (e.g. exercise intolerance or a fluctuating clinical course in patients with neuronal involvement).

LYSOSOMES

Lysosomes are small, single-membraned organelles, that act as the 'waste baskets' of the cell. They contain *hydrolytic enzymes* (e.g. cathepsins, ribonuclease, deoxyribonuclease, phosphatase, sphingomyelinase). It is advantageous to the cell to maintain such enzymes in a separate compartment so that intracellular structures are not degraded. Lysosomal enzymes are utilized in the digestion of:

- materials brought into the cell by *phagocytosis* or *pinocytosis*

- cell components after death

Lysosomes may be formed *de novo* from vesicles budding off from the golgi complex; these are known as *primary lysosomes*. Initiation of hydrolytic activity occurs only once they fuse with membrane-bounded vesicles known as *endosomes* that contain undigested material; they are then referred to as *secondary lysosomes*. Within lysosomes, an acidic pH (pH 5) is maintained although in the remainder of the cytosol the pH is 7. Specific ATP-dependent reactions are responsible for this acidic differential. Most of the lysosomal enzymes are unusually highly glycosylated. This may help to protect these proteins from lysosomal proteases in the lumen.

CHARACTERISTIC ENZYMES FOUND IN EACH OF THE MITOCHONDRIAL COMPARTMENTS	
Compartment	Enzyme
Outer membrane	Monoamine oxidase Cytochrome b5
Sucrose permeable space	Adenylate kinase
Inner membrane	Cytochromes a, a3, b, c, c1 NADH dehydrogenase - Succinate dehydrogenase
Matrix	Enzymes of the TCA cycle Glutamate dehydrogenase Enzymes required for fatty acid oxidation

Table 1.3

Clinical disorders associated with lysosomal defects

Lysosomes are involved directly, or indirectly, in any disease process in which there is cell death, cell involution, or cell injury. Inherited defects or deficiencies in lysosomal enzymes are known to give rise to over 20 different disease conditions referred to as *lysosomal storage diseases*. For example, *Tay-Sach's disease*, a rare, inherited neurological disease is due to a defect in *hexosaminidase A*, required for the catabolism of gangliosides, similarly, *Niemann-Pick disease* is due to a deficiency in *sphingomyelinase*, required for the catabolism of sphingomyelin. In *Sly syndrome* (*Mucopolysaccharidosis VII*), there is a deficiency of β-glucuronidase; this results in the pathological behaviour of a number of tissues (liver, spleen, brain, kidney and cornea) because proteoglycans are not being degraded.

Such enzyme abnormalities result in an accumulation of the substrate of that particular enzyme in the lysosome. The organelles become enlarged, and crowding interferes with cell function. In *gout*, the underlying disease is due to an accumulation of urate within cells, lysosomes become damaged, and their hydrolytic enzymes leak into the cell, resulting in injury to cells and tissues.

PEROXISOMES

Peroxisomes, are small, single-membraned vesicles that contain several oxidative enzymes (e.g. catalase, D-amino acid oxidase, and urate oxidase) that are associated with peroxide metabolism. For example, *catalase* catalyses the following reaction:

$$2H_2O_2 \rightarrow 2H_2O + O_2$$

Because H_2O_2 is toxic, its metabolism must be restricted as much as possible to a special compartment within the cell.

Peroxisomes also contain dihydroxyacetone phosphate acyltransferase and alkyl dihydroxyacetone phosphate synthase, which are involved in the synthesis of plasmalogans. Peroxisomes are also thought to participate in the biosynthesis of bile acids.

Clinical disorders associated with peroxisomal defects

Three genetic disorders, *Zellweger's syndrome, neonatal adrenoleucodystrophy,* and *childhood adrenoleucodystrophy* are associated with defective formation of peroxisomes, or deficiency of one or more constituent enzymes. In Zellweger's syndrome, there are no morphologically detectable peroxisomes, which is thought to be due to a deficiency of a 70 kDa peroxisomal protein with an as yet unknown function.

ENDOPLASMIC RETICULUM

The endoplasmic reticulum consists of a series of flattened membranous sacs and tubes extending throughout the cell cytoplasm, enclosing a large, intracellular space and structurally continuous with the outer membrane of the nuclear envelope. There are two types of endoplasmic reticulum – the *rough endoplasmic reticulum* (*RER*) has ribosomes associated with it externally, and the *smooth endoplasmic reticulum* (*SER*) is more tubular and lacks ribosomes.

The *RER* is mainly involved in the synthesis of proteins. The *SER* is involved in packaging and delivering proteins to the golgi complex. It is also a major site for lipid biosynthesis. Associated with the SER are enzymes responsible for the synthesis of sterols, triacylglycerols, and phospholipids. Other enzymes associated with it include those involved in the desaturation and elongation of fatty acids, hydrolysis of glucose-6-phosphate, and the detoxification of drugs. It also houses *cytochrome b_5* which serves as a limited electron carrier system in desaturation of fatty acids, and *cytochrome P450* which participates in the detoxification of drugs and other toxic compounds, especially in liver cells.

THE GOLGI COMPLEX

The golgi complex consists of a series of flat, single-membrane vesicles (cisternae) which are often stacked. The golgi apparatus receives newly synthesised proteins and lipids from the endoplasmic reticulum and distributes them to the plasma membrane, lysosomes, and secretory vesicles. Protein molecules passing through the golgi apparatus usually undergo various post-translational modifications. Initial modifications may include lipid additions or phosphorylations. This is followed by the addition of terminal sugars, by the many *glycosyl transferases* present in golgi to form glycoproteins. During the production of active secretory products, such as hormones, selected portions of the polypeptide chains may be removed from larger precursor molecules during their passage through golgi cisternae.

HUMAN CHROMOSOMES

In each eukaryotic species there is a characteristic number of chromosomes per cell. Each chromosome contains *genes* (the fundamental units of genetic information) arranged in a linear sequence along it. In a human diploid cell there are 23 pairs of chromosomes, giving a diploid number of 46, with half as many in a haploid cell. Of these, 22 pairs are alike in males and females and are called *autosomes*. The remaining pair, denoted by XX in females and XY in males, are referred to as *sex chromosomes*. One member of each pair of autosomal chromosomes is inherited from the mother, and the other from the father. Each of these autosomal chromosomes carries matching genetic information. Alternative forms of a gene are called *alleles*. If an individual has two identical alleles, he is *homozygous* for that gene or inherited characteristic; he is *heterozygous* if he has two different alleles.

Autosomal inheritance means inheritance of genes located on autosomes, while *X-linked inheritance* refers to inheritance of genes on the X-chromosome. If one copy of a gene is sufficient for the expression of a particular observable character in an individual, such a gene is said to be *dominant*. A gene is *recessive* if two copies of the gene are required for expression of an individual's phenotype. The gene responsible for *sickle cell anaemia* is an autosomal recessive type, while that responsible for *familial hypercholesteraemia*, for example, is an autosomal dominant type. *Haemophilia* is inherited in a sex-linked manner. Males with haemophilia genes are affected because they contain only one X-chromosome. In females, even if one of the two X-chromosomes contain a haemophilia gene, expression of the normal allele produces a normal phenotype.

Clinical conditions associated with chromosome changes

> *Down syndrome* — individuals with this condition possess three copies of chromosome 21 (trisomy 21).

> *Turner syndrome* — is characterised by an XO karytope and female protase.

> *Klinefelter syndrome* — individuals possess one Y-chromosome and at least two X-chromosomes.

> *Chronic myelogenous leukemia* — in about 95% of these individuals, chromosome 22 is shorter than normal because of a reciprocal translocation of segments between chromosomes 22 and 9. This abbreviated form of chromosome 22 is referred to as the *Philadelphia chromosome* and denoted Ph[1].

TRANSPORT OF MOLECULES AND IONS ACROSS CELL MEMBRANES

Three major mechanisms are responsible for the transport of water and other solutes in body fluids across cell membranes:

- simple diffusion

- facilitated diffusion via carriers or ion channels

- active mediated transport

SIMPLE DIFFUSION

The spontaneous movement of uncharged molecules or ions from a higher to a lower concentration is known as *diffusion*. Movement of molecules or ions by diffusion will occur until an equilibrium is reached. This process is energy independent, and the driving force for it is the *electrochemical gradient* across the membrane. Movement of molecules across membranes can occur in both directions (Figure 1.4).

FACILITATED DIFFUSION

Facilitated diffusion via carrier proteins — This type of diffusion is believed to depend upon the presence in the cell membrane of a relatively small number of *carrier proteins*. These carrier proteins ferry the solute molecules across the membrane by first binding to the solute molecule at the border of the membrane at which the solute concentration is higher. The solute-carrier protein complex then moves to the opposite border of the membrane where it dissociates to deliver the solute into the fluid on that side (Figure 1.5) As in simple diffusion, solutes can move in both directions in the membrane. Many solutes of physiological importance, such as sugars and amino acids are transported in this way. Seven different glucose transporters, each encoded by separate genes, have been identified.

Important features of facilitated diffusion systems are:

- transport of polar molecules occurs at a rate much faster than by simple diffusion

- they demonstrate saturation kinetics

- carrier molecules demonstrate structural specificity for the substrate (e.g. L-glucose cannot be transported by the D-glucose carrier)

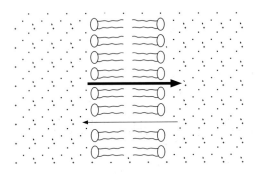

Figure 1.4 – Schematic representation of passive diffusion. The net flow of molecules occurs from the compartment with the higher to that with the lower concentration until the concentrations are equal in the two compartments.

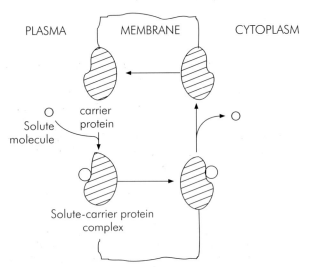

Figure 1.5 – Solute transport by facilitated diffusion via a carrier protein.

- they can be compeietively inhibited by structurally similar molecules (e.g. transport of D-glucose inhibited by D-galactose)

Facilitated diffusion through ion channels — The electrical charge on *small ions* such as Na^+, K^+, Ca^{2+} and Cl^- makes it very difficult for them to move across the lipid bilayer. Fast movements of such ions are, however necessary for certain cellular functions, (e.g. nerve action potential, muscle contraction, pacemaker function of the heart). Movement of small ions across cell membranes is made possible by the operation of selective *ion channels* in the cell membrane. Ion channels are intrinsic proteins spanning the width of the cell membrane and are normally composed of several homologous, polypeptide subunits (typically 4, 5, or

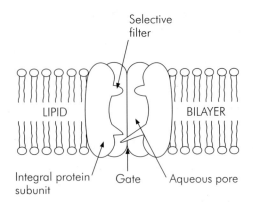

Figure 1.6 – A diagrammatic representation of an ion channel.

6). Certain specific stimuli cause the protein subunits to open a *gate* creating an aqueous channel through which the ions can move without having to interact with the lipid bilayer (Figure 1.6).

Ion channels are often selective. For example, there are specific channels for Na^+, K^+, Ca^{2+} and Cl^- as well as for other monovalent ions. The high degree of specificity of many channels depends on the type of interaction between the transported ion and residues lining the pore at a region called *the selectivity filter*. The degree of selectivity also depends upon the diameter of the narrowest part of the pore. The transition between the open and closed forms of a channel is allosterically regulated by voltage, the binding of another molecule or covalent modification.

According to the *gating mechanisms* (signals that make channels open) ion channels can be described as

- voltage gated

- ligand gated

Voltage gated ion channels open because changes in membrane potential beyond a certain threshold cause some charged amino acids in the channel to move and induce a conformational change in the protein.

Ligand gated or *chemically gated ion channels* cannot open unless they first bind specific agonist (e.g. an extracellular neurotransmitter or an intracellular second messenger). A conformational change in the protein induced by ligand binding opens the gate.

ACTIVE TRANSPORT

Active transport differs from both simple and facilitated diffusion in that it proceeds against a concentration gradient or electrical potential with consequent energy expenditure. Movement of solutes is also unidirectional. The energy source can be ATP, the electrochemical gradient of Na^+ or H^+ (sodium-motive force or proton-motive force respectively), or light. Active transport processes are important in:

- maintainance of Na^+ and K^+ gradients across plasma membranes

- the uptake of nutrients by the internal mucosa

- the reabsorption of solutes by the epithelia of the renal tubules

Intrinsic membrane proteins that directly use metabolic energy to transport ions against a concentration gradient or electrical potential are known as *ion pumps* or *ATPases*. Active transporters undergo a cycle of conformational changes that simultaneously changes the orientation and affinity of the binding site for the transported species. Two of the best known pumps are the *sodium pump* (Na^+– K^+ ATPase) in the plasma membrane and the *calcium pump* (Ca^{2+}-ATPase) in the plasma membrane, endoplasmic reticulum and the sarcoplasmic reticulum.

The Ca^{2+}-ATPase pumps Ca^{2+} from the cytosol of the cell into the extracellular space, so as to maintain a low cytosolic calcium concentration.

Other known pumps are the *proton pumps* (H^+ATPase) in the membranes of the lysosomes and golgi apparatus that pump H^+ from the cytosol into these organelles, and the H^+–K^+ATPase pumps found in the luminal membrane of the gastric parietal cells; they pump H^+ into the stomach lumen in exchange for K^+.

The Sodium pump — operates in all cells to maintain a high intracellular K^+ concentration and a low intracellular Na^+ concentration (Figure 1.7). This pump is an integral plasma membrane protein and consists of a tetramer of two large and two small subunits. Binding of intracellular Na^+ and phosphorylation by ATP inside the cell is thought to induce a conformational change that transfers Na^+ out of the cell. Subsequent binding of extracellular K^+ and dephosphorylation returns the protein to its original form and transfers K^+ into the cell. During each cycle, three Na^+ ions are exchanged for two K^+ ions and one ATP molecule is hydrolysed.

The sodium pump as a clinical drug target

The cardiotonic actions of steroids such as *digitalis* have

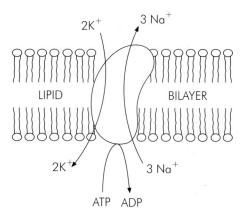

Figure 1.7 – The role of the sodium pump in the transport of Na^+ out of the cell and of K^+ into the cell.

been shown to be due to their inhibition of the Na^+–K^+ ATPase pump. They bind to an external site and inhibit dephosphorylation. The increased force of contraction of the heart following the administration of digitalis is caused by elevated levels of Ca^{2+}. The digitalis-mediated reduction in the Na^+ gradient across the plasma membrane leads to a lowered rate of Ca^{2+} extrusion via the Na^+/ K^+ ion exchanger.

Sodium-coupled transport (Secondary active transport)

The energy needed for the active transport of several compounds is provided by the movement of Na^+ down its concentration gradient. The coupled transport of glucose and Na^+ by the cells of the intestinal mucosa is a good example of this process (Figure 1.8).

The Na^+ gradient across the luminal surface is maintained by the action of the sodium pump at the serosal surface. Glucose passes from the intracellular fluid to the extracellular fluid by facilitated diffusion.

There are two types of secondary transport systems:

- *symport* or *co-transport systems* that transport the solute in the same direction as the Na^+ (e.g. Na^+-coupled glucose or amino acid transport in the gut and renal tubules)

- *antiport* or *exchange systems* that transport the solute in the opposite direction to Na^+ movement (e.g. Na^+/H^+ exchange and Na^+/ Ca^{2+} exchange systems in the plasma membranes of many cells)

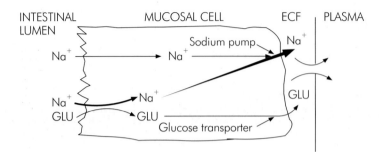

Figure 1.8 – The sodium-linked transport of glucose (GLU) across cells of the intestinal mucosa.

SELECTED READING

Becker, W.M. and Deamer, D.W. – The World of the Cell, 2nd ed., Benjamin/Cummings, Menlo Park, California, 1991.

Singer, S.J. and Nicholson, G.L. The Fluid Mosaic Model of the structure of the cell membrane. 1972 *Science*; **175**: 720–731.

Thompson, M.W., McInnes, R.R. and Willard, H.F. Genetics in Medicine, 5th ed., W.B.Saunders Company, Philadelphia, 1991.

Von Lichtenberg, F. – Cellular injury and adaptation, *In:* R.S. Cotran, V.Kumar and S.L. Robbins (eds), Pathologic Basis of Disease, 5th ed., W.B.Saunders Company, Philadelphia, 1989, 1–38.

2

CELLULAR ENERGETICS AND ENERGY PRODUCTION

Objectives

To understand:

- Basic facts about bioenergetics -free energy and relationship to cellular reactions, coupling of energy-requiring and energy-liberating reactions, energy release on ATP hydrolysis, high energy and low energy compounds

- Metabolic generation of ATP – roles played by the citric acid cycle, respiratory chain (oxidative phosphorylation) and factors controlling these pathways

- The mechanisms by which metabolites (mainly reducing equivalents) are transferred across the inner mitochondrial membrane

- How respiratory chain dysfunction can result in disease

- The consequences of incomplete reduction of oxygen (biological and clinical) and defence mechanisms against reactive oxygen and other free radicals

- The role of the electron transfer pathways in the endoplasmic reticulum

Energy is essential for living organisms to carry out the normal functions of the body. Energy is not only required for mechanical work, maintainance of body temperature and osmotic work, but also for driving synthetic reactions. Heat energy may be used by non-biological systems to perform work, but biological systems depend mainly on chemical energy provided by the oxidation of dietary food materials to power life processes.

BIOENERGETICS

Bioenergetics describes the energy changes that occur during biochemical reactions. A knowledge of the underlying thermodynamic concepts of bioenergetics aids the understanding of why some reactions occur within cells, while others do not.

FREE ENERGY

The free energy content (G) of a substance is a measure of the potential energy within the substance that is capable of doing the maximum amount of useful work under standard conditions (i.e. at a constant pressure, and temperature). For biochemical reactions, standard conditions also include a pH = 7.0.

If a substance, A, undergoes a chemical reaction to be converted to a product, B, there will be a *change in free energy* (ΔG).

For example, in the reaction A → B,

$$\Delta G = G_B - G_A$$

(where G_A and G_B represent the free energy in A and B respectively).

A negative ΔG indicates that energy has been released during the conversion of A to B. Such a reaction is said to be *exergonic*, and should proceed spontaneously, although many reactions may require the participation of catalysts (enzymes) to make them proceed at a faster rate. A positive ΔG indicates that a conversion of A to B has resulted in an increase in the free energy content of the system. Such a reaction is said to be *endergonic*. For such a reaction to proceed, energy must be supplied to drive it. If ΔG is zero, the system is at equilibrium and no net energy change is taking place.

Endergonic reactions can occur only when coupled to exergonic reactions. *Catabolic reactions* (reactions involved in the breakdown or oxidation of fuel molecules) are usually exergonic while *anabolic reactions* (biosynthetic reactions) tend to be endergonic. *Metabolism* describes the sum of all of the catabolic and anabolic processes.

ΔG depends on the concentrations of reactants and products. Under standard conditions, the DG of the reaction A → B can be represented as follows:

$$\Delta G = \Delta G° + RT \ln [B]/[A]$$

where ΔG^0 is the standard free energy change (see below)
R is the gas constant
T is the absolute temperature
[A] and [B] are the actual concentrations of the reactants and products
ln indicates the natural logarithm.

If $[A] = [B]$, $\Delta G = \Delta G^0$.

Standard free energy change

Standard free energy change (ΔG^0) is a term used to describe the changes that occur when the reactants and products in a reaction are kept at 1 mol/L concentration. ΔG^0 may be calculated from a knowledge of the equilibrium constant (K_{eq}) for the reaction by using the following equation:

$$\Delta G^0 = - RT \ln K_{eq}$$

For the reaction $A \rightarrow B$, $K_{eq} = [B]/[A]$, where [A] and [B] are the concentrations of A and B at equilibrium.

This equation may be used to predict the direction in which a reaction will proceed:

If $K_{eq} = 1$, then $\Delta G^0 = 0$, and the reaction will be at equilibrium ($A \leftrightharpoons B$).

If $K_{eq} > 1$, then $\Delta G^0 < 0$, and the reaction will proceed spontaneously and release energy that can perform work ($A \rightarrow B$).

If $K_{eq} < 1$, then $\Delta G^0 > 0$, and the forward reaction will not proceed spontaneously ($A \leftarrow B$). External energy must be added to drive the reaction forward from A to B. Such a reaction is endergonic or energy requiring. The reverse reaction will have a negative value of ΔG^0 and will tend to proceed spontaneously.

In a multi-sequence pathway, (e.g. $A \rightarrow B \rightarrow C \rightarrow D$), through which substrates must pass in a particular direction, the ΔGs of the reactions in the pathway will be additive. Even if some of the individual component reactions of the pathway have a positive ΔG, the pathway can proceed as written, as long as the sum of the ΔGs of the individual reactions is negative. The actual rates of the reactions may, however, depend on the activities of the enzymes that catalyse the reactions.

Redox potentials

In oxidation–reduction reactions, the free energy exchange is proportionate to the tendency of reactants to donate or accept electrons. Therefore, in addition to expressing the free energy change in terms of ΔG^0, it is also possible to express it numerically as an *oxidation-reduction* or *redox potential* (E^0). Table 2.1 shows the redox potentials of some physiologically important redox systems in mammals. The order in which the list of redox potentials is arranged in Table 2.1 allows prediction of the direction of flow of electrons from one redox couple to another. The oxidised form of a compound can oxidise the reduced form of any substance situated below it on the scale, while the reduced form of any compound will reduce the oxidized form of a compound situated above it.

REDOX POTENTIALS OF SOME MAMMALIAN OXIDATION SYSTEMS	
System	Redox potential (E^0) (volts)
Oxygen/water	+ 0.82
Cytochrome a; Fe^{3+}/Fe^{2+}	+ 0.29
Cytochrome c; Fe^{3+}/Fe^{2+}	+ 0.22
Ubiquinone; ox/red	+ 0.10
Cytochrome b; Fe^{3+}/Fe^{2+}	+ 0.08
Fumarate/succinate	+ 0.03
Flavoprotein; ox/red	– 0.12
Oxaloacetate/malate	– 0.17
Pyruvate/lactate	– 0.19
Acetoacetate/β-hydroxybutyrate	– 0.27
$NAD^+/NADH$	– 0.32
H^+/H_2	–0.42
Succinate/α-ketoglutarate	– 0.67

Table 2.1

COUPLING OF ENERGY-REQUIRING AND ENERGY-LIBERATING PROCESSES

In living cells, the passage of energy from one process to another has to occur through intermediate, 'energy-rich' molecules. *Adenosine triphosphate* (ATP) is the compound used most frequently to couple energy-requiring processes to energy-liberating processes. In some of these reactions (*anabolic reactions*) a phosphate will be transferred from ATP to another molecule, while in others (*catabolic reactions*) ATP will be synthesised by transfer of a phosphate from an energy-rich intermediate to *adenosine diphosphate* (ADP). The direct production of ATP from ADP occurs in only a few reactions. In most, energy liberated during the oxidation of complex molecules is used to synthesise the reduced forms of the nicotinamide (NADH) and flavin ($FADH_2$) coenzymes. The reduction of the coenzymes is coupled to the synthesis of ATP (Figure 2.1). Other nucleoside triphosphates that ATP helps to synthesise (e.g. UTP, GTP and CTP) can also participate in the transfer of high energy phosphate.

During the transfer of energy in metabolic reactions, varying proportions of the chemical energy are released as heat. This heat helps to maintain a relatively constant body temperature in different environmental conditions.

ENERGY RELEASED DURING ATP HYDROLYSIS AND THE INTERCONVERSION OF ADENINE NUCLEOTIDES

In an ATP molecule, there are three phosphate groups α, β and γ (Figure 2.2).

The free energy of hydrolysis of ATP (to ADP + P_i)

with removal of the γ-phosphate (step ① in Figure 2.2) is about -30 kJ /mol or -7.3 kcal /mol. Hydrolysis of an ADP molecule to AMP (removal of the β-phosphate, step ② in Figure 2.2) releases a similar amount of energy. ATP therefore has two energy-rich phosphoanhydride bonds. The hydrolysis of ATP with release of pyrophosphate (step ③ in Figure 2.2) releases more energy (about -10 kcal/mol). The hydrolysis of AMP releases only about -3.4 kcal/mol because the α-phosphate group is attached to the ribose residue by a phosphoester bond rather than a phosphoanhydride bond.

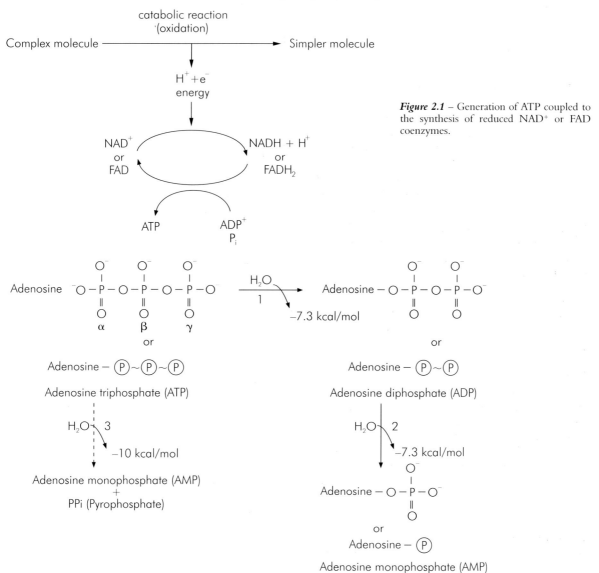

Figure 2.1 – Generation of ATP coupled to the synthesis of reduced NAD^+ or FAD coenzymes.

Figure 2.2 – Hydrolysis of ATP (~P represents a high energy phosphate group).

The interconversion of adenine nucleotides is catalysed by the enzyme *adenylate kinase (myokinase)* as follows:

$$\text{ATP} + \text{AMP} \xrightleftharpoons{\text{adenylate kinase}} 2\text{ADP}$$

HIGH- AND LOW-ENERGY COMPOUNDS

Compounds with a standard free energy of hydrolysis equal to or more negative than that of ATP (-30 kJ/mol or -7.3 kcal/mol) are said to be 'high-energy' compounds. Compounds with a standard free energy of hydrolysis less negative than -7.3 kcal/mol are said to be 'energy poor' or 'low-energy' compounds (Table 2.2).

Creatine phosphate found in muscle and brain is an example of a *phosphagen,* a compound that can act as a storage form of high energy phosphate. The presence in creatine phosphate of a phosphate bond of higher energy than ATP helps to maintain ATP concentrations in muscle when ATP is rapidly being utilised during muscular contraction. Conversely, when ATP is plentiful, the concentration of creatine phosphate can be built up to act as a store of high energy phosphate (Figure 2.3).

METABOLIC GENERATION OF ATP

Most of the ATP in cells is generated within mitochondria and involves the participation of two major sequences of reactions:

- the *citric acid cycle* (tricarboxylic acid (TCA) cycle or krebs cycle) that is located in the mitochondrial matrix

- the *respiratory chain* or electron transport chain that is located in the inner mitochondrial membrane.

Only a small amount of ATP is generated by direct transfer of energy from substrates to ADP.

CITRIC ACID CYCLE

(Tricarboxylic acid cycle; TCA cycle) — The citric acid cycle is a cyclic pathway located in the mitochondria, the central function of which is to oxidize acetyl coenzyme A (acetyl CoA) derived from the metabolism of fuel molecules such as amino acids, fatty acids and carbohydrates to carbon dioxide and water.

FORMATION OF ACETYL COA FROM PYRUVATE

The link between glycolysis and the citric acid cycle is provided by the decarboxylation of pyruvate in the mitochondrial matrix to form acetyl CoA. This reaction is irreversible and is catalyzed by a multienzyme complex known as the *pyruvate dehydrogenase complex.* This complex reaction may be written simply as follows:

STANDARD FREE ENERGY OF HYDROLYSIS OF SOME BIOCHEMICALLY IMPORTANT ORGANOPHOSPHATES		
Compound	**ΔG^0**	
	kJ/mol	kcal/mol
Energy-rich		
Phosphoenolpyruvate	– 61.9	– 14.8
Carbamoyl phosphate	– 51.4	– 12.3
1,3-Biphosphoglycerate	– 49.3	– 11.8
Creatine phosphate	– 43.1	– 10.3
ATP → ADP + P$_i$	– 30.5	–7.3
Energy-poor		
Glucose-1-phosphate	– 20.9	– 5.0
Fructose-6-phosphate	– 15.9	– 3.8
AMP	– 14.2	– 3.4
Glucose-6-phosphate	– 13.8	– 3.3
Glycerol-3-phosphate	– 9.2	– 2.2

Table 2.2

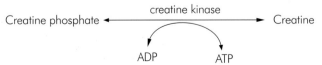

Figure 2.3 – Reversible conversion of creatine phosphate to ATP.

$$Pyruvate + CoA + NAD^+ \rightarrow Acetyl\ CoA + CO_2 + NADH + H^+$$

This enzyme complex contains three closely linked enzymes – *pyruvate decarboxylase, dihydrolipoyl transacetylase,* and *dihydrolipoyl dehydrogenase,* each catalysing a part of the overall reaction. This complex also contains five coenzymes (*thiamine pyrophosphate, lipoamide, FAD, NAD$^+$* and *coenzyme A*) that act as carriers or oxidants for the intermediates of the reaction. The oxidative decarboxylation of α-ketoglutarate dehydrogenase (Figure 2.4) is also catalyzed by an enzyme complex that is structurally similar to the pyruvate dehydrogenase complex.

The pyruvate dehydrogenase complex can be inhibited by its product, acetyl CoA, and by elevated levels of NADH in the cell. This enzyme complex can exist as an active, non-phosphorylated form or an inactive, phosphorylated form. The interconversion of the two forms can occur through the actions of a kinase and a phosphatase. An increase in the ratio of acetyl CoA / CoA or NADH/NAD$^+$ activates the kinase, while an increase in the ADP/ATP ratio inhibits the kinase activity and allows more of the active form of the enzyme complex to be produced.

REACTIONS OF THE CITRIC ACID CYCLE

The reactions of the citric acid cycle and the enzymes involved are shown in Figure 2.4 . The cycle begins by the transfer of the 2C acyl group from acetyl CoA to the 4C oxaloacetic acid to form a 6C citric acid molecule. By stepwise degradations and loss of two molecules of CO_2, accompanied by internal rearrangements, the citric acid is reconverted to oxaloacetic acid, which can then take up another acetyl group from acetyl CoA to form another citric acid molecule which goes through the whole cycle again.

Important points about the citric acid cycle

- a very small amount of oxaloacetate can convert a large number of acetyl units to CO_2. Oxaloacetate can therefore be considered to play a catalytic role.

- there are four dehydrogenation steps (reactions ④, ⑤, ⑦, ⑨ in Figure 2.4) in each cycle. During these dehydrogenation reactions, *reducing equivalents* in the form of hydrogen or electrons, are transferred to NAD$^+$ or FAD, which in turn pass them via the *respiratory chain (electron transport chain)* on to oxygen to form water. During the passage of electrons through the respiratory chain, ATP is synthesised

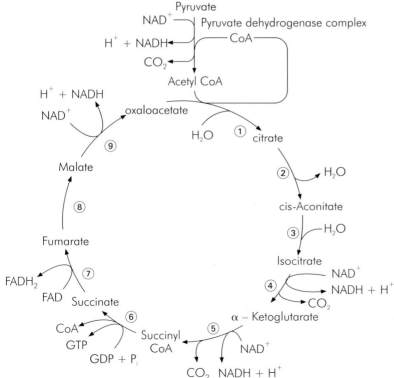

Figure 2.4 – The citric acid cycle enzymes : 1- *citrate synthase,* 2,3 – *aconitase,* 4 – *isocitrate dehydrogenase,* 5 – *α-ketoglutarate dehydrogenase complex,* 6 – *succinyl CoA synthetase,* 7 – *succinate dehydrogenase,* 8 – *fumarase,* 9 – *malate dehydrogenase.*

by a process of *oxidative phosphorylation*. The citric acid cycle enzymes are located in the mitochondrial matrix, either free or attached to the inner mitochondrial membrane. The proximity of these enzymes to the enzymes of the respiratory chain that are situated in the inner mitochondrial membrane helps in the transfer of reducing equivalents from the citric acid cycle to oxygen

• in each cycle, one molecule of high energy phosphate is also formed by *substrate level phosphorylation*. In reaction 6 of Figure 2.4, GTP is formed in this manner

• the participation of the respiratory chain is essential for the continuous operation of the citric acid cycle

• the condensation of oxaloacetate with acetyl CoA (①), the dehydrogenation of isocitrate (④), and the oxidative decarboxylation of α-ketoglutarate (⑤) are physiologically irreversible. The citric acid cycle therefore proceeds only in the forward direction

SIGNIFICANCE OF THE CITRIC ACID CYCLE

The citric acid cycle functions as a final common pathway for the oxidation of carbohydrates, proteins and lipids. Glucose, fatty acids, and many amino acids are metabolized to acetyl CoA. It is the mechanism by which most of the free energy liberated during the oxidation of carbohydrates, amino acids and lipids is made available. It has a dual or *amphibolic* role. While helping to oxidise carbohydrates, and amino acids and lipids, the citric acid cycle can also provide substrates for the synthesis of glucose, fatty acids, and amino acids, as well as for other biosynthetic pathways (Figure 2.5).

ENERGETICS OF THE CITRIC ACID CYCLE

As a result of oxidations catalysed by the dehydrogenase enzymes of the citric acid cycle, three molecules of NADH and one of $FADH_2$ are produced for each molecule of acetyl CoA catabolised in one revolution of the cycle. During the passage of electrons from these

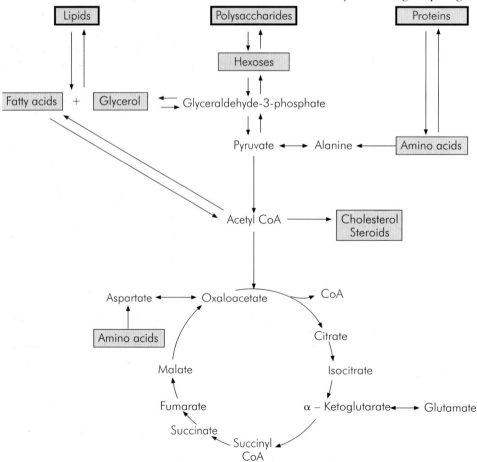

Figure 2.5 – Amphibolic nature of the citric acid cycle.

reduced nucleotides along the respiratory chain, a total of 11 molecules of ATP would be formed (three molecules/NADH molecule + two molecules from the $FADH_2$). An additional molecule of ATP would be generated from the GTP formed by substrate level phosphorylation. The total yield of energy generated would therefore be 12 molecules ATP/acetyl CoA metabolized in the citric acid cycle The conversion of a pyruvate molecule to an acetyl CoA molecule is also accompanied by the generation of one NADH molecule (= 3ATP). The oxidation of each pyruvate molecule via the citric acid cycle would therefore result in the generation of 15 molecules of ATP.

CONTROL OF THE CITRIC ACID CYCLE

The rate at which the citric acid cycle operates can be precisely adjusted to meet the cell's requirement for ATP. The cycle is controlled by:

- activation and inhibition of enzyme activities
- by the availability of ADP

Activation and inhibition of enzyme activities

The most important citric acid cycle enzymes that are regulated in this manner are citrate synthase, isocitrate dehydrogenase and α-ketoglutarate dehydrogenase complex (Figure 2.4). ATP allosterically inhibits activities of these enzymes. ADP allosterically activates isocitrate dehydrogenase while NADH decreases its activity (and also pyruvate dehydrogenase complex) by directly displacing NAD^+.

Availability of ADP

If ADP (or P_i) is present in limiting concentrations, the formation of ATP by oxidative phosphorylation will decrease. As a result, the oxidation of NADH and $FADH_2$ by the respiratory chain would also be inhibited, thereby causing a depletion of their oxidized forms. Inhibition of the citric cycle will occur due to the depletion of NAD^+ and FAD.

Conversely, an increase in the concentration of ADP will result in the acceleration of oxidative phosphorylation and other reactions that use ADP to generate ATP, and the citric acid cycle will operate at a faster rate. The increased rate of production of ATP will continue until it matches the rate of ATP consumption by energy requiring reactions.

THE RESPIRATORY CHAIN

The oxidation of carbohydrates, lipids and proteins results in the transfer of reducing equivalents (-H or electrons) to specialised coenzymes, NAD^+ and FAD, to form energy-rich reduced coenzymes, NADH and $FADH_2$. These reduced coenzymes can each donate a pair of electrons to a specialised set of electron carriers (located in the inner mitochondrial membrane) collectively called *the respiratory chain* or the *electron transport chain,* the composition of which is described below. At the end of their transfer along the components of the respiratory chain, the electrons are transferred to oxygen to form water; this process constitutes *respiration*. During the passage of electrons along the respiratory chain, they lose much of their free energy. The components of the respiratory chain are usually linked to a system that can trap most of the liberated free energy by formation of ATP from ADP and inorganic phosphate (P_i). This process of ATP formation linked to the transfer of electrons from NADH or $FADH_2$ to oxygen by a series of electron carriers is called *oxidative phosphorylation*.

ORGANISATION OF THE RESPIRATORY CHAIN

The respiratory chain is a complex of at least thirty proteins. These are arranged as four physically separate multi-subunit assemblies called "complexes" (Figure 2.6). These complexes are:

Complex I — *NADH-ubiquinone (coenzyme Q) reductase (NADH dehydrogenase)* Complex 1 transfers electrons from NADH to ubiquinone, has a tightly bound molecule of flavin mononucleotide (FMN, a coenzyme structurally related to FAD) that is reduced to $FMNH_2$ by acceptance of two hydrogen atoms ($2e^- + 2H^+$) and contains several iron atoms paired with sulphur atoms (iron-sulphur centres) which help in electron transfer from NADH to ubiquinone.

Complex II — *Succinate-ubiquinone reductase (succinate dehydrogenase)* This is a flavoprotein dehydrogenase that also contains iron-sulphur centres.

Complex III— *Ubiquinone-cytochrome c reductase* The main components are cytochrome b and cytochrome c.

Complex IV — *Cytochrome c oxidase* Major components are cytochromes

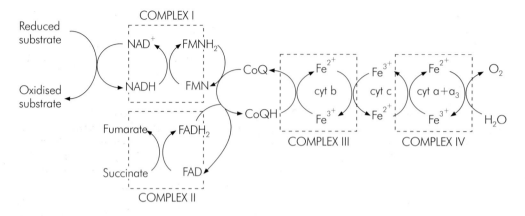

Figure 2.6 – Organisation of the respiratory chain.

a and a_3. Cytochrome a_3 can bind O_2 and is the terminal oxidase of the respiratory chain.

These complexes do not form stable associations with each other, and electron transfer occurs between them during interactions by random collisions. The relatively mobile electron carriers such as coenzyme Q and cytochrome c help the physical and functional interactions between these complexes to occur rapidly. Subdivisions of the respiratory chain into discrete complexes make it possible for the energy formed as a result of oxidations to be released in small 'parcels' instead of all at once.

The cytochromes

There are three main groups of cytochromes associated with the respiratory chain. These are cytochromes c (c_1 and c), b, and a (a and a_3). Each contains a haem group made of a porphyrin ring containing an iron ion.

During electron transfer, the cytochrome iron atom is reversibly converted from its ferric (Fe^{3+}) to its ferrous (Fe^{2+}) form. In addition to iron, cytochromes a and a_3 contain bound copper ions that are essential for its functions. The three groups of cytochromes also differ from each other in their redox potentials (which increase from b $\rightarrow$ c_1 $\rightarrow$ c $\rightarrow$ a and a_3).

Ubiquinone (Coenzyme Q)

This is a quinone derivative with a long isoprenoid tail. On acceptance of two electrons and two protons, it gets reduced to *ubiquinol.*

The various components in the respiratory chain are arranged sequentially in order of increasing redox

potential in Table 2.1. Electrons or hydrogen flow through the chain in a stepwise manner from the more electropositive components to the more electronegative oxygen. The major route of electron transfer in the respiratory chain proceeds from the NAD^+-linked dehydrogenase system through flavoproteins and cytochromes to molecular oxygen. Some substrates (e.g. fumarate, succinate) are not linked to the respiratory chain through NAD^+-specific dehydrogenases, but are linked through flavoprotein dehydrogenases directly to the cytochromes because their redox potentials are more positive than those of the $FMN/FMNH_2$ redox couple.

ATP production during electron transfer in the respiratory chain

When substrates are oxidised via an NAD^+-linked dehydrogenase and the respiratory chain, three molecules of inorganic phosphate are incorporated into three molecules of ADP to form three molecules of ATP per ½ molecule of O_2 consumed, i.e. P/O ratio = three (Figure 2.7). On the other hand, when a substrate is oxidised via a flavoprotein-linked dehydrogenase, only two molecules of ATP are generated, i.e. P/O ratio = 2. As stated before, ATP synthesis utilising the free energy release accompanying the passage of reducing equivalents along the respiratory chain is referred to as *oxidative phosphorylation.* ATP synthesis by *substrate level phosphorylation* occurs without help from the mitochondrial respiratory chain. The energy from the substrate molecule is transferred directly to an ADP or other molecule such as GDP (e.g. in the phosphoglycerate kinase and pyruvate kinase reactions in glycolysis and the succinate thiokinase reaction in the citric acid cycle).

MECHANISMS OF OXIDATIVE PHOSPHORYLATION

Many different theories have been advanced to explain how the oxidation of NADH is coupled to the phosphorylation of ADP. The theory that is presently accepted is Peter Mitchell's *chemiosmotic hypothesis*. According to this hypothesis, oxidation of components in the respiratory chain generates protons (hydrogen ions). The transfer of electrons along the respiratory chain is tightly coupled to the expulsion of these protons from the matrix side of the inner mitochondrial membrane to the intermembrane space. The respiratory chain therefore acts as a complex proton pump. The inner mitochondrial membrane is impermeable to ions in general, and particularly to protons which accumulate outside the membrane, resulting in the generation of an electrochemical potential differ-

ence across the membrane or *proton-motive force* (difference in pH and electrical charge). In the respiratory chain there are three sites (Figure 2.8) where such proton ejection takes place : between F_p and CoQ, between cytochromes b and c, and between cytochrome a and oxygen.

The inner mitochondrial membrane contains a second proton pump, the enzyme *ATP synthetase* which is composed of three parts – the catalytic part, F_1, made up of five subunits (located in the spherical particles), a hydrophobic complex of three or four proteins, the F_0 complex, located in the inner mitochondrial membrane, and a *stalk* that connects F_0 to F_1. This enzyme is also called an ATPase because it can hydrolyse ATP to ADP and inorganic phosphate. However, the proton-motive force generated by the respiratory chain forces this second pump to work in reverse, allowing protons to re-enter the matrix (via the proton channel F_0) and

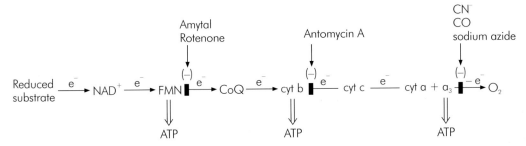

Figure 2.7 – Sites of ATP synthesis and action of inhibitors in the respiratory chain.

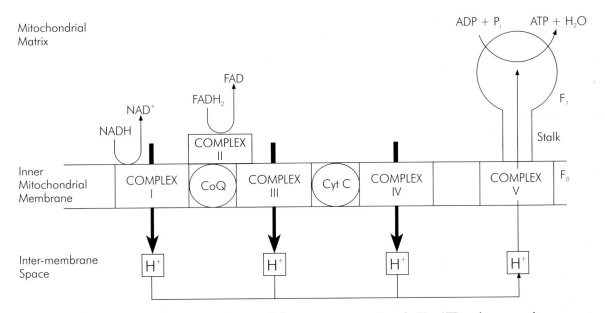

Figure 2.8 – Electron transfer in the respiratory chain coupled to proton transport. Complex V = ATP synthetase complex.

cause synthesis of ATP, at the same time dissipating the pH and electrical gradients. Proton movements through F_0 into F_1 is thought to induce conformational changes in the ATP synthetase resulting in movement of tightly bound ADP and P_i into a hydrophobic pocket within the complex. In the absence of water molecules, ADP and P_i can link to form ATP without energy input.

RESPIRATORY CONTROL

Under normal circumstances, sufficient O_2, NADH, $FADH_2$, and P_i are available in cells and they do not therefore, influence the rate of electron transport. The rate controlling factor in electron transport via the respiratory chain is the availability of ADP. The regulation of the respiratory rate by the availability of ADP is referred to as *respiratory control*. When the level of cellular ADP decreases, the rate of respiration will also be gradually decreased until it reaches an 'idling' or 'resting' state. An increase in the ADP concentration due to utilization of ATP by cellular processes will increase the respiratory rate until it reaches a maximum.

INHIBITION OF RESPIRATION

Site-specific inhibitors of electron transport (and therefore respiration) have been identified (Figure 2.7). Since electron transport and oxidative phosphorylation are tightly coupled, inhibitors of respiration will also inhibit ATP synthesis. There are two main types of inhibitors:

- *inhibitors of respiratory chain proper* - e.g. *rotenone* inhibits electron transport in complex I; *antimycin* inhibits in complex II; *CO, H₂S* and *CN* inhibit cytochrome oxidase, and can therefore totally arrest respiration

- *inhibitors of adenine nucleotide* or *proton transport* – e.g. *Atractyloside, barbiturates*, and *oligomycin*

UNCOUPLING OF OXIDATIVE PHOSPHORYLATION

The normal tight coupling of respiration and phosphorylation can be disrupted by several compounds known as *uncouplers*. Classic uncouplers include *2,4-dinitrophe-*

nol (2,4-DNP), dicumarol, and *m-chlorocarbonyl cyanide phenylhydrazone (CCCP)*. Uncouplers such as DNP bring protons across the mitochondrial membrane and disrupt the proton gradient required for oxidative phosphorylation. When the respiratory chain is dissociated from phosphorylation, respiration cannot be controlled by the concentration of ADP or P_i, and will continue at a slightly faster rate than normal, but without synthesis of ATP. The energy released in electron transport by uncoupled mitochondrial respiration is liberated as heat.

A partial uncoupling of oxidative phosphorylation occurs in aspirin overdose and in this condition, there is an increase in body temperature as a result of consequent heat production. An excess of thyroid hormone also partially uncouples oxidative phosphorylation.

TRANSFER OF METABOLITES ACROSS THE INNER MITOCHONDRIAL MEMBRANE

The inner mitochondrial membrane, being impermeable to most charged or hydrophilic substances, contains numerous proteins that permit passage of specific molecules from the cytosol into the mitochondrial matrix or in the reverse direction. Examples include *carnitine*, which helps to transport fatty acylCoA from the cytosol into the mitochondrial matrix and the *adenine translocase*, which transports one molecule of ADP from the cytosol into mitochondria while transporting one ATP molecule from the matrix back into the cytosol.

TRANSPORT OF REDUCING EQUIVALENTS

NADH generated in the cytosol is unable to cross the inner mitochondrial membrane due to the lack of an NADH transport protein. NADH therefore uses several 'shuttles' to transfer its electrons into the mitochondria. In the *glycerophosphate shuttle* (Figure 2.9), glycerol-3-phosphate is used to convey an electron pair from NADH into the mitochondrion. Glycerol-3-phosphate is reoxidized to dihydroxyacetone phosphate (DHAP) by the *glycerophosphate dehydrogenase* on the inner membrane. During this process, the two electrons are transferred to the *flavoprotein dehydrogenase* which in turn passes them onto the respiratory chain in a manner similar to that of succinate dehydrogenase (Figure 2.6). The glycerophosphate shuttle therefore results in the synthesis of two ATP molecules for each cytosolic NADH oxidised.

The *malate shuttle* employs malate to carry electrons into mitochondria. Once inside, malate reduces NAD+ to NADH while malate gets oxidized to oxaloacetate (Figure 2.9). This NADH is oxidized by the *NADH dehydrogenase* to yield three molecules of ATP per molecule of cytoplasmic NADH oxidised.

RESPIRATORY CHAIN DYSFUNCTION AND DISEASE

Deficiencies in components of the respiratory chain have been implicated in the pathogenesis of several neuromuscular diseases. Deficiency of cytochrome oxidase is associated with the inherited conditions myoclonic epilepsy and ragged red fibre (MERRF) disease and mitochondrial encephalomyopathy, lactic acidosis and stroke-like episodes (MELAS).

CONSEQUENCES OF INCOMPLETE REDUCTION OF OXYGEN

During normal mitochondrial respiration, oxygen simultaneously accepts four electrons and gets reduced to water, and the release of oxygen intermediates with unpaired electrons is prevented. The stepwise transfer of electrons to oxygen will, however, result in the formation of *oxygen-derived free radicals* (e.g. *superoxide radicals* and *hydroxyl radicals*) and other reactive oxygen metabolites (e.g. H_2O_2), collectively termed *reactive oxygen intermediates* (ROIs). A *free radical* is any molecule containing an odd number of electrons. A simplified scheme of ROI formation is outlined in Figure 2.10.

Reactive oxygen intermediates are generated in the body as by-products of normal metabolism. They can also be formed when cells are exposed to ionising radi-

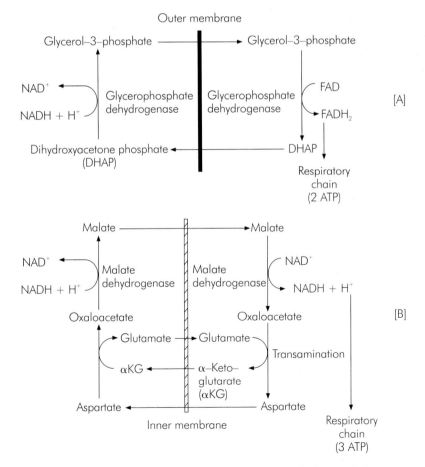

Figure 2.9 – Shuttle systems used for transporting reducing equivalents across the inner mitochondrial membrane. [A]- Glycerophosphate shuttle; [B] – Malate shuttle.

ation, drugs capable of redox cycling, or xenobiotics that can form free radical metabolites in-situ (e.g. *paraquat, halothane, CCl_4*).

ROIs and other free radicals, being highly reactive, can cause cell injury, chiefly due to their actions on:

- cell membranes – peroxidation of membrane lipids (Figure 2.11), and cross-linking of proteins by disulphide bond formation

- DNA nucleotides (may cause mutations and even cell death). Hydroxyl radicals are the most reactive in this manner

In addition to toxic effects within cells, ROIs released extracellularly promote tissue injury by several other mechanisms. ROIs can inhibit the anti-protease effect of α-antitrypsin, and thereby promote the action of locally released serine proteases, particularly elastin. ROIs can react directly with matrix macromolecules, which can potentially cause degradation of extracellular matrix. They can also react with locally available arachidonate, forming derivatives with potent chemo-attractant properties for neutrophils, which in turn amplify local inflammatory reactions and tissue injury.

DEFENCE MECHANISMS AGAINST REACTIVE OXYGEN RADICALS

Detoxication of reactive oxygen radicals is one of the prerequisites of aerobic life, and many antioxidant defence systems that can prevent, intercept and repair reactive radical-mediated damage have evolved. These consist of *enzymatic systems* including *superoxide dismutase,* and hydroperoxidases such as *glutathione peroxidase,*

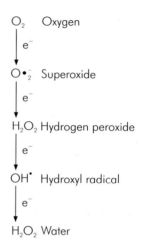

Figure 2.10 – Formation of reactive oxygen intermediates. e^- = Addition of one electron.

catalase and other *haemoprotein peroxidases* as well as *non-enzymatic scavengers* and *quenchers* known as *antioxidants* (Table 2.3).

Certain radical scavenging compounds present in dietary plant material (e.g. β-*carotene, flavonoids*) may also contribute to the antioxidant pool in the body.

ELECTRON TRANSFER PATHWAYS IN THE ER

Endoplasmic reticulum possesses short electron transfer pathways that do not transfer protons or are

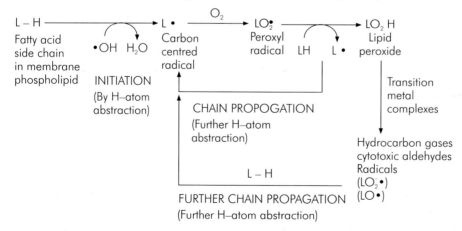

Figure 2.11 – Lipid peroxidation by free radicals. The organic free radicals ($L\bullet$) generated react with O_2 to form peroxides which in turn can act as free radicals initiating an autocatalytic chain reaction.

involved with ATP production. They are primarily concerned with:

- hydroxylation of drugs and steroids
- the production of ions and radicals toxic to micro-organisms (in neutrophils)
- the desaturation of long-chain fatty acids

The cytochromes P-450 and b_5 are involved in electron transfer associated with the endoplasmic reticulum. Both NADH and NADPH donate reducing equivalents for the reduction of these cytochromes (Figure 2.12).

Enzymes involved in the hydroxylation of drugs catalyze the incorporation of only one atom of an oxygen molecule into the substrate (*monooxygenases*) while reducing the other oxygen atom to water as shown below:

$$\text{Drug-H} + O_2 + 2Fe^{2+}\text{-(P-450)} + 2H^+ \xrightarrow{\text{Hydroxylase}}$$
$$\text{Drug-OH} + H_2O + 2Fe^{3+}\text{-(P-450)}$$

These enzymes, being involved in a simultaneous reduction and an oxidation, are sometimes referred to as *mixed function oxidases*. Cytochrome P-450-dependent monooxygenase systems are also found in mitochondria of steroidogenic tissues such as adrenal cortex, testes, ovary and placenta, and are involved in the biosynthesis of steroid hormones.

SELECTED READING

Haliwell, B. and Gutteridge, J.M.C. – *Free radicals in biology and medicine*, 2nd ed., Oxford: Clarendon Press, 1989.

Katz, M. – The expanding role of oxygen-free radicals in clinical medicine. *West J Med* 1986; 144: 441.

ANTIOXIDANT DEFENCE SYSTEMS IN THE BODY	
System	Mechanism of action
Enzymatic	
Superoxide dismutase (SOD) cytoplasmic enzyme containing Cu^{2+} and Zn^{2+}; mitochondrial enzyme contains Mn^{2+}	Converts superoxide to H_2O_2
Catalase in peroxisomes	Decomposes H_2O_2 ($2H_2O_2 \rightarrow O_2 + 2H_2O$)
Glutathione peroxidase in erythrocytes; selenium containing enzyme	Helps to detoxify H_2O_2 or $OH^\cdot$ by GSH ($H_2O_2 + 2GSH \rightarrow 2H_2O + GSSG$) or ($2OH^\cdot + 2GSH \rightarrow 2H_2O + GSSG$)
Non-enzymatic	
Vitamin E (α-tocopherol) very important for much of the lipid-soluble chain breaking antioxidant capacity in human plasma and erythrocyte membrane	Free radical scavenger (inactivates free radicals, e.g. peroxyl radicals) ($ROO^\cdot + vitE\text{-}OH \rightarrow ROOH + Vit\text{-}O^\cdot$)
Vitamin C	Free radical scavenger
Glutathione in many cells	Substrate for glutathione peroxidase; radical $OH^\cdot$ and single oxygen scavenger
Caeruloplasmin (Cu-binding protein) Transferrin (Fe^{3+} binding β-globulin)	Block initiation of free radical formation by binding free copper or iron in circulation

Table 2.3

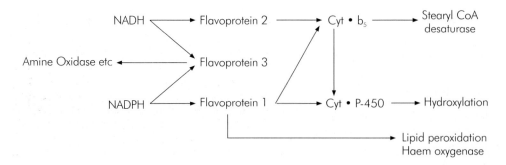

Figure 2.12 – Electron transport chain in microsomes. (With kind permission from Mayes, P.A. In *Harper's Biochemistry,* 24th ed., page 113. Appleton and Lange, California, 1996).

Mitchell, P.- Keilin's respiratory chain concept and its chemiosmotic consequences. *Science*, 1979; **206:** 1148.

Murray, R.K., Granner, D.K., Mayes, P.A. and Rodwell, V.W. (eds). – *Harper's Biochemistry*, 24th ed., Appleton and Lange, California, 1996.

Stryer, L. – *Biochemistry*, 4th ed., W.H. Freeman and Co., N.Y.,1995.

3

INFORMATION STORAGE AND TRANSMISSION

Objectives
To understand:

- How genetic information in cells is stored (DNA double helix) and the biological importance of the nucleotide arrangement in the DNA molecule

- The organisation of DNA in chromosomes

- DNA replication

- The types, consequences and repair of DNA damage

- Biological importance of genetic recombination in cells

- Recombinant DNA technology

All genetically relevant information in a cell resides in the base sequences of genomic DNA. This information can be retrieved as an RNA copy that can either function directly (e.g. ribosomal RNA) or act as a template for synthesis of proteins (e.g. messenger RNA). The nucleotide sequences in DNA are organised into a series of functional units known as *genes*, each of which carries the information for a single function. A *structural gene* carries the information corresponding to a specific RNA or protein. A *regulatory gene* or *element* is a nucleotide segment that alters the expression of the structural gene.

INFORMATION STORAGE – THE DNA DOUBLE HELIX

DNA is a polymer of thousands of residues, containing the purine bases adenine and guanine, and the pyrimidine bases cytosine and thymine.

According to the 3-D model put forward in 1953 by Watson and Crick, DNA consists of two helical chains of polynucleotides coiled around the same axis to form a right handed *double helix* with a pitch of 3.4 nm or 10 base pairs per turn (Figure 3.1). The two strands of the DNA duplex coil in such a way that they cannot be separated except by unwinding. In the helix, the two chains or strands are *antiparallel* (Figure 3.1). Their hydrophobic backbones which consist of alternating deoxyribose and negatively charged phosphate groups, are on the outside of the double helix facing the aqueous environment.

The hydrophobic purine and pyrimidine bases of both strands are stacked inside the double helix. The bases of the two chains pair by intermolecular hydrogen bonding such that the purines always pair with the pyrimidines, i.e. (A–T), (G–C). This type of specific bonding arises from spatial constraints imposed by the physical structure of DNA. The two strands are therefore *complementary*, and the base sequences on one strand predetermine the base sequence in the other strand. The sequence of bases along the sugar-phosphate backbone makes up the *primary structure of DNA*, and the specific sequences distinguish the DNA of one gene from another. *The sequence of bases express the information content of DNA.*

The individual hydrogen bonds are weak, but the large numbers in a double helix and the partial overlapping of the hydrophobic parts of bases of successive nucleotides provide additional stability to the structure. Associated proteins, mainly histones, also stabilize the helical structure by interacting with the phosphate groups in the molecule.

BIOLOGICAL IMPLICATIONS OF THE DNA DUPLEX STRUCTURE

The complementary nature of the DNA duplex and its mode of replication is important when explaining the predictable inheritance between generations. Watson and Crick argued that, if the strands of a double helix are separated and serve as a template for the synthesis of their complement, two identical DNA duplexes would result. The daughter cells would then each receive a complete set of genetic instructions.

DNA IN CHROMOSOMES

The DNA of all eukaryotes is organised into morphologically distinct units called chromosomes. Each chromosome contains only a single folded DNA molecule.

Chromosomal DNA is bound to one of five classes of basic proteins called *histones* which are extremely rich in the positively charged amino acids arginine and lysine, allowing binding to the negatively charged phosphates of DNA. Under electron microscopy, chromosomes appear like a 'string of beads'. The beads called *nucleosomes* consist of a segment of duplex DNA wound round a set of eight molecules of histones (two each of H_2A, H_2B, H_3 and H_4). The nucleosomes are connected to each other.

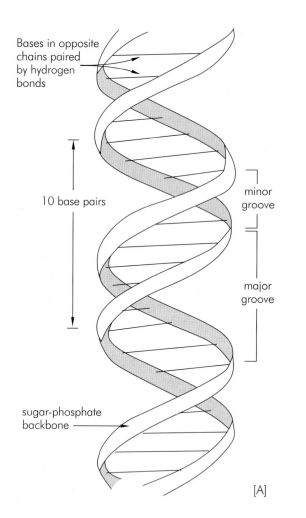

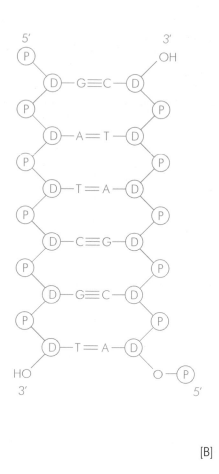

Figure 3.1 – Diagrammatic representation of [A] the DNA (B-form) double helix, and [B] the antiparallel arrangement of the two chains in the DNA double helix: (P – phosphate; D – deoxyribose; A – adenine; T – thymine; C – cytosine; G – guanine).

While most of the DNA in cells is in the nuclei, some DNA is found in mitochondria where it may have a different molecular structure, including circular molecules as in prokaryotes. *Circular DNA* may be relaxed or supercoiled. *Supercoiled DNA* is formed when a closed circle is twisted around its own axis, or when a linear piece of duplex DNA whose ends are fixed, is twisted. The latter type of supercoiling is also seen in human DNA, segments of which are tethered to nuclear matrix proteins. Enzymes that catalyze topologic changes of DNA are called *topoisomerases;* the best characterized being *bacterial DNA gyrase.*

Topoisomerases are also implicated as antigens in some 'autoimmune' human diseases such as *scleroderma.* Bacterial and mitochondrial DNA lack histones and

nucleosome structure. Sperm contains *protamine*, a basic protein in place of histones.

Supercoiling is biologically important because:

- it makes DNA more compact so that it can be easily packed within a cell

- it affects the capacity of the double helix to unwind and thereby affects its interactions with other molecules

Analysis of eukaryotic DNA shows the presence of *non-repetitive* or *unique sequences* interspersed with *repetitive sequences.* The highly repetitive sequences include *interspersed sequences* and *satellite sequences.*

Satellite DNA consists of short sequences of 6–8 base pairs that are repeated many times. These sequences are composed of *tandem repeats*. The presence of satellite sequences provides the basis for *DNA fingerprinting*. This technique is also useful in determining parentage.

Interspersed sequences include the *Alu* sequences which are dispersed throughout the chromosome and comprise about 4% of total DNA. In forensic testing, the presence of *Alu* sequences is diagnostic of tissues of human or higher primate origin.

TRANSMISSION OF INFORMATION

The primary function of DNA is to provide progeny with the genetic information possessed by the parent. During cell division, this is achieved by *replication of DNA*.

DNA REPLICATION

Replication is the process by which each strand of the parental DNA duplex is copied precisely, by base pairing with complementary nucleotides. This base selection is accomplished by *(DNA-dependent) DNA polymerase* that adds nucleotides to the end of a growing strand.

FACTORS NECESSARY FOR REPLICATION

Several other factors, apart from the DNA template, are required for successful replication:

- an RNA primer

- nucleoside triphosphates

- energy in the form of ATP

- unwinding enzymes, primase (a special type of RNA polymerase), DNA polymerase, DNA ligase, topoisomerases)

- cytoplasmic factors needed for initiation of replication

- a supply of new histones to reform the replicated DNA into nucleosomes for packaging into chromosomes

ORIGIN OF REPLICATION

Replication does not start randomly on a DNA molecule. In eukaryotic chromosomes there are multiple initiation sites of replication, referred to as 'ori' sites. Replication occurs usually in a bidirectional

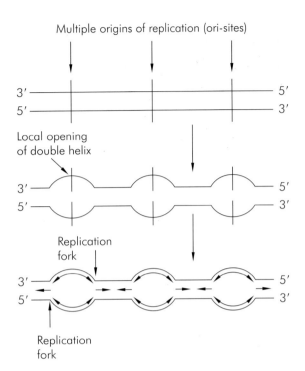

Figure 3.2 – Semi-conservative replication of DNA.

mode (Figure 3.2). Coalescence of the 'eyes' of replication (*replicons*) occurs at the completion of the synthesis of the daughter strands.

During replication, each of the two strands of parental DNA becomes one of the two strands in the two daughter DNA molecules. The DNA in the offspring therefore contains one parental strand and a newly synthesised strand (Figure 3.3). There are three major stages in DNA replication:

- initiation

- elongation

- termination

Initiation of replication

For initiation, the two strands of the double helix are unwound by a *DNA helicase* enzyme; one ATP molecule is expended for every base pair separated by it. During unwinding, the topology of the DNA is maintained by *DNA gyrase*. The helix is prevented from reforming until replication is complete by specific *helix destabilising proteins (single stranded DNA binding proteins)*. As the strands separate, a *replication fork* is formed (Figure 3.3). A complex of 6–7 initiation proteins called a *primosome* provides a starting point for the binding of *primase,* which creates a short, complementary *RNA primer* of about 10 – 30 bases for each DNA strand. These primers are necessary because *DNA polymerases* are incapable of initiating DNA synthesis and require a 3′-hydroxyl residue for the formation of the first phosphodiester bond.

Elongation of the DNA strand

After primer formation is complete, the elongation process is initiated by a *DNA-dependent DNA polymerase (DP).* Five different DPs have been isolated from mammalian cells (*DPα, β, γ, δ and ε*).

DPs catalyse the extension of the existing RNA primer. During elongation, the free 3′-hydroxyl group of the primer attacks the α-phosphorus atom of the incoming deoxyribonucleoside ·triphosphate. Pyrophosphate is displaced, and a new phosphate ester formed . Elongation of the DNA chain occurs only in the 5′ → 3′ – direction. Since the two chains in the DNA duplex are antiparallel, only one strand, the *leading strand,* can be elongated continuously; the other, the *trailing* or *lagging strand* is synthesized discontinuously, 3′ → 5′-,

in pieces called *Okazaki fragments* (Figure 3.3). Each fragment consists of 400 – 2000 nucleotides.

Termination of DNA replication

Termination involves the removal of the RNA primers, filling in of the resulting gaps, and joining together of the DNA fragments. The gaps left by the removal of the primers is filled by the proper base-paired deoxyribonucleotides by the DPs. The fragments are then sealed by *DNA ligases.* In mitochondria, the small piece of RNA primer remains as an integral part of the closed, circular DNA structure.

The fidelity of copying by the DNA-template-directed RNA polymerase ultimately depends on accurate hydrogen bonding between base pairs in the template and the newly formed DNA chain.

THE CELL CYCLE

In man, cell division occurs in an orderly cycle which varies considerably in total duration from minutes to months. The cell cycle has four distinct phases: G_1, S, G_2

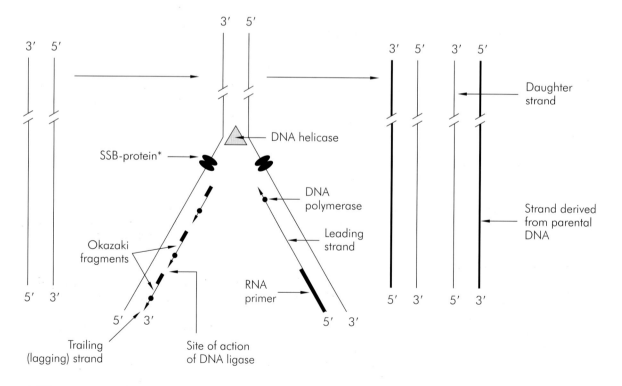

* SSB-protein – single-stranded DNA-binding protein

Figure 3.3 – Diagrammatic representations of the different phases of the cell cycle.

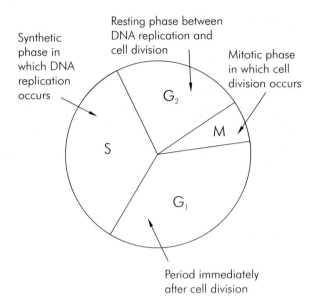

Synthetic phase in which DNA replication occurs

Resting phase between DNA replication and cell division

Mitotic phase in which cell division occurs

G₂

M

S

G₁

Period immediately after cell division

Figure 3.4 – The cell cycle.

and M (Figure 3.4). DNA synthesis and cell division are key events in this cycle.

G_1 phase is the period beginning immediately after a cell division when cells are diploid. In the *S-* or *synthetic phase,* replication of the DNA genome takes place. At the end of the S-phase, the cells have twice the amount of chromatin, and pass to G_2-phase which is the gap between DNA replication and cell division. From G_2, the cells pass to the *M-phase*, during which they actually divide. During M-phase, the nuclear envelope breaks down, the contents of the nucleus condense to visible chromosomes and the cytoskeleton undergoes extensive reorganisation to form the *mitotic spindle* that will separate the chromosomes. In most cells, M-phase takes about 1 hour. The long period of time between this and the next phase is known as the *interphase*.

The cell cycle control system

A *cell cycle control system* cyclically triggers the essential processes of cell reproduction such as DNA replication and chromosome segregation. This system is based on two key families of proteins: the *cyclin-dependent protein kinases* (*cdk proteins*), and the activating proteins called *cyclins* that bind to the *cdk* molecules and control their ability to phosphorylate appropriate target proteins. In cancer cells, products of certain oncogenes help to bypass these check points and thus promote continuous cell proliferation.

DNA DAMAGE AND ITS REPAIR

DNA DAMAGE

DNA is a stable compound compared with other biomolecules. However, it can undergo a variety of covalent alterations both spontaneously (due to replication errors) and induced by external agents. Cells are constantly exposed to physical (e.g. UV rays, ionising radiation), and chemical agents (e.g. environmental and industrial pollutants) that disrupt the genetic information in DNA. Such deleterious agents can cause four major types of damage to DNA (Table 3.1)

Although ionising radiation is a physical agent, many of its effects are chemical in nature, because ionising radiation generates highly reactive chemical species such as hydroxyl radicals from water.

DNA REPAIR

All cells have developed DNA repair mechanisms to maintain the correct base sequences. Two major types are recognised:

- *light-induced repair* (*photoreactivation*)
- *light-independent repair* (*dark repair*)

LIGHT-INDUCED REPAIR

This involves a photolyase and corrects UV-induced thymine dimers, cytosine dimers and cytosine-thymine (C-T) dimers.

LIGHT-INDEPENDENT REPAIR

This is achieved by three distinct mechanisms:

- excision of the damaged nucleotides (*excision repair*)
- reconstruction of a functional DNA molecule from undamaged fragments (*recombination* repair)
- disregard of the damage (*SOS repair*)

Excision repair is a highly versatile repair pathway that removes a wide variety of DNA lesions, including those induced by UV-radiation and bulky carcinogens, by the sequential activities of four enzymes:

- an *endonuclease* that can make an incision at a damaged or incorrect base (detected by the 5′ 3′ nuclease activity of DNA polymerase

- an *exonuclease* that can remove the damaged or incorrectly incorporated base

TYPES OF DAMAGE TO DNA	
Type of damage	Mechanism
Single base alteration	Depurination or depyrimidation Deamination or alkylation of bases Insertion or deletion of nucleotides Base-analogue incorporation.
Two-base alteration	UV-light induced thymine-thymine dimer formation. Cross-linkage by bifunctional alkylating agents.
Chain breaks	Backbone breakage or inhibition of DNA replication by ionising radiation (e.g. X-rays) or radioactive elements.
Cross-linkage	Linking between bases in the same or opposite strands. Base linkage between DNA and protein molecules such as histones.

Table 3.1 – Types of damage to DNA.

- *DNA polymerase* activity that fills the gap created during removal of the damaged base

- *DNA ligase* activity that makes the final phosphodiester bond after DNA synthesis by DNA polymerase action

Defective excision repair activity results in several diseases including *xeroderma pigmentosum* and *Fanconi's anaemia,* both associated with malignancy.

Recombination repair involves a replacement of a large segment of one strand of damaged duplex DNA by the corresponding intact segment of another DNA molecule. Recombination repair occurs, for example, after damage to a viral chromosome in the host cell.

SOS repair includes a bypass system that allows DNA chain growth across damaged segments at the cost of fidelity of replication. The mechanism of induction of the SOS process is not fully understood.

CONSEQUENCES OF INABILITY TO REPAIR DNA DAMAGE

There are three possible consequences of damage to cellular DNA:

- there will be *no apparent effect*

- *DNA replication will be inhibited*

- *mutation* may occur

NO EFFECT

This may be due to one or more of the following reasons:

- damage causes a change in a "non-essential" part of the cell's DNA

- damage occurs in an essential part of the cell's DNA, but does not alter the cell's information

- damage causes a change which is repaired by cellular mechanisms before it can exert any harmful effect

CELL DEATH

Some damage to DNA is reversible, but if the damaging stimulus persists, or is very severe, cell death may occur.

MUTATIONS

A *mutation* is a change in the base sequence of the genetic code). The most common changes are *substitutions, additions,* or *deletions* of one or more bases. A physical or chemical agent that causes a mutation is a *mutagen.*

Mutations in germ cells could result in the birth of offspring with various defects. Women of child-bearing age should particularly avoid exposure to DNA-damaging agents (e.g. ionising rays). The higher incidence of various birth defects in children of women >35 years of age is thought partly to be due to the accumulation of damage to ova.

Cell mutation, whether spontaneous or induced, is a major cause of the initiation of cancer. For example, mutations in the *p53* gene are important for the development of many different types of cancers. The importance and characterisation of mutagens implicated in human disease encompasses all areas of medicine.

TYPES OF MUTATIONS

Mutations can be classified in several ways:

According to the nature of the change

A single base change is a *point mutation*; a change in two or more bases is a *multiple mutation*. A point mutation may occur in one of three ways: (1) *a base substitution,* (2) *a base-insertion,* or (3) *a base deletion.* Of these, base substitution is the most frequent.

According to the consequence of the change

A *silent mutation* has no detectable effects because of the degeneracy of the genetic code. Silent mutations are most likely if the mutation occurs in the third nucleotide of a codon.

A *missense mutation* involves an amino acid substitution resulting in the production of a different protein which may or may not carry out normal functions. A change in the second base of a codon usually results in a partially acceptable mutation (best exemplified by sickle cell haemoglobin, HbS). HbS differs from HbA in having a glutamate residue in the 6th position of the β-globin chain replaced by valine.

Chain-termination mutation (nonsense mutation) causes a codon which normally codes for an amino acid to be changed to a nonsense codon and termination of protein synthesis occurs at that point.

Frame-shift mutation occurs when a deletion or insertion of a nucleotide to a gene results in an altered reading frame in the base sequence in that gene.

Dynamic (unstable) mutation is a recently identified type of mutation characterised by an increased copy number of certain triplet repeat sequences in their DNA, known as *triplet amplification* or *expansion*. This has been identified as the mutational basis for inherited disorders, including *Huntington's disease* and *Fragile X syndrome.*

RECOMBINATION OF DNA

DNA replication and repair are mechanisms by which DNA sequences are maintained with very little change. Although such genetic stability is crucial for survival, genetic variation may help in the adaptation to changing environments.

Recombination of DNA results in genetic exchange between DNA duplexes, and can occur between different DNA molecules, or between different parts of the same DNA.

RECOMBINANT DNA TECHNOLOGY AND ITS IMPACT ON MEDICINE

DNA recombination has been used by scientists to manipulate genes artificially. This process, which involves the covalent joining of two molecules of DNA from any source and propagation of the hybrid molecule is known as *recombinant DNA (rDNA) technology* or *genetic engineering*.

BASIS OF RECOMBINANT DNA TECHNOLOGY

Recombinant DNA technology is based on several important findings:

- the availability of enzymes that can cut, join, and replicate DNA and reverse transcribe RNA

- the ability to recognise specific nucleotide sequences in DNA by using complementary DNA or RNA probes (see below)

- the ability to use vectors such as plasmids, viruses and cosmids to insert a DNA fragment into cells in which it can be cloned and amplified

Enzymes of recombinant DNA technology

The principal types of enzymes employed in recombinant DNA technology are *restriction endonucleases, polymerases* and *ligases*.

Restriction endonucleases (*restriction enzymes)* are bacterial enzymes that recognize a specific palindromic sequence (typically of 4–8 nucleotides) in double-stranded DNA, and hydrolyse a phosphodiester bond in each strand in this region, creating two restriction fragments.

The restriction fragments can be separated by electrophoresis. The pattern can serve as a *'fingerprint'* of a DNA molecule. The pattern of DNA fragments produced by a particular enzyme digest of DNA will sometimes differ from person to person. Such restriction fragment length polymorphisms are useful in clinical medicine for the detection of defective genes in several members of the same family and prenatally, in fetal tissues.

- Terminal transferases add nucleotide sequences to the 3′ ends of DNA.

- Ligases are used to join various DNA fragments together.

- *Reverse transcriptase* or *RNA-dependent DNA polymerase* transcribes the base sequence of an RNA molecule into a *complementary DNA (cDNA)* strand.

This cDNA contains only the nucleotide sequence of the mRNA. Such cDNAs can readily be converted to double-stranded DNA for cloning (see below). Reverse transcriptase can also be used to synthesise *cDNA probes,* single stranded DNA molecules containing a sequence of bases complementary to a protein of interest. Such probes will hybridise with the complementary base sequence in either DNA or RNA and can be used to detect sequences of interest.

Identification of specific restriction fragments

A restriction fragment can be identified by *hybridising* it with a labelled, complementary DNA strand (Figure 3.5). Restriction fragments separated by gel electrophoresis are heat-denatured to form single-stranded DNA, and transferred to a nitrocellulose sheet. DNA fragments in the nitrocellulose sheet are located by hybridization with a single-stranded *DNA probe.* Hybridised fragments are then visualised, for example, by autoradiography for a ^{32}P-labelled probe. This technique of identification of the DNA fragments is known as *Southern blotting.* An analogous technique for analysis of RNA molecules is termed *Northern blotting.* *Western blotting* refers to a technique for detecting a protein by staining with a particular antibody.

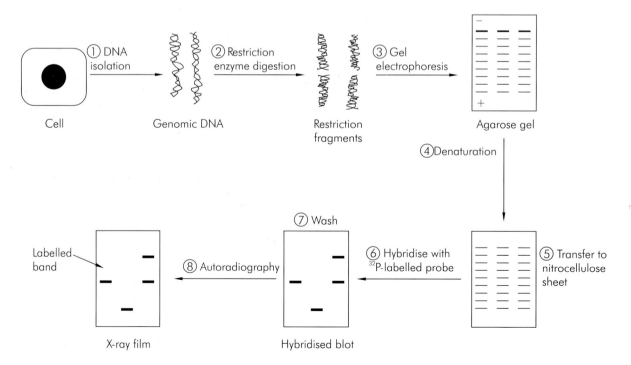

Figure 3.5 – The principles of Southern blotting.

POLYMERASE CHAIN REACTION (PCR)

This is an *in vitro* method that allows selective amplification of small quantities of DNA. DNA isolated from the desired source is incubated with three other components:

- *heat stable polymerase (Taq polymerase)* isolated from the thermophilic bacterium *Thermus aquaticus*

- an excess of two short, *synthetic DNA primers* with complementary sequences to the two ends of the opposite strands of the target DNA

- an excess of *deoxyribonucleoside triphosphates*

PCR consists of repetitive cycling of three reactions – *denaturing, annealing,* and *synthesis* (Figure 3.6). Twenty cycles amplify DNA by about 10^6; the technique can also be used, with modifications, to amplify target RNA sequences. PCR has found wide applications in genetic analysis, such as forensic pathology, identification of infectious agents and diagnosis of inherited diseases.

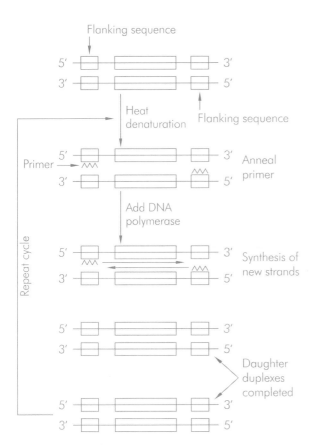

Figure 3.6 – The polymerase chain reaction (PCR).

GENE CLONING

Cloning is an *in vitro* technique used for the production of a large number of identical DNA molecules. DNA fragments are manipulated into *vectors* (DNA plasmids, viruses of bacteria). The host bacteria are selected by culture by an antibiotic, a condition under which only cells containing the recombinant plasmid which confers antibiotic resistance will grow (Figure 3.7).

A *genomic clone* is the recombinant DNA molecule of interest in a culture of host bacterial cells derived from a single bacterium. A *genomic library* is a set of clones representing all the cellular DNA of the organism, prepared by digesting total cellular DNA with restriction enzymes and cloning each of the resulting fragments in one culture as described. A *cDNA clone* is a culture in which all bacteria contain an identical fragment of cDNA. A *cDNA library* is a set of cDNA clones representing all of the mRNAs expressed in a particular cell type.

DNA SEQUENCING

The segments of specific DNA molecles obtained by recombinant DNA technology can be analysed for their nucleotide sequence by employing chemical methods (e.g. Maxam and Gilbert) or enzymatic methods (e.g. Sanger's). Details can be found in molecular biology text books.

Application of DNA sequencing in clinical medicine

Cystic fibrosis (CF) affects 1 in 2000 Caucasian children. Affected children have abnormal pancreatic and pulmonary secretions resulting in malabsorption and severe lung disease. Analysis of the *CF* gene on chromosome 7 has shown its product to be *cystic fibrosis transmembrane conductance regulator*[*] (CFTR), a protein involved in chloride (Cl-) ion transport. The most common mutation involves deletion of a phenylalanine residue at position 508 and accounts for about 75% of all cases.

GENE THERAPY

Over the past decade, several attempts have been made to ameliorate diseases caused by a deficiency of a gene product by replacement gene therapy. The strategy is to clone a gene into a vector that will be taken up readily and incorporated into the genome of a host cell. Gene therapy protocols have been developed for

[*]*cystic fibrosis transmembrane conductance regulator*

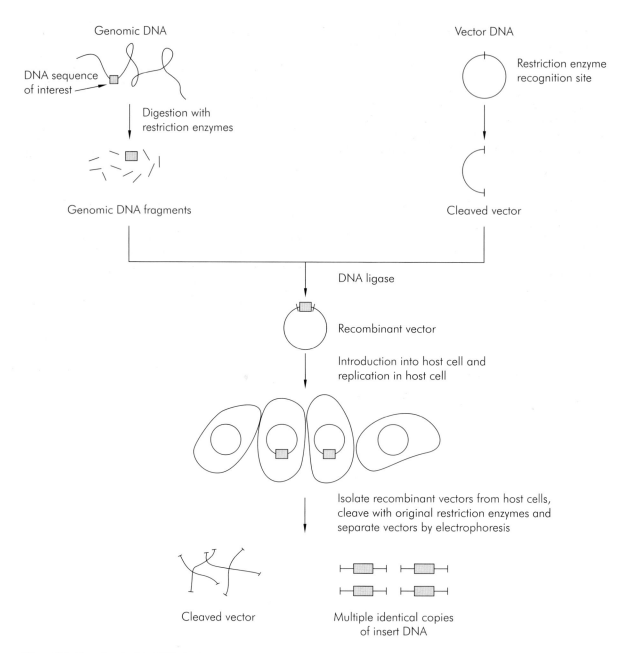

Figure 3.7 – Steps involved in DNA cloning.

adenosine deaminase deficiency, using T-lymphocytes, *LDL-receptor deficiency (familial hypercholesterolaemia),* using liver cells and *cystic fibrosis* using airway epithelial cells. The introduced gene would begin to direct the expression of its protein product, and this would correct the deficiency in the host cell.

A weakened form of virus (*adeno-, herpes*) containing

the gene is often used as the vector (e.g. *adenoviruses* target the lungs; *herpes viruses* target the neural tissues). However, there is the danger of the targeted gene being switched off by the body's antiviral responses. Direct delivery of DNA by charged lipid droplets called *lipo-somes* has been attempted to overcome inflammation/ immunity associated with the use of viral vectors. Liposomes transfer genes to the target cells by fusing with the plasma membrane but are not as efficient as viral vectors at delivering the DNA to the nucleus. Aerosols of such vesicles containing a healthy *cystic fibrosis gene* have been administered to the lungs of patients suffering from the disease, with some success. Attempts have also been made to shoot DNA molecules directly into cells at high velocity. Strategies to alter germ cell lines have also been devised, but so far have been tested only in animals *(transgenic animals)*.

CLINICAL APPLICATIONS OF RECOMBINANT DNA TECHNOLOGY

The process of recombinant DNA technology, together with improvements in techniques for extensive mapping and sequencing of human and other genomes, has revolutionised:

• the understanding of the molecular basis of many diseases

• methods for the diagnosis of diseases

• means of producing large quantities of products with therapeutic value (e.g. insulin, factor VIII), and vaccines.

• the potential to replace defective genes in the somatic cells of the human body to correct genetic diseases (gene therapy)

SELECTED READING

Alberts, B., Bray, D., Lewis, J., Raff, A.M., Roberts, K. and Watson, J.D. – *Molecular Biology of the Cell*, 3rd edn. Garland Publishing Inc., London, 1994.

Kornberg, A. and Baker, T.A. – *DNA replication.*, 2nd edn. W. H. Freeman and Co., New York, 1992.

Mueller, R.F., Young, I.D. – *Emery's Elements of Medical Genetics*. Churchill Livingstone, London, 1995.

Mullis, K.B. An unusual origin of the polymerase chain reaction, *Scientific American* 1990; **262**: 56–65.

Roskoski, R. (Jr) – Biochemistry. W.B.Saunders Company, London, 1996.

Thompson, C.B. – Apoptosis in the pathogenesis and treatment of disease. *Science* 1995; **267**: 1456–1462.

Wetherall, D.J. – *The New Genetics and Clinical Practice*, 3rd edn. Oxford University Press, Oxford, 1991.

4

INFORMATION EXPRESSION

Genetic information in chromosomes when transferred to daughter cells by DNA replication, is expressed through *transcription* to RNA, and in the case of messenger RNA (mRNA), subsequent *translation* into proteins:

$$\text{DNA} \xrightarrow{\text{transcription}} \text{RNA} \xrightarrow{\text{translation}} \text{Protein}$$

This flow of information from DNA to RNA to protein is true of all organisms with the exception of some retroviruses (e.g. HIV) that have genetic information stored in RNA. Retroviral RNA in infected cells has to be first transcribed into DNA by an RNA-directed DNA polymerase (reverse transcriptase).

TRANSCRIPTION

Transcription describes the synthesis of complete RNA molecules from DNA templates. It occurs from specific regions of the genome and is, therefore, highly selective; many transcripts are made from some regions of the DNA, while few or no transcripts are made from other regions.

COMPONENTS REQUIRED

Transcription requires the essential participation of the following components:

- a DNA template

- a Mg^{2+} or Mn^{2+}-dependent *DNA* directed *RNA polymerase* (*RNA* polymerase)

- the nucleoside triphosphates ATP, GTP, UTP and CTP

- accessory protein factors (*transcription factors)*

- energy supplied by ATP and GTP

RNA polymerases

Unlike prokaryotes, in which a single series of RNA polymerase (RP) is found, eukaryotes have three distinct classes of RP, differing in template specificity, localization, and susceptibility to inhibitors. (Table 4.1).

MECHANISM OF TRANSCRIPTION

Transcription begins by the binding of an RP to a specific *promoter* site on the DNA, which helps to open the DNA double helix in that region (Figure 4.1). The RP is capable of both initiation of transcription and elongation of the RNA chain. This enzyme helps sequentially to add on and join (by phosphodiester bonds), ATP, UTP, GTP and CTP in a $5' \rightarrow 3'$- direction to create an RNA strand that is complementary to one of the strands of the DNA template (Figure 4.1). RP can transcribe only one of the DNA strands (known as the *template strand*) at a time. The basis for the selection of which DNA strand will be transcribed has yet to be understood completely, but in eukaryotes there is evidence that the binding of certain supplemental transcription factors to distinct sites on the DNA (see below) either within the promoter region or some distance from it, helps the RP to determine which genes are to be transcribed.

As successive nucleotides are added to the RNA chain, the 5' end of this RNA retains its original triphosphate group, which provides one terminus of the RNA. Elongation of the RNA continues until a termination signal is reached, and the newly formed RNA transcript is released from the DNA template near the terminator region thereby slowing down the progress of the RP.

Recognition of the promoter region in DNA by the RNA polymerase

To transcribe a gene correctly, RP must recognise the correct transcriptional start site in a gene (Figure 4.2). RP must bind 'upstream' of the start site and then proceed 'downstream' until the termination site is reached. Sequence recognition by an RP during transcription is a complex process and involves two major elements:

THE GENETIC CODE					
First nucleotide	Second nucleotide				Third nucleotide
	U	C	A	G	
	Phe	Ser	Tyr	Cys	U
	Phe	Ser	Tyr	Cys	C
U	Leu	Ser	CT*	CT*	A
	Leu	Ser	CT*	Trp	G
	Leu	Pro	His	Arg	U
	Leu	Pro	His	Arg	C
C	Leu	Pro	Gln	Arg	A
	Leu	Pro	Gln	Arg	G
	Ile	Thr	Asn	Ser	U
	Ile	Thr	Asn	Ser	C
A	Ile	Thr	Lys	Arg	A
	Met	Thr	Lys	Arg	G
	Val	Ala	Asp	Gly	U
	Val	Ala	Asp	Gly	C
G	Val	Ala	Glu	Gly	A
	Val	Ala	Glu	Gly	G

First, second and third nucleotide refer to the individual nucleotides of a triplet codon. AUG, which codes for methionine, is the chain initiator codon; CT is the chain terminator.

Table 4.1

- specific sequences on the DNA template, e.g. Figure 4.3

- transcription factors that bind to these sequences in a sequence specific manner

Unlike prokaryotes, sequence recognition in eukaryotes is not carried out by the RP, but by certain other transcription factors, before the RP arrives at the promoter region. Eukaryotic RP therefore recognizes not a sequence of DNA, but a pre-existing DNA-protein complex at the gene promoter. The binding of RP to the promoter region has been shown to depend on the ability of transcription factors to recognise the following concensus sequences that lie upstream from the transcription site that codes for the initial base of the mRNA:

- the *TATA* or *Hogness box* has a sequence of nucleotides that is almost identical to that of the Pribnow box in prokaryotes, and lies about 25 nucleotides upstream of the transcriptional start site

- the *CAAT box* lies between 70 and 80 nucleotides upstream from the transcriptional start site

- the *GC box* contains a sequence GGGCGG and is located 50–60 nucleotides upstream of the transcription start site

Certain other controlling nucleotide sequences called *enhancers* may lie at variable distances upstream or downstream of the transcription start site and assist in the initiation of transcription. Genes also contain *silencers* or *negative enhancers* that can decrease the rate of initiation of transcription by RP.

TRANSCRIPTION FACTORS

Any protein needed for the initiation of transcription, but which is not itself a part of the RP, is a transcription factor (TF). TFs function by recognising specific sites on promoters or enhancers, as well as by binding to other TFs. Several initiator TFs form a complex through which the RP interacts with the promoter region and do not act as a part of the RP itself (these TFs are also released following initiation). The binding of RNA polymerase II (RPII) to a promoter during assembly of a transcription complex by TFs is outlined in Figure 4.3. There are characteristic domains or

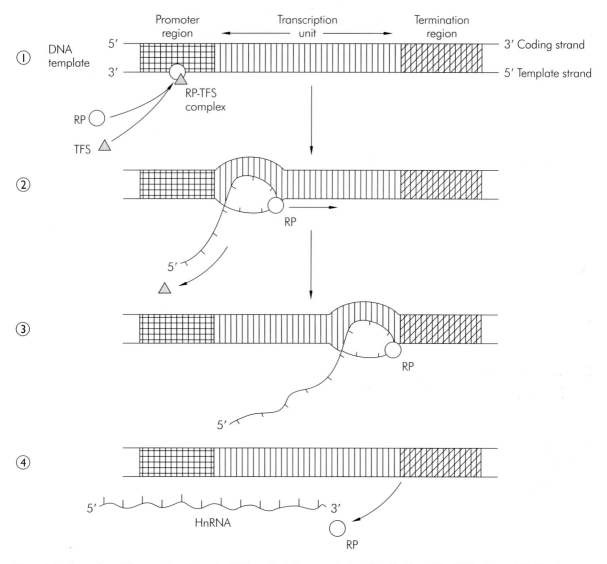

Figure 4.1 – An outline of the steps in eukaryotic RNA synthesis by transcription. ① – Binding of the DNA -directed RNA polymerase (RP)-transcription factor (TF) complex to the promoter region; ② – RP begins to synthesize RNA while the TFs are recycled; ③- Elongation continues till the termination region is reached; ④ – The nascent protein is released from the DNA template.

motifs common to most TF proteins and other proteins that bind to DNA. Examples include the *zinc-finger motif, leucine-zipper motifs* and *helix-turn-helix motif.* *Zinc-fingers* are regions of a protein that consist of two histidines and two cysteines bound to zinc. The *leucine-zipper* contains a stretch of amino acids rich in leucine that may be involved in dimerisation of TFs. *Helix-turn-helix motifs* contain a combination of antiparallel β-sheets and α-helices.

Action of antibiotics on transcription

Actinomycin D blocks cell division by binding to guanine in DNA and interfering with movement of RNA polymerase along the DNA template. It is used in the treatment of some malignancies.

Rifampicin inhibits the initiation of transcription by binding to the β-subunit of bacterial RP. It does not inhibit human RP, and therefore is not toxic.

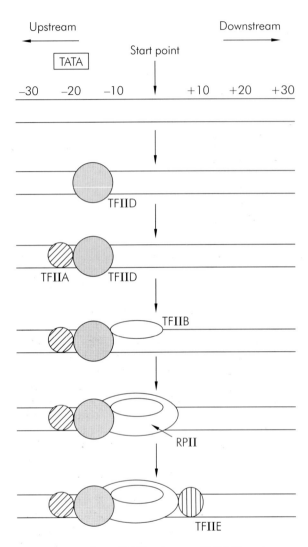

Figure 4.2 – Binding of RNA polymerase II (RP II) to the promoter region as a transcription complex that contains several transcription factors. TFIID first recognizes the TATA sequence. TFIIA TFIIB and TFIIE then assemble sequentially to form a transcription complex which helps RP II to bind correctly to the DNA template for initiation of transcription.

MAJOR TYPES OF RNA

Three major types of RNA transcribed from DNA, participate in protein synthesis:

- *messenger RNA (mRNA)*
- *ribosomal RNA (rRNA)*
- *transfer RNA (tRNA)*

These RNA molecules are synthesised as long polynucleotide chains, but they differ from DNA in having ribose instead of deoxyribose, having uracil instead of thymine and being smaller in size. mRNA, rRNA and tRNA differ from each other in terms of size, function and special post-transcriptional, structural modifications they undergo.

Ribosomal RNA (rRNA)

Transcription and processing of rRNA occur in the nucleolus. rRNA comprises approximately 80% of cellular RNA and 60% of the mass of ribosomes (the complex structures that serve as the sites for protein synthesis). In ribosomes, rRNA is associated with different proteins. Immature ribosomal subunits assembled from processed rRNA and ribosomal proteins imported from the cytoplasm are passed through the pores in the nuclear membrane into the cytoplasm where they become mature, functional units.

In mitochondria, there are three distinct size species of rRNA (23S, 16S, and 5S). In eukaryotic cell cytosol, there are four rRNA species (28S, 18S, 5.8S and 5S; s refers to a Svedberg unit which is related to the molecular weight of the compound). RP I produces a single pre-RNA transcript that contains 18S, 5.8S and 28S rRNA joined by transcribed spacers. Post-transcriptional processing involves hydrolytic separation of these three types of rRNA, and alterations to bases (e.g. methylation or conversion of uridine to pseudouridine).

Transfer RNA (tRNA)

tRNA is the smallest (4S) of the three major types of RNA and each molecule has between 74–95 nucleotide residues. Each pre-tRNA transcript must be activated first by the removal of 20 to 30 nucleotides, and by the addition of a cytidine-cytidine-adenine trinucleotide (CCA unit) to the 3′-end (amino acid acceptor end). Many of its nucleotides undergo alterations by methylation, reduction or sulphation. The primary structure of all tRNA molecules allows extensive folding and intrastrand and complementarity to generate a 'clover-leaf' shaped secondary structure (Figure 4.3).

There is at least one specific type of tRNA molecule for each of the 20 amino acids used in protein synthesis. Each tRNA molecule serves as an 'adaptor' that carries its specific amino acid to the site of protein synthesis. In all tRNA molecules, starting from the 3′ end, the first loop (7-membered) always contains a nucleotide triplet TΨC (Ψ = pseudouridine). The second or middle loop contains a triplet of nucleotides

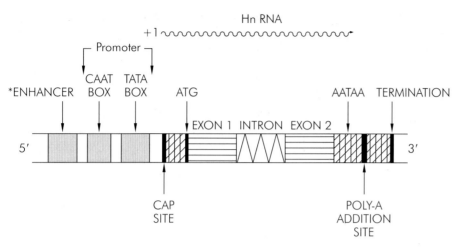

Figure 4.3 – A diagrammatic illustration of the typical structure of a gene transcribed by RNA polymerase II. *-Enhancers may also be found internally or downstream of the gene.(Hn RNA – heteronuclear RNA).

called the *anticodon* which recognises a complementary codon on mRNA. The third loop which has a variable number of nucleotides, consisting of mainly dihydrouracil (DHU) and purines, is important for the proper recognition of the tRNA molecule by its specific enzyme (*aminoacyl tRNA synthetase*) that helps a specific amino acid to bind to tRNA.

Messenger RNA (mRNA)

mRNA comprises only about 5% of the cellular RNA, but is the most heterogeneous in terms of size. Its primary function is to transfer the genetic information passed on to it from DNA during transcription to the cytosol.

The primary mRNA transcript synthesized by RPII is sometimes referred to as *heterogeneous nuclear RNA* or *hnRNA*. This transcript is extensively modified after transcription. Post-transcriptional changes include:

- *addition of a poly A tail* (a chain of up to 200 adenylic acid residues) at the 3′-end by a nuclear enzyme *poly A polymerase*. This tail is thought to help stabilize mRNA and facilitate its exit from the nucleus into the cytosol; in the cytosol, the poly A tail is gradually shortened

- addition at the 5′-end, of a 7-methylguanosine residue attached by a 5′-5′-pyrophosphate link; the next two nucleotides may also be methylated. This modified end is known as the *methyl cap*. The addition of this methyl cap facilitates initiation of translation, and helps stabilise the mRNA

- *splicing* or removal of specific sequences (splice sites) along the length of the modified pre-mRNA molecule. The sections of mRNA removed in this way (*introns* or *intervening sequences*) do not code for proteins from the primary transcript. The remaining *coding sequences*, the *exons*, are joined together to form the mature mRNA. The snRNAs, in association with small nuclear ribosomal protein particles (snRNPs), help in the splicing of some exons by forming base pairs with each end of an intron. This binding brings the sequences of the neighbouring exons into the correct alignment for splicing

Splicing is very important – a single pre-mRNA transcript can be spliced in more than one way to generate two or more mature mRNAs. These can therefore be translated to yield different, but related polypeptides from a single gene.

THE GENETIC CODE

The genetic information required for synthesis of a protein is stored in mRNA as the *genetic code*. A sequence of three consecutive bases on a mRNA molecule forms each 'word' in the code, referred to as a *codon*. Each codon leads to the addition of one particular amino acid during translation or protein synthesis. The various codons found in mRNA and the amino acids which are represented by each of them are shown in Table 4.1.

4^3 (or 64) possible trinucleotide sequences formed

from the four nucleotides in mRNA are required to code for the 20 amino acids used in protein synthesis. Three codons, UAA, UAG and UGA, do not represent any amino acid, but act as *stop signals* to indicate the point of polypeptide termination.

Most amino acids are coded for by more than one codon. The genetic code is therefore said to be *redundant* or *degenerate,* but a single codon always codes for a specific amino acid. The presence of 'WOBBLE' at the 3′ end of most codons enables non-standard base pairing between 3′ position of the codons and 5′ positions anticodons in tRNA; thus enabling a tRNA to interact with more than one codon. The DNA strand used as a template for a particular mRNA has base triplets that are complementary to the codons on the mRNA. Any change in the DNA base sequence (mutation) will therefore be transmitted in both DNA replication and transcription (see Chapter 3).

TRANSLATION

COMPONENTS REQUIRED

The components required for translation are:

- amino acids found in the completed polypeptide chain

- the mRNA to be translated

- tRNAs for the respective amino acids

- functional ribosomes

- energy in the form of ATP and GTP and enzymes

and other accessory protein factors (*initiation, elongation* and *termination factors*) required for the various steps in the process.

Ribosomes

Ribosomes are the sites of protein synthesis. They are found either free in the cytoplasm, or bound to the endoplasmic reticulum. Each is a complex assembly of 60% rRNA and 40% protein. A functional ribosome is made up of 2 subunits, a smaller and a larger. A functional eukaryotic ribosome (80S) is composed of a 40S small subunit and a 60S large subunit, each of which contains a distinctive set of RNA and protein molecules (Figure 4.4). Ribosomes of a 70S type (as in prokaryotes) are found in mitochondria.

ACTIVATION OF AMINO ACIDS

Activation of an amino acid occurs before it binds to its specific tRNA. This process, as well as the formation of the amino acyl-tRNA complex, is catalysed by *aminoacyl tRNA synthetase.*

Amino acid + ATP $\longleftrightarrow$ Aminoacyl-AMP + PP, tRNA Aminoacyl-tRNA + AMP
$\longleftrightarrow$

The activated amino acid is joined covalently by an ester linkage through its carboxyl group to the CCA-sequence at the 3′ terminus of the tRNA. After it has given up its amino acid for protein synthesis, tRNA can be re-used. The aminoacyl tRNA synthetase has two main functions: to ensure the loading of the correct amino acid to its cognate tRNA, and to activate the carboxyl group for peptide bond formation.

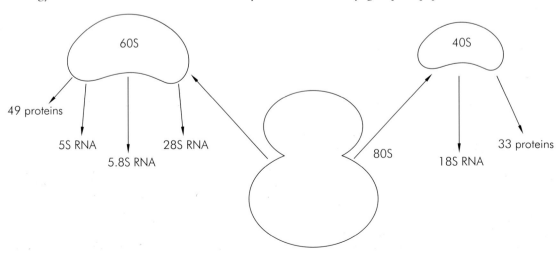

Figure 4.4 – Composition of a eukaryotic 80S ribosome. (S = Sedimentation coefficient in Svedberg units).

Accessory protein factors

Several initiation, elongation, and termination factors are required for protein synthesis. Some of these perform a catalytic function while others appear to stabilize the protein synthesising machinery.

TRANSLATION OF mRNA

Translation of the mRNA begins at the 5′ end. Three stages can be recognized in the process of translation:

- initiation of polypeptide chain formation

- chain elongation

- chain termination

Initiation of polypeptide chain formation involves the formation of a complex between the ribosomal subunits, mRNA and the aminoacyl-tRNA specified by the first codon in the message (*initiator codon*). At least ten different iniatiation factors have been identified. The tRNA that transfers the first amino (formylated methionine in prokaryotes, and methionine in eukaryotes) to the initiator codon is referred to as the *initiator tRNA*. Initiator tRNA is structurally different from the tRNA that inserts methionine to internal positions in the polypeptide chain being synthesised.

Initiation occurs in four stages (Figure 4.5):

Stage I – Binding of initiation factors to the 40S ribosomal subunit

Stage II – Formation of a ternary complex, including the initiator tRNA, which binds to the 40S ribosomal subunit to form the *40S pre-initiation complex*.

Stage III – Binding of mRNA (facilitated by the methyl Cap sequence at its 5′ end) to the 40S pre-initiation complex with the assistance of several initiation factors to form a *40S initiation complex*. Following this association, and the melting of the secondary structure near the 5′ end of mRNA, the complex scans the mRNA for the initiator codon (usually AUG nearest the 5′ end); the precise initiation codon is determined by a specific nucleotide sequence (*Kozak concensus*) that surrounds the AUG.

Stage IV – Binding of the 60S ribosomal subunit to the 40S initiation complex to form the 80S initiation complex. The ribosome has two binding sites for tRNAs carrying amino acids (A - and P - sites); each of which extends over both subunits. At the completion

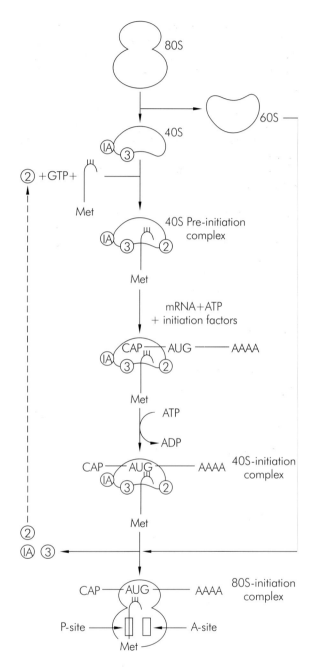

Figure 4.5 – A schematic representation of the initiation of protein synthesis in eukaryotes. (IA) (2) and (3) represent the initiation factors eEF-1a, eEF-2, and eIF-3 respectively.

of the 80S complex, the initiator tRNA will be occupying the P-site on the ribosome, leaving the A-site free.

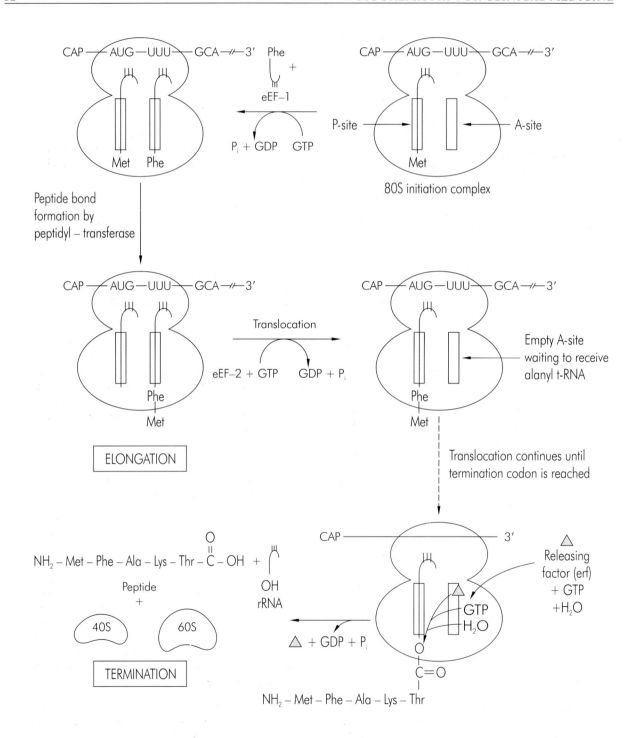

Figure 4.6 – A schematic representation of the steps involved in the elongation and termination processes of eukaryotic protein synthesis. eEF-1 and eEF-2 are elongation factors.

ELONGATION OF THE POLYPEPTIDE CHAIN

Elongation involves three main events (Figure 4.6):

- *binding of an aminoacyl-tRNA to the A-site*, as dictated by the codon adjacent to that occupied by tRNA carrying the growing polypeptide chain, occupying the P-site. Proper binding of the incoming aminoacyl-tRNA requires assistance from GTP and certain elongation factors. It is noteworthy that these elongation factors do not interact with the initiator met-tRNA. Hence, the initiator tRNA is not delivered to the A-site, and internal AUG codons cannot be read by the initiator tRNA

- *peptide bond formation*. A component (23S rRNA) of the 60S ribosomal subunit known as *peptidyl transferase* catalyses the transfer of the amino acid at the P-site to the A-site, and a peptide bond is formed between the two amino acids. Peptidyl transferase is an example of a *ribozyme* (an RNA molecule acting as an enzyme). Upon removal of the peptidyl moiety from the tRNA at the P-site, the discharged tRNA dissociates from the P-site

- *translocation*. This involves a movement of the ribosome and mRNA in relation to one another in such a manner that the ribosome will move along each time, by one codon, towards the 3′ end of the mRNA. Elongation factor eEF-2 and GTP are responsible for the transfer of the peptidyl-tRNA from the A-site to the empty P-site, leaving the A-site free for another cycle of aminoacyl-tRNA codon recognition and elongation

Termination occurs when one of the three terminator codons, UAA, UAG or UGA, moves into the A-site; there is no tRNA with an anticodon that recognises these codons. Hydrolysis of the bond between the peptide and the tRNA occupying the P-site then occurs, releasing the nascent polypeptide chain and the tRNA from the P-site.

Polyribosomes

Because of the length of most mRNAs, more than one ribosome can translate the same mRNA molecule simultaneously. Such a complex of a single mRNA with a number of bound ribosomes is referred to as a *polyribosome* or *polysome*.

POST-TRANSLATIONAL MODIFICATIONS OF PROTEINS

Many polypeptide chains undergo covalent modifications either while they are still attached to the ribosome, or after their synthesis has been completed. They are referred to as *post-translational modifications*. The more common types of modifications undergone by polypeptides are removal of initiator methionine, removal of a part of the translated sequence (e.g. pancreatic islet cell hormones) vitamin C-dependent hydroxylations (e.g. collagen) or covalent alterations such as *glycosylation* (e.g. membrane proteins) and *phosphorylation*.

PROTEIN FOLDING TO FORM A FUNCTIONAL MOLECULE

Nascent polypeptide chains must undergo folding to form the native three-dimensional structures that are functionally active. The process probably begins while the polypeptide chain is still being synthesised on the ribosome and is usually assisted by catalysts such as *molecular chaperones* (e.g. heat-shock proteins) that assist protein folding by inhibiting improper attachments and separating unwanted liaisons.

ANTIBIOTIC INHIBITORS OF PROTEIN BIOSYNTHESIS

Antibiotics have the ability to inhibit the growth of various disease-causing micro-organisms. Most achieve this by interfering with one or more steps in protein biosynthesis (usually by combining with one or both of the ribosomal subunits of the micro-organisms). For example erythromycin binds to the 50S subunit while streptomycin binds to the 30S subunit. These antibiotics, with a few exceptions (e.g. puromycin and cycloheximide), do not interfere with the host protein biosynthesis because eukaryotic ribosomal subunits have proteins different from those in prokaryotic ribosomal subunits.

The antibacterial action of *β-lactam antibiotics* (e.g. *penicillins* and *cephalosporins*) is due to an interference with bacterial cell wall biosynthesis. Thus penicillins and cephalosporins inhibit cell wall synthesis by binding to a *transpeptidase* that normally transfers a D-alanyl-D-alanine peptidyl group to other amino acids of the cell wall peptidoglycan core; the β-lactam ring resembles the D-alanyl–D-alanine peptidyl group.

INHIBITION OF EUKARYOTIC PROTEIN SYNTHESIS BY BACTERIAL AND PLANT TOXINS

Some bacterial and plant toxins inhibit eukaryotic protein synthesis by inactivating protein factors involved in the elongation process or their binding to ribosomes (e.g. *corynebacterium diphtheriae* toxin and *toxic plant lectins* such as *abrin, ricin* and *modecin*).

PROTEIN TARGETING

Cells contain several 'compartments'. Mechanisms must therefore operate to ensure that proteins are transported to the correct locations within cells and, in eukaryotes, to various extracellular locations such as the blood stream. *Protein targeting* is the process by which polypeptides are delivered to their correct intra- and extracellular destinations.

TARGETING OF NASCENT PROTEINS

The ultimate destination of a nascent protein is determined by the presence or absence of a *signal sequence* or *signal peptide sequence*. All proteins (except those encoded by mitochondrial DNA) begin on free ribosomes in the cytosol. However, ribosomes involved in the synthesis of proteins that are destined to be (1) delivered to the membranes of the endoplasmic reticulum, golgi bodies, lysosomes and plasma membrane, or (2) secreted, are directed to the endoplasmic reticulum by special *signal sequences* in the proteins being synthesized, and the synthesis of the protein is completed while the ribosome is attached to the endoplasmic reticulum membrane. Proteins that lack this signal sequence, are synthesised completely on free ribosomes, and are finally delivered to the cytosol. Depending on the presence of certain other special signals (see below), the proteins delivered to the cytosol are directed into mitochondria, nuclei and peroxisomes; those that lack a signal, remain in the cytosol.

Targeting of membrane and secretory proteins

Soon after initiation of proteins bound for membranes or for secretion on free ribosomes, the signal peptide sequence, also called the *leader sequence*, is joined at the N-terminal end of each of the growing polypeptide chains.

As the leader sequence emerges from the larger ribosomal subunit, it is recognised by a ribonucleoprotein assembly known as a *signal recognition particle* (SRP) that blocks further translation after about 70 amino acids have been polymerised. The SRP-imposed block is not released until the SRP-leader sequence-ribosome complex has bound to a receptor for SRP (*docking protein*) on the endoplasmic reticulum membrane (Figure 4.7). The endoplasmic reticulum also contains a receptor for the ribosome itself. By guiding the leader sequence to the SRP receptor site, SRP prevents premature folding and expulsion into the cytosol of the protein being synthesised. On binding of the SRP to the docking protein, a GTP-GDP cycle releases the signal sequence from the SRP and then detaches the latter from its receptor. The interaction of the ribosome and the growing polypeptide chain with the endoplasmic reticulum also results in the opening of a pore in the endoplasmic reticulum membrane, through which the polypeptide chain is transported into the endoplasmic reticulum. During transport, the leader sequence of most polypeptides is removed by *signal peptidase*. As translation proceeds, the protein is either inserted into, or translocated across, the endoplasmic reticulum membrane where secondary sorting signals in the polypeptide chain are responsible for directing it to particular intracellular or extracellular locations.

Many secretory and membrane proteins contain covalently attached carbohydrate moieties; N-glycan chains are usually added on as these proteins traverse through the endoplasmic reticulum by the carrier *dolichol phosphate* (a long lipid of about 20 isoprene (C5) units). Subsequently, the proteins enter the lumen of the golgi bodies, where further changes in glycan chains occur prior to intracellular distribution or secretion. The transport of proteins between the endoplasmic reticulum and golgi, and between golgi and subsequent destinations, is mediated by small, membrane bound compartments called *transport vesicles* (*transfer vesicles*). The correct folding and stabilisation of proteins prior to exit from the endoplasmic reticulum is carried out by various molecular chaperones.

The presence of special *stop-transfer sequences* ensures the insertion of proteins into the correct membrane. Mannose-6-phosphate is the marker that normally directs many hydrolytic enzymes from the golgi into lysosomes. Most of these special sequences are cleaved after translocation.

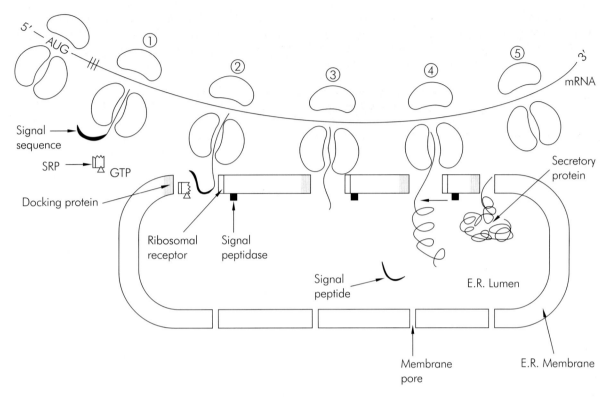

Figure 4.7 – Schematic representation of the stages in the synthesis of secretory and membrane proteins.
① Binding of SRP (signal recognition particle) to signal peptide shortly after initiation of protein synthesis.
② Binding of the SRP-bound polypeptide to the docking protein in the endoplasmic reticulum (ER) membrane.
③ Release of signal peptide from SRP as the ribosome binds to the ribosome receptor on the ER membrane.
④ Release of signal peptide from polypeptide by the signal peptidase, after the polypeptide has moved through the E.R.membrane pore.
⑤ Completion of protein synthesis and release of ribosome.

Targeting of proteins synthesized on free ribosomes

Targeting of proteins into mitochondria, nuclei or peroxisomes is achieved primarily by post-translational modifications of the cytoplasmic precursors. For example, most *proteins targeted to the mitochondrial matrix* contain a special amino acid sequence (15–35 residues long, and rich in positively charged residues and in serine and threonine) at their N-terminal ends. At least two types of short peptides called *nuclear localisation signals* that target *proteins that enter nuclei,* have been identified.

Clinical importance of protein targeting

Targeting defects have been shown to be responsible for the development of certain inherited disorders. Defects in targeting have also been implicated in the development of lysosomal storage diseases.

CONTROL OF GENE EXPRESSION

The expression of genetic information must be regulated during differentiation of an organism and its cellular components. Genetic expression must also be responsive to extrinsic signals in order for an organism to adapt to its environment. When a particular protein has to be synthesised in increased amounts, the expression of the gene corresponding to that protein has to be *positively regulated;* when protein production has to be decreased, the expression of the gene coding for that protein has to be *negatively regulated.*

TRANSCRIPTIONAL CONTROL

The expression of some genes is *constitutive* (i.e. they are expressed at a reasonably constant rate all the time, and not subject to regulation). There are also many other *inducible* genes whose activities can be regulated. Positive or negative regulation of an inducible gene involves the interaction of specific, regulator molecules with promoter regions of the DNA. Regulator molecules that increase gene expression are called *inducers,* while those that decrease gene expression are referred to as *repressors.* Some inducer molecules (*de-repressors*) increase gene expression indirectly by inter-acting with a repressor molecule and preventing the latter binding to the promoter region of the DNA. Many regulated systems that appear to be induced are in fact *de-repressed* at the molecular level.

The principles of induction and repression are easily understood by reference to the regulation of the *lac*-

operon in *E. coli*. Glucose is the preferred substrate for the growth of *E. coli*. The genes for the *lac*-operon (Figure 4.8) code for proteins required to transport the disaccharide lactose into the cell in the absence of glucose, and catabolize it to glucose. When *E. coli* are grown in the presence of glucose or glycerol, the *lac*-operon genes are *repressed* because there is no need to produce lactose metabolising enzymes. Repression involves the binding of a repressor protein, generated constitutively by a repressor gene (*i-gene* in Figure 4.8), to the operator locus, thus preventing subsequent tran-scription of the *lac*-operon genes by the DNA-depen-dent RNA polymerase. When *E. coli* are grown in the absence of glucose (a starvation situation), and the presence of lactose, the latter can act as an *inducer* and

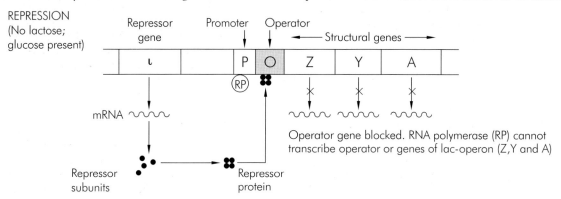

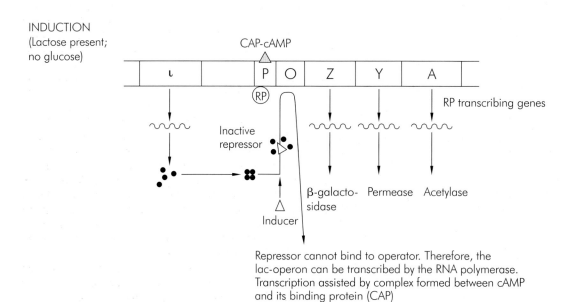

Figure 4.8 – A schematic representation of induction and repression of the lactose operon (*lac* operon) of *Escherichia coli* (*E. coli*).

cause the *lac*-operon to be expressed. In addition to lactose, a complex formed between cyclic AMP (cAMP) and a *catabolite gene activator protein (CAP)*, is also required for the full expression of the *lac*-operon. CAP enables bacteria to use alternative carbon sources such as lactose when glucose is unavailable for growth. When glucose is available, CAP cannot bind to the DNA. In the absence of glucose, there is a high concentration of cAMP in the cells; cAMP binds to CAP and promotes binding of CAP to the promoter and alters the DNA conformation to induce expression of the *lac*-operon. This arrangement enables the *lac*-operon to respond to and integrate two different signals, so that it is expressed only when two conditions are met: (1) lactose is present, and (2) glucose is absent. In any other conditions, the *lac*-operon is kept switched off; it would be wasteful for CAP to induce expression of the *lac*-operon if lactose were absent.

As evident from the example of the *lac*-operon, bacteria generally 'shut down' unwanted genes with help from repressor proteins and then induce them in response to some specific stimulus. In eukaryotes, due to the complexity of the genome, there are important differences in the control of transcription:

- activators and repressors of gene expression operate by altering the rate of formation of transcription complexes at specific DNA sequences such as the TATA box rather than by influencing only the RNA polymerase action. In this context, transcription activators contain a DNA binding domain that recognizes a particular DNA sequence, and an activation domain that aids the assembly of the transcription complex at the TATA box. Different combinations of activators switch on different sets of genes

- most genes are controlled by multiple proteins rather than by just one or two. For example, the serum albumin gene in mice contains six binding sites for regulatory proteins near its TATA box. Additional control sites (*enhancer* and *silencer sequences*) are also present several kilobases away. Proteins bound to enhancer or silencer sequences can regulate transcription. It is thought that each type of cell in higher eukaryotes contains a specific combination of gene regulatory proteins that ensures the expression of only those genes appropriate to that cell type

- control of gene expression occurs mostly in a positive direction. Many genes appear to be normally expressed at low or basal levels and activated to increase the rate of transcription by one or more transcription activation protein factors in response to various chemical signals (e.g. hormones)

OTHER METHODS UTILISED BY EUKARYOTES FOR CONTROLLING GENE EXPRESSION AT THE TRANSCRIPTIONAL END

Gene amplification and rearrangement are two other mechanisms utilised to increase quantitatively the concentration of specific RNA transcripts involved in protein synthesis.

Gene amplification

Under selective pressure (e.g. in response to hormones during early development, or to drugs), certain pre-existing genes that usually code for only single copies of specific RNA molecules are amplified to provide multiple sites for gene transcription. Gene amplification has been implicated in the development of *drug resistance* in cancer patients.

Gene rearrangement

Gene rearrangement involves the formation of new arrangements of genes by the movement of DNA segments from different parts of the same chromosome or from different chromosomes. *Gene rearrangement plays an important role in the formation of active immunoglobin genes that generate a diversity of antibodies* (e.g. IgG, IgA, IgE, IgM and IgD). Each immunoglobulin molecule is composed of two types of polypeptide chains – a heavy or H-chain and a light or L-chain. Three unlinked families of genes are responsible for the generation of these chains. Two families are responsible for the generation of the two types of light chains (λ and κ) found in immunoglobulin molecules, while the third family is responsible for the five different types of heavy chains. The heavy and light chains are coded for by several widely separated genes in the germ line DNA. During the development of somatic cells, and also later during B-cell differentiation, genes encoding the various segments of the heavy and light chains (variable or V, constant or C, and joining or J segments) undergo several rearrangements so as to bring the C,V and J genes of a particular immunoglobulin chain closer together so that they can all be transcribed as a single mRNA precursor that can subsequently undergo various post-transcriptional modifications to yield mRNA that produces a particular heavy or light chain required for the formation of a specific immunoglobulin molecule.

Translational control

The overall rate of protein synthesis is controlled by the rate of translation, which in turn is regulated by changes in activities of initiation and elongation factors. Similarly, the rate of translation can be controlled by regulating the activity of the elongation factor complex that guides the mRNA to the small ribosomal subunit to form the 40S initiation complex. Insulin and mitogenic growth factors can activate this elongation factor complex by mediating the phosphorylation of eIF-4E, an elongation factor involved in the formation of this complex.

SELECTED READING

Alberts, B., Bray, D., Lewis, J., Raff, M., Roberts, K., and Watson, J.D. – *Molecular Biology of The Cell*, 3rd ed. Garland Publishing Inc., London, 1994.

Lewin, B. – *Genes IV*, Oxford University Press, Oxford, 1990.

Moldave, K. – Eukaryotic protein synthesis. *Annual Review of Biochemistry* 1985; **54**: 1109–1149.

Murray, R.K., Granner, D.K., Mayes, P.A. and Rodwell, V.W. – Harper's Biochemistry, 24th ed. Prentice Hall International (UK) Ltd., London, 1996.

Rapoport, T.A. – Protein transport across the ER membrane. *Trends in Biochemical Sciences* 1990; **15**: 355.

Roskoski, R (Jr). – *Biochemistry*. W.B. Saunders Co. Ltd., London, 1996.

Wilkinson, J.H. (ed) – *The Principles and Practice of Diagnostic Enzymology*, Edward Arnold, London, 1976.

Zylva, J.F., Pannall, P.R. and Mayne, P.D. – *Clinical Chemistry in Diagnosis and Treatment*, 5th ed. Edward Arnold, London, 1992.

5

CARBOHYDRATES

Carbohydrates may be defined as *polyhydroxy aldehydes* or *ketones*, or as substances that yield one of these compounds on hydrolysis. Most of them have an empirical formula $(CH_2O)_n$.

TYPES OF MONOSACCHARIDES		
Monosaccharide class	Aldoses	Ketoses
Trioses $(C_3H_6O_3)$	Glycerose	Dihydroxyacetone
Tetroses $(C_4H_8O_4)$	Erythrose	Erythrulose
Pentoses $(C_5H_{10}O_5)$	Ribose	Ribulose
Hexoses $(C_6H_{12}O_6)$	Glucose	Fructose

Table 5.1

BIOLOGICAL FUNCTIONS OF CARBOHYDRATES

- *a major source of energy* – the carbohydrate most commonly used for this purpose is *glucose*

- *energy storage* – in animals and humans, excess glucose is stored as *glycogen* while in plants, it is stored as *starch*. Starch is the major dietary carbohydrate for man

- *structural function* – carbohydrates (as *proteoglycans, glycolipids,* and *glycoproteins*) provide the skeletal framework for tissues and organs of the human body and serve as lubricants and support elements of connective tissue

- *cell-surface function* – glycoproteins and glycolipids on cell membrane surfaces are involved in a variety of receptor activities associated with cell signalling, cell-cell interactions and recognition

- *sources of building blocks* – metabolic intermediates derived from glucose may be diverted for use in the biosynthesis of a variety of molecules including amino acids, fatty acids, and nucleotides

CLASSIFICATION OF CARBOHYDRATES

Carbohydrates may be classified as *monosaccharides, disaccharides, oligosaccharides and polysaccharides.*

MONOSACCHARIDES

Monosaccharides are simple sugars that cannot be hydrolysed into smaller units under reasonably mild conditions. They are the basic units from which larger carbohydrate polymers are assembled. According to the number of carbon atoms they possess, monosaccharides may be referred to as *trioses* (3C), *tetroses* (4C), *pentoses* (5C), *hexoses* (6C) and *heptoses* (7C). They may also be classified as *aldoses* or *ketoses* depending on whether the functional carbonyl group in the molecule is an aldehyde or ketone (Table 5.1).

STEREOISOMERISM IN SUGARS

All sugar molecules contain *asymmetric carbon atoms* (carbon atoms connected to four different atoms or groups) and can exist as *isomers* having the same structural formula, but differing in spatial configuration. The simplest monosaccharide that possesses an asymmetric carbon atom, *glyceraldehyde* or *triose glycerose* can exist in the following isomeric forms designated *D* – and *L* - forms (Figure 5.1) which differ in the configuration of the penultimate carbon atom and differ in the direction in which they rotate polarised light. The isomer that rotates light in the clockwise direction is said to be *dextrorotatory*, and identified by the symbol (+); the isomer that rotates light in an anti-clockwise direction is said to be *laevorotatory*, and represented as (–). Because there are a large number of optical isomers of carbohydrates, glyceraldehyde is used as a reference compound. Those whose penultimate carbon atom configuration resembles that of D-glyceraldehyde (with the hydroxyl group on the right hand side) are referred to as D-sugars (e.g. *D-glucose*, Figure 5.2). The natural monosaccharides are, with a few exceptions, D-sugars.

D-Glyceraldehyde L-Glyceraldehyde

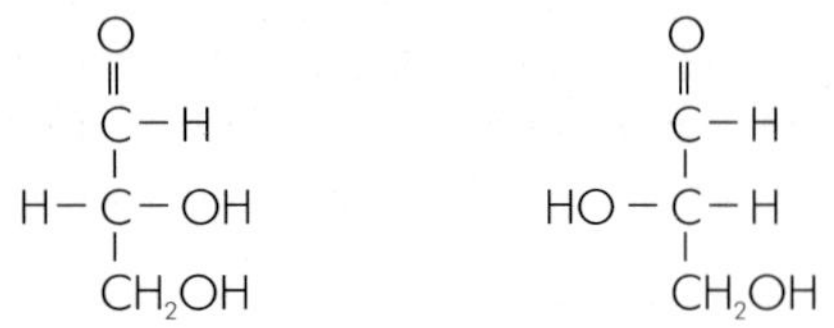

Figure 5.1 – D- and L- forms of Glyceraldehyde.

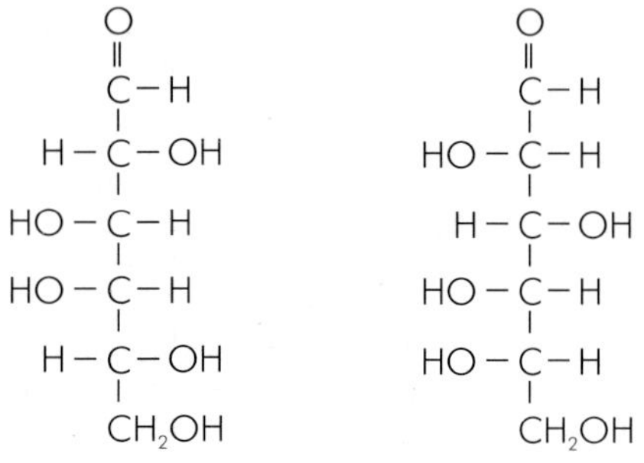

D-Galactose L-Glucose

Figure 5.2 – The structures of D- and L-Glucose.

RING STRUCTURE OF SUGAR MOLECULES.

Many carbohydrates, including glucose, can exist either in an *open chain form* or in a *ring form*. Monosaccharides with 5 or more carbon atoms, for thermodynamic reasons, exist predominantly in the ring or cyclic form.

The asymmetric carbon atom at the first carbon atom (C1) of the ring is referred to as the *anomeric carbon*. Depending on whether the H at C1 is above the OH or below it, there can be two isomeric forms referred to as the *α-anomer* and *β-anomer* respectively. Very closely related sugars which differ in the configuration of a single carbon atom other than the anomeric carbon (C3 and C4 in glucose) are structural isomers referred to as *epimers*. Biologically, the most important epimers of glucose are *galactose* and *mannose formed* by epimerisation at C4 and C2 respectively (Figure 5.3).

REDUCING PROPERTIES OF SUGARS

Sugars that contain a free carbonyl functional group (CHO or C=O) are reducing agents. In dilute alkali, monosaccharides tend to exist predominantly in the open chain form; the aldehyde and keto groups in the molecule are free to exhibit strong reducing properties. This property is exploited in the estimation of sugars in body fluids.

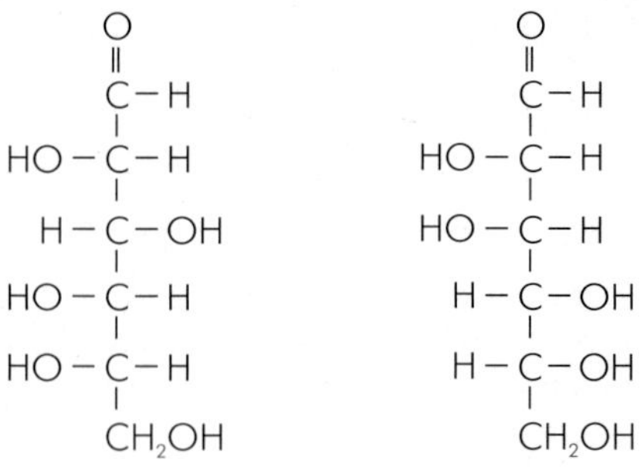

L-Glucose D-Mannose

Figure 5.3 – The structures of D-Galactose and D-Mannose.

IMPORTANT MONOSACCHARIDE DERIVATIVES

Sugar alcohols

The carbonyl group of both aldoses and ketoses can be reduced chemically or biologically to yield polyhydric alcohols. Examples of sugar alcohols and their biomedical importance are shown in Table 5.2.

Sugar acids

Sugar acids are formed when the carbonyl group or a hydroxyl group in a sugar molecule is oxidised to a carboxylic acid. Both C1 and C6 of aldoses can undergo oxidation (e.g. glucose can give rise to *gluconic acid* and *glucuronic acid* respectively), while in keto sugars, only C6 (or C5) can be oxidised.

Glucuronic acid is important as a constituent of complex polysaccharides, and as a conjugating agent. For example, bilirubin, many hormones, drugs, and environmental pollutants are eliminated from the body as soluble glucuronide conjugates. In animals other than guinea pigs and primates, glucuronic acid can be used to synthesise *ascorbic acid*.

Gluconic acid can be converted to ribose that is used in the synthesis of nucleotides. Salts of gluconic acid, because of their solubility, are often used to fortify the diet with essential elements such as iron and calcium

SUGAR ALCOHOLS AND THEIR BIOMEDICAL IMPORTANCE.		
Sugar alcohol	**Mechanism of formation**	**Importance**
Glycerol	Reduction of glyceraldehyde or dihydroxyacetone	Component of triglycerides and phospholipids
D-Sorbitol (D-Glucitol)	Reduction of carbonyl group at C1 of glucose, or C2 of fructose	Causes pathological changes in certain conditions (e.g. in diabetes mellitus, galactosaemia), by accumulation in lens, peripheral nerves, renal papillae etc.
*Mannitol	Reduction of carbonyl group at C2 of fructose or C1 of mannose	Used as an osmotic diuretic in acute renal failure, or raised intracranial pressure.
Xylitol	Reduction of carbonyl group at C1 of D-xylose or C2 of D-xylulose	Sucrose substitute; can help prevent dental caries as oral microorganisms cannot utilize these sugar alcohols.

*Administered intravenously. It is not metabolised appreciably, is filtered by the glomerulus, and is not reabsorbed by the renal tubules.

Table 5.2

(ferrous gluconate and calcium gluconate respectively).

Amino sugars (Hexosamines)

Amino sugars are formed when a hydroxyl group of a monosaccharide is replaced by an amino group. The amino sugars usually occur as N-acetyl derivatives. *Glucosamine* (the hexosamine formed from glucose) in the N-acetylated form is a major component of many complex polysaccharides. N-acetyl derivatives of *galactosamine* and *mannosamine* are important constituents of glycoproteins and glycolipids.

Neuraminic acid is another important amino sugar. Acetyl derivatives of neuraminic acid, also known as *sialic acids* are important constituents of glycoproteins in bone, cartilage, and connective tissue and of glycolipids in the nervous system. Several antibiotics (e.g. *erythromycin, carbomycin*) contain amino sugars. These amino sugars are thought to be related to the antibiotic activities of these drugs.

Glycosides

These are sugar derivatives formed by a reaction between the hydroxyl group of a sugar at the anomeric carbon, and the hydroxyl group of a second compound referred to as the *aglycone*. If the sugar is glucose, the product formed is called a *glucoside*, and if it is a galactose, a *galactoside*. The aglycone can be another sugar or a non-sugar molecule (e.g. methanol, glycerol, sterol, phenol).

Glycosidic linkages are very important in the formation of disaccharides, polysaccharides, and other complex glycosides. Many important drugs (e.g. the antibiotic *streptomycin* and *digoxin* used in the treatment of heart failure) are glycosides.

Deoxysugars

In deoxysugars, one or more hydroxyl groups of the pyranose or furanose ring is substituted by hydrogen for example, *deoxyribose* used in the synthesis of DNA, and *L-fucose* (6-deoxy-L-galactose), a constituent of cell membrane glycoproteins.

DISACCHARIDES

Disaccharides are formed by the condensation of two monosaccharide units with the elimination of one molecule of water. The two monosaccharide units may be of the same type (e.g. *maltose*), or of different types (e.g. *lactose, sucrose*). The three disaccharides of physiological importance are *sucrose, maltose* and *lactose* (Figure 5.4).

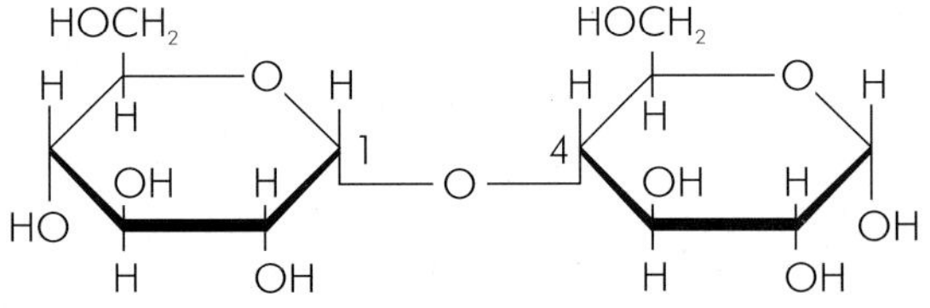

Sucrose is an important dietary carbohydrate. **Maltose** is produced in the intestine from the breakdown of dietary polysaccharides such as starch. **Lactose** is a constituent of milk, and is synthesised in the mammary gland.

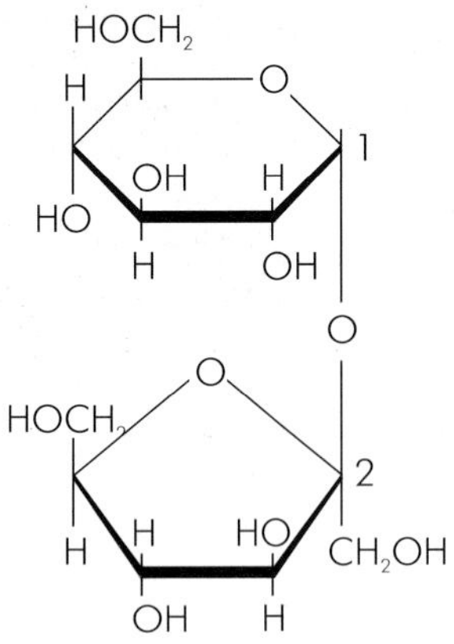

OLIGOSACCHARIDES

The condensation of 3–6 monosaccharide units results in the formation of an oligosaccharide (e.g. *maltotriose*). Oligosaccharides are very important for the synthesis of glycoproteins.

POLYSACCHARIDES

Polysaccharides (e.g. *starch, cellulose, glycogen*) are formed by the condensation of a large number of monosaccharide units. If the polymer is made up of a single type of monosaccharide, it is a *homopolysaccharide* (e.g. starch, glycogen). If different monosaccharides are involved, it is known as a *heteropolysaccharide* (e.g. hyaluronic acid, chondroitin). According to the function they perform,

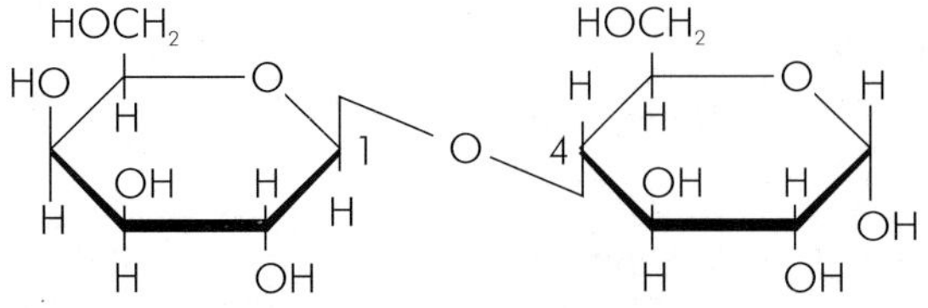

Figure 5.4 – Sucrose, maltose and lactose.

polysaccharides may be classified as *storage polysaccharides* or *structural polysaccharides*.

Storage polysaccharides

Glycogen (Figure 5.5) is the most abundant storage polysaccharide in animals (mainly in the liver and muscle). It is a large, highly branched polymer of glucose in which linear chains of glucose residues are linked by α-1,4 glycosidic bonds and branches are created through the formation of α-1,6 glycosidic linkages.

Liver glycogen serves as a store of glucose to maintain the normal level of blood glucose. Muscle glycogen constitutes a reserve of energy which is used in the early stages of exercise.

Starch, the most abundant polysaccharide in plants, is present as a mixture of two forms – *amylose*, a long, unbranched glucose polymer with α-1,4 bonds, and *amylopectin*, an α-1,4 linked polymer with branches formed by α-1,6 linkages. Both forms of starch are nutritionally useful for animals.

Structural polysaccharides

Glycosaminoglycans (*mucopolysaccharides*) are unbranched heteropolysaccharide chains consisting of repeating disaccharide units (Table 5.3) that contain (i) glucosamine or galactosamine, (ii) a uronic acid residue (except keratan sulphate) and (iii) covalently attached sulphate groups (except in hyaluronic acid). They make up the carbohydrate content of the ground substance in connective tissue.

Free *hyaluronic acid* is mainly responsible for the viscosity of the synovial fluid. Glycosaminoglycan chains also serve as docking sites for fibroblast growth factor and other proteins that stimulate cell proliferation. Most of the glycosaminoglycans, with the exception of hyaluronic acid occur as *proteoglycans*.

Proteoglycans have a small fraction (about 5% by weight) of protein covalently attached to the carbohydrate chains. They are very large molecules that have a *core protein* non-covalently attached to molecules of *hyaluronic acid* through small *link protein* molecules. In addition, smaller glycosaminoglycans, *keratan sulphate, heparan sulphate, chondroitin sulphate* or *dermatan sulphate* are attached covalently to the core protein. The best characterised proteoglycan is in the extracellular matrix of cartilage.

The presence of a large number of hydroxyl groups and negative charges on proteoglycan molecules help in holding large quantities of water and occupying space, thus cushioning or lubricating other structures. Interwoven among the proteoglycans of the ground

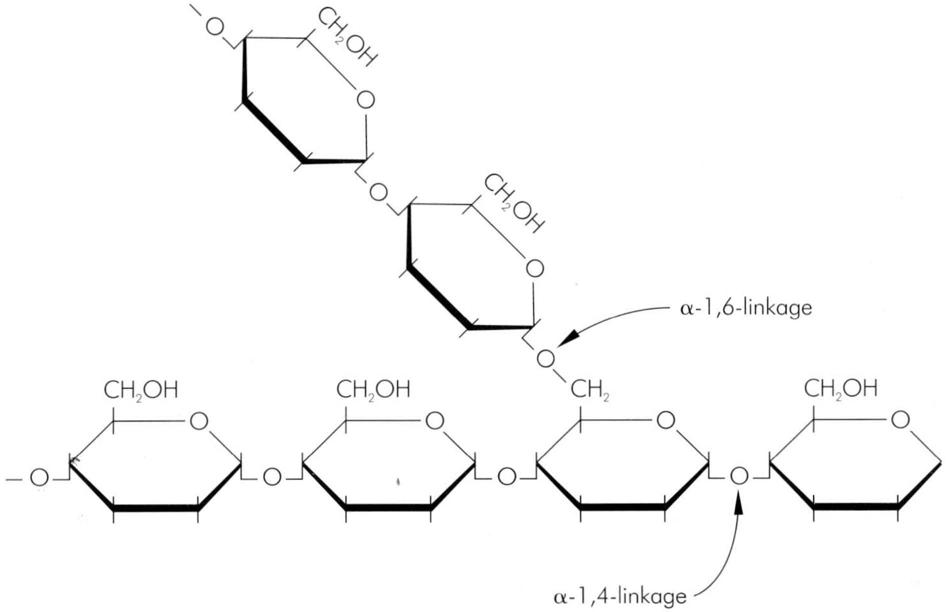

Figure 5.5 – The structure of glycogen showing the α-1,4 glycosidic bonds linking linear chains of glucose residues and α, 1,6-linkages at branch points.

MAJOR GLYCOSAMINOGLYCANS IN THE BODY		
Polysaccharide	Constituents of repeating units	Occurrence
Hyaluronic acid	N-Acetylglucosamine, Glucuronic acid	Synovial fluid, skin, cartilage, umbilical cord
Chondroitin sulphate	N-Acetylgalactosamine 4-sulphate, Glucuronic acid	Cartilage, cornea and other connective tissue
Chondroitin	N-Acetylgalactosamine, Glucuronic acid	Cornea, skin and bony tissue
Keratan sulphate	Galactose 6-sulphate, N-Acetyl D-glucosamine 6-sulphate	Cornea, skin and bony tissue
Dermatan sulphate	N-Acetyl D-galactosamine 4-sulphate, Iduronic acid*	Skin
Heparan	Glucosamine 6-sulphate, Glucuronic acid 2-sulphate, Iduronic acid*	Mast cells lining blood vessels, especially in lungs and liver

* Iduronic acid is the C5 epimer of D-glucuronic acid.

Table 5.3

substance are fibres of collagen and elastin, which strengthen the structure and help in the adhesion of connective tissue cells to the extracellular matrix.

Disorders of proteoglycan metabolism

The metabolism of proteoglycans involves many different types of lysosomal enzymes. Inherited deficiencies of these result in connective tissue disorders known as *mucopolysaccharidoses*. These are rare in occurrence.

These include *Hunter* and *Hurler syndromes* in which metabolism of dermatan and heparan sulphates is defective, and *Marquio syndrome* in which keratan sulphate metabolism is defective.

Disintegration of connective tissue can also occur due to the action of *hyaluronidase*, an enzyme secreted by pathogenic bacteria that hydrolyses β-1,4 linkages, and provides them with a mechanism for invasion of the host tissues.

Glycoproteins are proteins to which are covalently attached relatively small amounts of carbohydrates, generally as monosaccharides or oligosaccharides. The oligosaccharide chains may contain neutral sugars, N-acetylated amino sugars (N-acetyl galactosamine and N-acetyl glucosamine) and sialic acid, but no uronic acid. The connection between the oligosaccharide and the peptide chain may be by an *O-glycosidic link* (e.g. in *mucin, collagen, blood group antigens*), or by a *N-glycosidic link*.

The human *blood group proteins* contain oligosaccharide side chains with residues of L-fucose, D-galactose, N-acetylgalactosamine and N-acetyl D-glucosamine; blood group specificity is determined by these side chains.

SELECTED READING

Lehninger, A.L. – *Biochemistry: The molecular basis of cell structure and function*. 3rd ed. Worth Publishers Inc., N.Y., 1993.

Murray, R.K., Granner, D.K., Mayer, P.A. and Rodwell, V.W. (eds.) – *Harper's Biochemistry*, 24th ed. Appleton and Lange, California, 1996.

Stryer, L – *Biochemistry*, 4th ed. W.H. Freeman and Co., N.Y., 1995.

6

CARBOHYDRATE METABOLISM AND RELATED DISORDERS

Objectives
To understand:

- Carbohydrate metabolism
- Control of blood glucose concentration
- Disorders of carbohydrate metabolism

DIFFERENCES IN THE PROPERTIES OF HEXOKINASE AND GLUCOKINASE	
Hexokinase	Glucokinase
Broad specificity for hexoses	Specific for glucose
Inhibited by the product G6P	Not inhibited by G6P
High affinity for glucose (K_m < 0.1 mM)	Low affinity for glucose (K_m = 10 mM)
Not inducible	Inducible by insulin in the liver

Table 6.1

ENTRY OF BLOOD GLUCOSE INTO TISSUES

Entry of blood glucose into *liver cells* occurs through an insulin-independent, low affinity transporter, GLUT 2. Transport into most other tissues appears to be by specific insulin-activated glucose transporters. The primary form of transporter found in *skeletal muscle* and *adipose tissue* is GLUT 4, whose numbers are increased by insulin.

METABOLIC FATE OF GLUCOSE IN TISSUES

Glucose in tissues cannot be further metabolised until it has been converted to glucose-6-phosphate (G6P) by a reaction with ATP (Figure 6.1) catalysed by the non-specific *hexokinase* and also by the specific *glucokinase* present only in hepatic and pancreatic islet β-cells. Differences in the properties of hexokinase and glucokinase are shown in Table 6.1.

IMPORTANCE OF THE TISSUE SPECIFIC DISTRIBUTION OF HEXOKINASE AND GLUCOKINASE

The tissue specific distribution of hexokinase and glucokinase ensures the following:

- in tissues other than the liver, phosphorylation of glucose will occur only if it is being further metabolised, because an accumulation of G6P will inhibit hexokinase

- even when the blood glucose concentration is low, the liver will not compete with other tissues for the supply of glucose. The high affinity of hexokinase for glucose in glucose-dependent tissues such as brain and erythrocytes ensures that they will be supplied with glucose before other tissues; because of the relatively low affinity of glucokinase for glucose, the liver is prevented from utilizing glucose until the nutrient requirements of other tissues are satisfied

- at high blood glucose concentrations, an increased amount of glucose will enter the liver and reach a concentration sufficient to drive the glucokinase reaction, and excess glucose will be converted to and stored as glycogen or fat. Although glucokinase

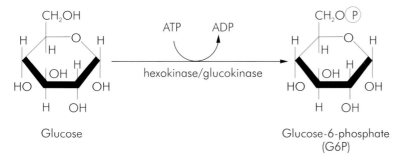

Glucose → hexokinase/glucokinase → Glucose-6-phosphate (G6P)

Figure 6.1 – Conversion of glucose to glucose-6-phosphate.

is not inhibited by G6P, it can be controlled by the levels of fructose-6-phosphate (F6P) and fructose-1-phosphate (F1P) in the cell. F6P promotes binding of an inhibitory protein and inhibits glucokinase activity. F1P inhibits the interactions between the inhibitory protein and glucokinase. This control mechanism enables glucokinase to monitor the utilisation of glucose through the later stages of glycolysis. Because glucokinase is an inducible enzyme, it is influenced by the nutritional state, being low in starvation and high after carbohydrate feeding. In *diabetes mellitus* this enzyme activity is low and is returned to normal by insulin

FURTHER METABOLISM OF PHOSPHORYLATED GLUCOSE (G6P)

The phosphorylated glucose can be utilised by body tissues in three ways:

* oxidised for purposes of obtaining energy

* converted to and stored as glycogen or fat

* used in the synthesis of other carbohydrates

OXIDATION OF GLUCOSE FOR PROVISION OF ENERGY

The complete oxidation of glucose to $CO_2 + H_2O$:

$$C_6H_{12}O_6 + 6O_2 \rightarrow 6CO_2 + 6H_2O$$

producing maximal energy requires the participation of two major pathways:

* *glycolysis (Embden-Meyerhof pathway)*

* *the citric acid cycle* (also known as the *tricarboxylic acid* (TCA) *cycle* and the *Krebs' cycle*)

The *pentose phosphate pathway* or *hexose monophosphate shunt* is an alternative pathway by which glucose is oxidized. It is important for the biosynthesis of other biologically important compounds.

GLYCOLYSIS

Glycolysis is the chief pathway for carbohydrate metabolism, (i.e. in this pathway a six-carbon glucose molecule gets split into two molecules of pyruvate). Pyruvate may be converted to lactate, or enter the citric acid cycle for further oxidation. The reactions of the glycolytic pathway and the enzymes involved are shown in Figure 6.2.

IMPORTANT POINTS TO NOTE ABOUT THE GLYCOLYTIC CYCLE

It is important to note that:

* *three reactions in this sequence (reactions ①, ③ and ⑩ in Figure 6.2) are irreversible* under physiological conditions because a considerable loss of free energy occurs during these reactions. Because of their irreversibility, the rate at which glycolysis occurs may be regulated by controlling the activities of the enzymes concerned

* *the formation of ATP in the glycolytic sequence alone (in reactions ⑦ and ⑩ of Figure 6.2) does not involve the participation of the mitochondrial respiratory chain.* These are therefore examples of ATP production by *substrate level phosphorylation*

* *the NADH formed in reaction ⑥ has to be reoxidised if glycolysis is to continue.* In anaerobic conditions, this is achieved by conversion of pyruvate to lactate (reaction ⑪). In aerobic conditions, the NADH in the cytosol is reoxidized in mitochondria. However, because NADH cannot freely enter mitochondria, it transfers reducing equivalents to other substrates which can enter the mitochondria for further oxidation

* *the amount of energy produced differs in aerobic and anaerobic conditions.* In anaerobic glycolysis there is a net formation of two molecules each of ATP and NADH per molecule of glucose metabolized (Figure 6.2). In aerobic conditions, a total of 36 – 38 molecules of ATP will be formed (2 ATP by substrate-level phosphorylation in the glycolytic pathway + 4 – 6 ATP by the oxidation of the 2 NADH molecules via the respiratory chain; the amount of ATP will depend on the shuttle used by NADH + 30 ATP from the complete oxidation to CO_2 and H_2O, of pyruvate formed from each glucose molecule)

* *fluoride ions can inhibit glycolysis.* The enzyme *enolase* (reaction ⑨ in Figure 6.2) is magnesium-dependent. Fluoride ions can complex with Mg^{2+} and phosphate to form a magnesium fluorophosphate complex and thereby inhibit enolase activity. Since this inhibition can stop the entire glycolytic sequence, sodium fluoride is added to samples of blood collected for glucose estimations

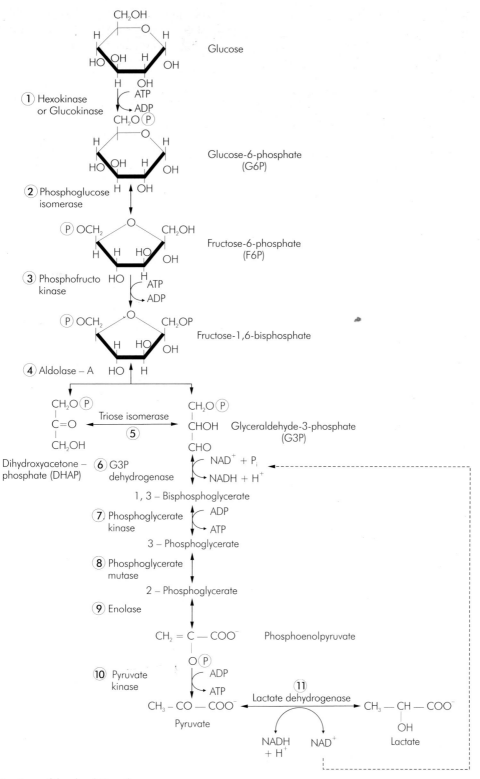

Figure 6.2 – Reactions of the glycolytic pathway.

PHYSIOLOGICAL IMPORTANCE OF GLYCOLYSIS

Provision of energy

Although the net amount of energy produced by glycolysis is small, this pathway is very important in certain specific tissues and conditions:

- *mature red blood cells* have no mitochondria and depend solely on glycolysis for their energy. The lactic acid produced in these cells will be released into the blood to be further oxidized to pyruvate by other tissues such as heart, liver, or resting muscle

- *in hypoxia* or anaerobic conditions (e.g. after strenuous exercise or in traumatic shock) glycolysis will occur at an increased rate to provide extra energy

Synthesis of other biologically important compounds

Intermediates of the glycolytic cycle can be utilised to synthesise other biologically important compounds in the body. Examples include the synthesis of amino acids serine and glycine from 3-phosphoglycerate; 2,3- bisphosphoglycerate from 1,3-bisphosphoglycerate; Various amino acids (e.g. alanine and serine) from pyruvate; neuraminic acid from phosphoenolpyruvate; and glycerol phosphate from dihydroxyacetone phosphate.

THE PENTOSE PHOSPHATE PATHWAY

The pentose phosphate pathway or hexose monophosphate (HMP) shunt is an alternative pathway for the oxidation of glucose that operates in many tissues, especially in the liver, lactating mammary gland, adipose tissue and red blood cells. The enzymes of this pathway are also located in the cytoplasm.

REACTION SEQUENCE IN THE PENTOSE PHOSPHATE PATHWAY

The pentose phosphate pathway (Figure 6.3) can be considered to be a multicyclic process in which three molecules of G6P are converted to three molecules each of CO_2 and 5C residues (pentoses). The latter eventually rearrange to form two molecules of G6P and one molecule of glyceraldehyde 3-phosphate, which can enter the glycolytic cycle and be reconverted to G6P. The overall pathway may be summarised:

$$3G6P + 6NADP^+ \rightarrow 3CO_2 + 2G6P + \text{glyceraldehyde } 3\text{-phosphate} + 6NADPH + 6H^+$$

Nicotinamide adenine dinucleotide phosphate ($NADP^+$) and *thiamine pyrophosphate* (TPP) are cofactors in this sequence of reactions.

As shown in Figure 6.3, in the pentose phosphate pathway, there is an oxidative and a non-oxidative phase.

Oxidative phase

In this phase, G6P undergoes dehydrogenation followed by decarboxylation to yield the pentose ribulose-5-phosphate. These changes are accompanied by the reduction of $NADP^+$ to NADPH.

Non-oxidative phase

In this phase, ribulose-5-phosphate is first converted to the pentose xylulose-5-phosphate or ribose-5-phosphate (R5P) by the action of an epimerase or an isomerase respectively. This is followed by a series of reactions catalysed by the enzymes *transketolase* and *transaldolase* which transfer C-3 and C-2 units respectively from one 5C sugar to another to generate a series of C-3, C-4 and C-7 sugars including F6P and glyceraldehyde 3-phosphate which can enter the glycolytic pathway.

PHYSIOLOGICAL SIGNIFICANCE OF THE PENTOSE PHOSPHATE PATHWAY

The pentose phosphate pathway does not generate ATP but has two major functions:

- generation of NADPH for reductive synthesis of biologically important molecules (e.g. fatty acids, steroids, sorbitol, reduced glutathione)

- provision of pentoses (mainly ribose) for nucleotide and nucleic acid synthesis

An inherited deficiency of glucose 6-phosphate dehydrogenase (and therefore NADPH required to maintain the reduced glutathione concentration is responsible for the haemolysis observed in certain individuals, especially when under conditions of oxidative stress.

GLUCOSE CONVERSION TO STORAGE FORMS

Excess dietary glucose has to be stored in some form because tissues would otherwise be flooded with glucose immediately after a meal and starved of it at all other times. Glucose is usually stored as *fat* or *glycogen*

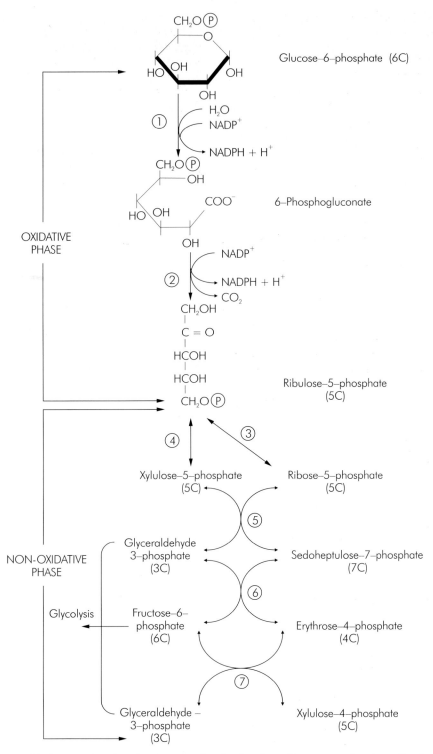

Figure 6.3 – Reactions of the hexose monophosphate (pentose phosphate) pathway. Enzymes numbered are: ① – glucose-6-phosphate dehydrogenase and 6-phosphoglucanolactone, hydrolase ② – 6-phosphogluconate dehydrogenase, ③ – phosphopentoisomerase, ④ – phosphopentose epimerase, ⑤ and ⑦ – transketolase (thiamine pyrophosphate is the coenzyme), and ⑥ – transaldolase.

since these compounds have a high molecular weight and low osmotic pressure.

GLUCOSE CONVERSION TO FAT

Excess glucose obtained from the diet is stored mainly as fat (triacylglycerols). The conversion of glucose to fat in the adipose tissue occurs by the sequence of reactions outlined in Figure 6.4.

GLUCOSE CONVERSION TO GLYCOGEN

Glycogen synthesis involves a polymerisation of several glucose molecules, and it occurs in almost every tissue (especially in liver and skeletal muscle). An outline of the reactions involved in the processes of *glycogenesis* (glycogen synthesis) and *glycogenolysis* (glycogen breakdown) are shown in Figure 6.5.

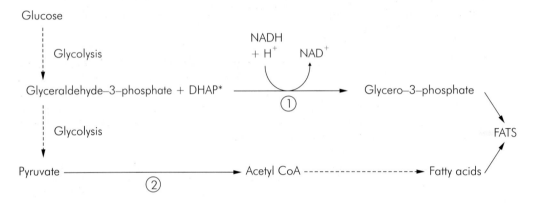

DHAP* – Dihydroxyacetone phosphate

Figure 6.4 – An outline of the sequence of reactions by which glucose is converted to fat in the adipose tissue. Enzymes are : ① – glycerol phosphate dehydrogenase, ② – pyruvate dehydrogenase complex.

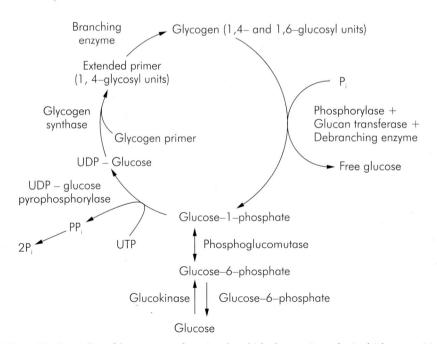

Figure 6.5 – An outline of the sequence of reactions by which glycogen is synthesized (glycogenesis) and degraded (glycogenolysis).

Glycogenesis

Glycogen molecules are built up (Figure 6.5) from units of uridine diphosphoglucose (UDP glucose). A molecule of UDP glucose transfers the glucose molecule to the end of an existing glycogen primer (at least four glucose units long). UDP is then reconverted to UTP by transfer of a phosphate group from ATP. In this way, an existing glycogen chain is repeatedly extended by one unit. Two enzymes participate in glycogenesis; *glycogen synthase* promotes the formation only of the α-1,4 linkages while the *branching enzyme* helps to form the α-1,6 linkages required for the branched structure of glycogen.

Glycogenolysis

Phosphorylase is the principal enzyme involved in glycogenolysis. It requires *pyridoxal phosphate* (a derivative of vitamin B_6) as a coenzyme. The phosphorylase helps to add on a phosphate group to the terminal glucose units in the branches, and then removes each glucose as glucose 1-phosphate. This process continues until about four glucose residues remain on either side of a branch point. The further degradation of the chains involves two additional enzymes, a *transferase* and a *debranching enzyme* (Figure 6.5).

Glycogen breakdown within lysosomes occurs by the action of the lysosomal enzyme α-*glucosidase*. Although the amount of glycogen degradation by this pathway is only a fraction of that carried out by phosphorylase in muscle cell cytosol, its importance is indicated by the fact that its deficiency results in severe glycogen storage disease, and even death within the first year of life.

THE METABOLISM OF FRUCTOSE, GALACTOSE AND LACTOSE

FRUCTOSE METABOLISM

Dietary fructose transported to the liver gets rapidly converted to glucose. In humans, some fructose can also be converted to glucose in the intestine. The steps involved in the metabolism of fructose are summarized in Figure 6.6. *Essential fructosuria* results from a lack of fructokinase in the liver.

In mild, or treated, diabetes, fructose is considered to be a suitable source of energy because its metabolism is insulin-independent, and the oxidation of fructose via glycolysis and the TCA cycle is favoured (Figure 6.6). In severe diabetes, however, the flux is towards the synthesis of glucose, and fructose instead of being helpful will be detrimental to the patient, and in the eye lens, sorbitol (a polyol) synthesised from the excess glucose may promote cataract development.

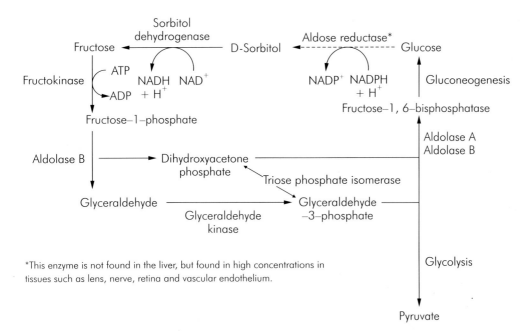

*This enzyme is not found in the liver, but found in high concentrations in tissues such as lens, nerve, retina and vascular endothelium.

Figure 6.6 – Metabolism of fructose.

GALACTOSE METABOLISM

Galactose derived usually from the intestinal hydrolysis of lactose (milk sugar) is also converted to glucose in the liver. The ability of the liver to carry out this conversion is sometimes used as a hepatic function test known as the *galactose tolerance test*. The steps involved in galactose metabolism are outlined in Figure 6.7.

LACTOSE METABOLISM

Lactose is synthesized from UDP-galactose (Figure 6.7) by *lactose synthase (UDP-galactose: glucose galactosyltransferase)* which is a complex of two proteins, A(*β-D-galactosyltransferase*) and B (*α-lactalbumin*). Protein A is found in many tissues and helps to transfer galactose from UDP-galactose to N-acetyl-D-glucosamine to produce N-acetyllactosamine that is a component of structurally important N-linked glycoproteins. Protein B is found only in lactating mammary glands. During pregnancy, the steroid hormone *progesterone* inhibits the synthesis of protein B. After birth, the drop in the progesterone level stimulates the synthesis of the peptide hormone *prolactin,* which in turn stimulates synthesis of protein B. The complexing of the proteins B and A changes the specificity of that transferase so that lactose, instead of N-acetyllactosamine, is synthesised.

GLUCONEOGENESIS

Gluconeogenesis is the process by which glucose is synthesised from non-carbohydrate sources. It involves the conversion of 3- and 4-carbon compounds to the 6-carbon glucose. In mammals, the liver and kidney are the principal organs responsible for gluconeogenesis. The fuels for gluconeogenesis are the sugar alcohol glycerol and non-carbohydrates such as lactate and the α-keto acids pyruvate and oxaloacetate derived from glucogenic amino acids (e.g. alanine, serine, glutamate, aspartate). This process can occur always, but markedly increases during periods of low blood glucose concentration (e.g. between meals and during fasting). This is important for the following reasons:

- to maintain blood glucose concentration, and provide energy for glucose-dependent tissues (e.g. red blood cells, brain, and renal medulla); in anaerobic conditions, glucose is the only fuel to supply energy to the skeletal muscle

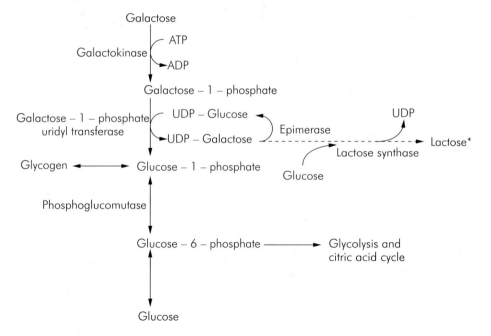

*Lactose synthesis occurs only in mammary glands

Figure 6.7 – Metabolism of galactose.

- glucose is the source of glyceride glycerol in the adipose tissue. Since there is no *glycerokinase* in adipose tissue, free glycerol cannot be utilized readily in this tissue for triacylglycerol synthesis

- in the mammary gland, glucose is required for lactose synthesis.

- the gluconeogenic pathway helps to clear from the blood metabolic products of other tissues (e.g. lactate produced by muscle and red blood cells, and glycerol produced by adipose tissue).

THE GLUCONEOGENIC PATHWAY

The central pathway of gluconeogenesis from the α-keto acids is the conversion of pyruvate to glucose. This occurs essentially by a reversal of glycolysis with the exception of the three physiologically irreversible glycolytic enzymes pyruvate kinase, phosphofructokinase and hexokinase. In gluconeogenesis, four new enzymes (*pyruvate carboxylase, phosphoenolpyruvate carboxykinase, fructose-1,6-bisphosphatase*, and *glucose-6-phosphatase*) have been used to bypass the above reactions (Figure 6.8).

The conversion of pyruvate to phosphoenolpyruvate (PEP) involves the participation of the two enzymes pyruvate carboxylase and phosphoenolpyruvate carboxykinase.

Pyruvate carboxylase (located in the mitochondria) converts pyruvate to oxaloacetate. Biotin, a member of the B-group of vitamins, is essential for the activity of this enzyme. It functions as a component of specific multisubunit enzymes (e.g. *pyruvate carboxylase, acetyl CoA carboxylase, propionyl CoA carboxylase*) that catalyse carboxylation reactions. It is attached to the apoenzyme through the e-amino group of a lysyl residue. This enzyme activity is stimulated by acetyl CoA and inhibited by ADP.

Phosphoenolpyruvate carboxykinase (PEPCK) converts oxaloacetate to PEP using guanosine triphosphate (GTP) or inosine triphosphate (ITP) as the energy source. In man this enzyme is located in the mitochondria as well as in the cytosol although in rat and mouse it is exclusively cytosolic.

PEP is converted to fructose 1,6-bisphosphate by a reversal of glycolysis, which is converted to glucose by *fructose-1,6-bisphosphatase* and *glucose 6-phosphatase* (Figure 6.8) which are located in the cytosol. The synthesis of one molecule of glucose requires the utilisation of two molecules of pyruvate.

EFFECT OF ETHANOL ON GLUCONEOGENESIS

About 90% of ethanol absorbed in the stomach and intestine is metabolised in the liver (Figure 6.9). An excessive intake of ethanol may result in decreased gluconeogenesis, mainly due to a reduction in the level of NAD^+. The NAD^+ is required for the conversion of gluconeogenic substrates lactate and glycerol to pyruvate and dihydroxyacetone phosphate respectively (Figure 6.8) and for the oxidation of fatty acids to acetyl CoA, with the release of energy required for gluconeogenesis. The decrease in acetyl CoA will also decrease pyruvate carboxylase activity allosterically.

CONTROL OF CARBOHYDRATE METABOLISM

A complex set of controls exist in cells to ensure that the pathways involved in the metabolism of carbohydrates are closely co-ordinated. Such co-ordination will ensure that in an energy deficient state, carbohydrates will be metabolised to produce energy, but in high energy conditions, they will be stored as fat or glycogen. In high-energy states, glycolysis and glycogenolysis will be inhibited while glycogenesis and lipogenesis will be stimulated. In low energy states, the flux through glycolysis will be increased and glycogenolysis and lipolysis will be favoured.

The rates at which carbohydrate metabolic pathways operate maybe achieved through:

- allosteric regulation of key enzymes in the pathways; or

- hormonal regulation of the pathways

ALLOSTERIC REGULATION

The allosteric modulation of key enzymes involved in carbohydrate metabolism is shown in Figure 6.10.

Fructose 2,6-bisphosphate (F2,6 BP), an allosteric stimulator of key glycolytic enzymes, is a signal molecule derived by phosphorylation of fructose-6-phosphate (F6P) by *phosphofructokinase 2*, an enzyme different from phosphofructokinase 1. The level of F2,6 BP is high in the fed state and low in starvation because of the antagonistic effects of insulin and glucagon in the production and degradation of this molecule.

A decreased availability of ADP and inorganic phosphate (P_i) in high-energy states would also cause a reduction in activities of the reactions which require

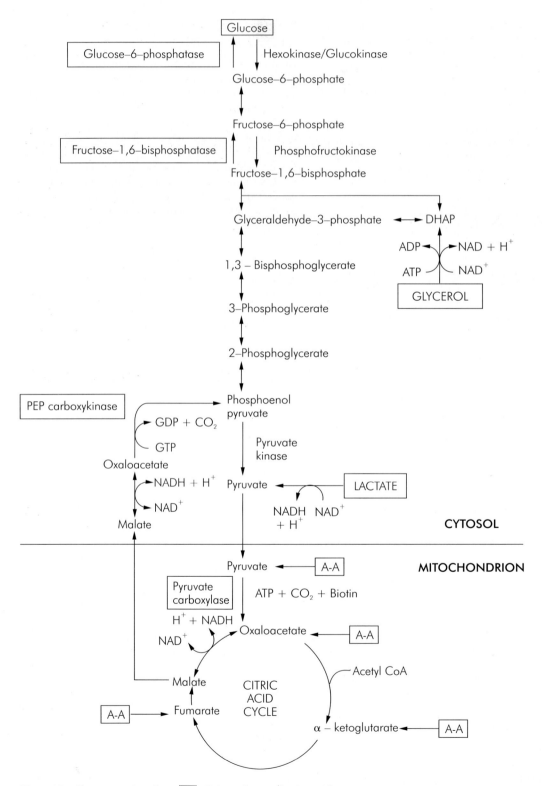

Figure 6.8 – Gluconeogenic pathway. A-A – Points of entry of amino acids.

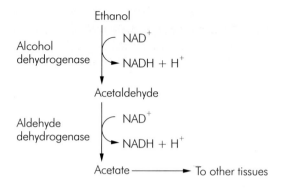

Figure 6.9 – Major route of ethanol metabolism in the liver.

their participation (e.g. the glycolytic enzymes phosphoglycerate kinase and enolase that require ADP, and glyceraldehyde-3-phosphate dehydrogenase that requires ADP and P_i).

HORMONAL REGULATION

The chief hormones that participate in the regulation of carbohydrate metabolism, and their effects on the individual pathways involved are summarized in Table 6.2.

In addition, *thyroxine* increases the tissue oxidation of glucose and can also increase the intestinal absorption of carbohydrates. These hormonal effects are mediated through one or more of the following mechanisms:

- alteration in substrate availability

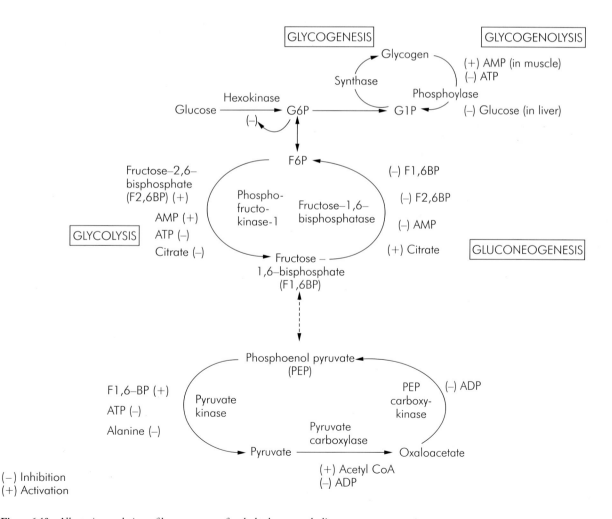

Figure 6.10 – Allosteric regulation of key enzymes of carbohydrate metabolism.

PRINCIPAL ACTIONS OF HORMONES INVOLVED IN THE CONTROL OF CARBOHYDRATE METABOLISM			
	Liver	Adipose tissue	Muscle
Insulin	Increased Glucose utilisation Glycogen synthesis Fatty acid synthesis Protein synthesis	Increased Glucose uptake Triacylglycerol synthesis	Increased Glucose uptake Glycogen synthesis Protein synthesis
	Decreased Gluconeogenesis Ketogenesis	Decreased Lipolysis	Decreased Proteolysis
Glucagon	Increased Glycogenolysis Gluconeogenesis Ketogenesis	Increased Lipolysis	Increased Protein catabolism
	Decreased Glycogen synthesis		
Growth hormone	Increased Protein synthesis Gluconeogenesis	Increased Lipolysis	Increased Protein synthesis
	Decreased Glucose utilisation in extrahepatic tissues		
Glucocorticoids	Increased Gluconeogenesis Glycogenesis		Increased Protein catabolism
Adrenaline*	Increased Glycogenolysis Gluconeogenesis Ketogenesis	Increased Lipolysis	Increased Glycogenolysis
	Decreased Glycogenesis		Decreased Glycogen synthesis

*Adrenaline also inhibits secretion of insulin and promotes secretion of adrenocorticotrophic hormone.

Table 6.2

- alteration in the concentration or activities of key enzymes

- alterations in the availability of energy for the operation of the pathway

For example, *insulin* promotes lipogenesis in adipose tissue by increasing the availability of glucose which can be converted to glycerol, fatty acids, and energy required (by increasing glycolysis). On the other hand, it inhibits gluconeogenesis by reducing the availability of the substrates amino acids and glycerol; the availability of fatty acids for provision of energy; and the pyruvate carboxylase and PEPCK concentrations by repression at the gene level. Pyruvate carboxylase activity will also be reduced due to the decreased availability of the activator acetyl CoA as a result of the reduction in fatty acids available for oxidation.

Glucagon and *adrenaline* stimulate lipolysis and glycogenolysis by influencing the activities of the lipolytic enzyme, hormone sensitive lipase, and the glycogen-metabolising enzymes respectively through cAMP-dependent or -independent mechanisms. *Growth hormone* also increases the activity of hormone sensitive lipase through a similar mechanism.

With respect to glycogen metabolism, glucagon, adrenaline and insulin exert their control on the glycogen synthase and phosphorylase in a reciprocal manner. Thus, when the rate of glycogenolysis is increased that of glycogenesis is decreased, and vice versa. This is possible because the synthase and the phosphorylase enzymes can each exist in two forms, active and inactive. Phosphorylation (either via a cAMP dependent or Ca^{2+} calmodulin dependent protein kinase) results in the formation of active phosphorylase (phosphorylase a) while the synthase (by a protein phosphatase) is converted to an inactive form. Dephosphorylation activates the synthase while inactivating the phosphorylase (phosphorylase b).

BLOOD GLUCOSE CONCENTRATION

FACTORS DETERMINING BLOOD GLUCOSE CONCENTRATION

The blood glucose level at any time is determined by the balance between the amount of glucose entering the blood stream and the amount leaving it. The principal determinants are therefore:

- the dietary intake

- the rate of entry of glucose into the cells of muscle, adipose tissue and other organs

- the amount of glucose released from the liver due to glycogenolytic and gluconeogenic activities

In normal individuals, glucose derived from the diet and liver glycogenolysis are sufficient to maintain the blood glucose level. In prolonged starvation or fasting, however, gluconeogenesis plays a major role in maintainance of blood glucose level.

CONTROL OF BLOOD GLUCOSE CONCENTRATION

After ingestion of a carbohydrate meal, there is a rise in the blood glucose concentration, until a maximum is reached about 1 hour post-prandially. The blood glucose concentration returns to the fasting level within a few hours, the time taken to return to this level depending on the nature of the carbohydrate ingested.

In the human body, the efficient control of the blood glucose concentration requires the participation of the liver, extrahepatic tissues and several hormones. The chief hormones involved are insulin (tending to decrease glucose concentration) and the counter-regulatory hormones (glucagon, adrenaline, glucocorticoids and growth hormone).

In hyperglycaemia (high blood glucose concentration) insulin secretion from the pancreas will be stimulated and through the actions shown in Table 6.2, insulin will help to lower the blood glucose level. The glucose stimulates the pancreatic glucokinase resulting in an accelerated production of ATP in the β-cells. The influence of this ATP on membrane ion channels results in an increase in intracellular calcium ion concentration which is thought to be the immediate signal for secretion of insulin from the pancreatic β-cells.

In hypoglycaemia (low blood glucose concentration) glucagon, adrenaline, glucocorticoids and growth hormone will, through the actions shown in Table 6.2, increase the blood glucose concentration. In normal conditions, glucose is the preferred energy source for tissues. In hypoglycaemic conditions (and in starvation), the increased amount of ketones synthesised in the liver (due to increased oxidation of fatty acids) is used as energy by most tissues including the brain and muscle tissue. The increased utilisation of ketone bodies for energy in the above conditions helps to spare the non-obligatory oxidation of glucose in muscle and also helps to conserve muscle by reducing the need for protein catabolism for gluconeogenesis.

DISORDERS OF CARBOHYDRATE METABOLISM

ABNORMALITIES IN GLUCOSE METABOLISM

Diabetes mellitus is the most common endocrine disorder. It arises from an insufficiency of insulin, or the presence of factors which oppose its action.

Primary diabetes

Type 1 or insulin-dependent diabetes (IDDM) arises as a result of an inadequate production of insulin due to the destruction of the pancreatic β-cells, most commonly by autoimmune disease or viral infection. In a few cases, due to a genetic reason, the structure of insulin or the structure of the insulin receptor may be abnormal so that the hormone cannot be recognised by the receptor.

Type 2 or non-insulin dependent diabetes (NIDDM) is most commonly associated with obesity in middle-aged individuals. It is due to a reduction in the number or affinity of insulin receptors on the plasma membrane of cells in target tissues, or an abnormal binding of insulin to the receptors. In obese individuals, persistent dietary excess may cause excessive secretion of insulin, resulting in hyperinsulinaemia which leads to a reduction in the number of insulin receptors. This type of diabetes may be reversed by dietary alterations; a weight loss regime can help at least to reverse partially the down regulation of receptors.

SECONDARY DIABETES

Diabetes may occur secondary to pancreatic disease, endocrine diseases such as Cushing's syndrome and acromegaly and drug therapy, eg. with thiazides. It may also occur in certain rare genetic disorders that cause abnormalities in insulin or insulin receptors. In the tropics young individuals present with diabetes secondary to malnutrition related pancreatitis.

The secretion of insulin may be reduced due to generalised pancreatic disease. In diabetes secondary to other endocrine disorders, ineffective insulin action is caused by abnormal secretion of hormones with 'diabetogenic' activity.

Gestational diabetes develops during pregnancy but, in the majority of cases, reverts to normal after pregnancy. Such patients have an increased risk of developing diabetes mellitus in the future.

DIAGNOSIS OF DIABETES

Biochemical tests are used for the diagnosis of diabetes mellitus and its monitoring. The diagnosis of diabetes mellitus depends upon the demonstration of *hyperglycaemia*.

1. Diabetes symptoms (i.e. polyuria, polydipsia and unexplained weight loss) plus:
   random venous plasma glucose
   concentration $\geq$ 11.1 mmol/L or
   fasting plasma glucose
   concentration $\geq$ 7.0 mmol/L or
   2 hour plasma glucose
   concentration $\geq$ 11.1 mmol/L

(after 75g anhydrous glucose in an oral glucose tolerance test)

2. With no symptoms diagnosis should not be based on a single glucose determination but requires confirmatory plasma venous determination. At least one additional glucose test result on another day with a value in the diabetic range is essential, either fasting, from a random sample or from the two hour post glucose load. If the fasting or random values are not diagnostic the 2-hour value should be used.

MONITORING

The efficacy of treatment in diabetes is monitored by ensuring that the patient's symptoms are controlled and by biochemical tests. Most patients with diabetes test their own blood glucose concentration using specific reagent strips.

- *glycated haemoglobin (haemoglobin A_{1c}) measurement*: glycated haemoglobin reflects the mean glycaemia over 2 months prior to its measurement. In normal individuals the proportion of haemoglobin in the glycated form is < 7%, but may exceed 12% in poorly controlled patients.

- *fructosamine measurement*: glycation may also be assessed by measuring fructosamine, the ketoamine product of non-enzymatic glycation of plasma proteins, albumin being the major contributor.

- *microalbuminuria estimations* are found to be very useful for the early detection of diabetic nephropathy. Microalbuminura may be defined as an albumin excretion rate intermediate between 20-200μg/min/24hr This small increase in albumin cannot be detected by simple albumin stick tests and requires careful quantitation.

Biochemical basis of metabolic complications of diabetes mellitus

Diabetic patients may develop metabolic complications.

Diabetic ketoacidosis is a presenting feature in about one-third of new IDDM patients.

There are four major mechanisms which predispose to ketoacidosis:

- insulin deficiency
- counter-regulatory hormone excess
- fasting

• dehydration

Of these, insulin deficiency is the most important.

In uncontrolled diabetes, there is a marked increase in circulating ketone bodies (acetoacetate, 3-hydroxy-butyrate, and acetone) derived from fatty acid metabolism in the liver). This results in metabolic acidosis as the liver and other tissues cannot, in general, completely metabolise the excessive amounts of the ketone bodies that are being formed; ketogenic amino acids aggravate the derangement in lipid metabolism The acidosis causes H^+ to move into cells and K^+ to move out. The increase in plasma K^+ may also result from the lack of insulin action that normally promotes K^+ entry into cells. Excess ketone bodies are also excreted in the urine. During excretion, the charge on the ketone bodies is balanced by the loss of cations (mostly Na^+) except to the extent that the kidney can substitute NH_4^+ for Na^+. Thus, the loss of glucose in urine is accompanied by water and electrolyte loss, the individual suffers ion imbalances and becomes dehydrated, and the loss of water from cerebral cells is probably the reason for the confusion and coma that may develop in this condition. About 20% of acetone produced in human diabetic ketosis is also converted to glucose or lactate. Acetone may also be detectable in the breath of patients suffering from diabetic ketoacidosis.

Non-ketotic hyperosmolar coma is found only in NIDDM. Severe hyperglycaemia may develop with extreme dehydration and very high plasma osmolality, but with no ketosis and minimal acidosis.

Lactic acidosis is an uncommon complication of diabetes mellitus previously associated with the drug phenformin.

Long-term complications include *microvascular complications* such as retinopathy, nephropathy and neuropathy, *macrovascular complications* such as ischaemic heart disease and peripheral vascular disease. Glycosylation of membrane proteins is thought to be important in the pathogenesis of basement membrane thickening that cause alterations in vascularity of many tissues including, kidney, retina and nerve. Excessive accumulation of sorbitol in hyperglycaemia has also been implicated in the pathogenesis of diabetic neuropathy and cataract.

Hypoglycaemia

Hypoglycaemia may be biochemically defined as a venous plasma glucose concentration < 2.5 mmol/L. Hypoglycaemia occurs when the rate of delivery of glucose into the blood is less than the rate of its uptake into tissues. A low blood glucose concentration normally leads to the stimulation of catecholamine secretion and correction of hypoglycaemia through suppression of insulin secretion and stimulation of glucagon, cortisol and growth hormone.

'Whipple's triad' consisting of symptoms of hypoglycaemia in the presence of a low plasma glucose concentration and symptoms relieved by administration of glucose may be useful in the diagnosis of hypoglycaemia. The brain is particularly vulnerable to the decrease in glucose fuel that occurs in hypoglycaemia.

Causes of hypoglycaemia

Specific causes. Over 99% of all episodes of hypoglycaemia occur in insulin-dependent diabetic patients due to one or more of the following causes:

• insufficient carbohydrate intake

• excess of insulin

• strenuous exercise or excessive alcohol intake

Hypoglycaemia may also occur in non-insulin-dependent diabetic patients due to excess sulphonylurea administration.

Other causes may conveniently be considered in two groups:

• those that produce hypoglycaemia in the fasting patient (*fasting hypoglycaemia*)

• those in which the low blood glucose is due to a stimulus (*reactive hypoglycaemia*)

Neonatal hypoglycaemia

Important causes of neonatal hypoglycaemia are as follows:

• *Intra-uterine growth retardation.* Babies, more particularly if premature, may have inadequate liver glycogen stores if growth has been retarded, as glycogen stores are laid down in the last part of pregnancy. These conditions are made worse by perinatal asphyxia or sepsis

• *Babies of mothers with uncontrolled diabetes.* These babies have pancreatic cell hyperplasia and therefore inappropriately high insulin levels at birth

• *Inborn errors of metabolism.* For example, *galactosaemia* and certain *glycogen storage diseases* (see below)

GLYCOGEN STORAGE DISEASES

In these conditions, increased glycogen storage occurs either due to the production of glycogen in abnormal amounts or with an abnormal structure. The inheritance of these disorders is autosomal recessive except for type VI that is X-linked. At least ten different enzyme defects that lead to the accumulation of glycogen in tissues have been described.

Children with *type I glycogen storage disease* (due to a deficiency of glucose-6-phosphatase) are prone to severe fasting hypoglycaemia because their only source of glucose is dietary carbohydrate. Blood glucose may be maintained by constant intragastric infusion of glucose or frequent ingestion of glucose or corn starch.

ABNORMALITIES IN THE METABOLISM OF OTHER SUGARS

Galactosaemia

This is most commonly due to an inherited deficiency of *galactose 1-phosphate uridyl transferase* (Figure 6.7). Excessive galactose 1-phosphate accumulates in cells with consequent deleterious effects. Affected infants exhibit vomiting, diarrhoea, failure to thrive, deranged hepatic function and increased susceptibility to sepsis by *E. coli*. Patients frequently develop cataract before one year of age because of the accumulation of galactitol (a polyol), formed by a reduction of galactose by aldose reductase in the eye. Treatment is the removal of galactose from the diet.

Fructose intolerance

This inherited disorder is caused by lack of fructose 1-phosphate aldolase B (Figure 6.6), leading to accumulation of fructose 1-phosphate in the liver; this causes hypoglycaemia due to inhibition of glucose production from glycogenolysis and gluconeogenesis. Clinical effects include convulsions, an enlarged liver and jaundice, symptoms which disappear rapidly after the withdrawal of fructose (and sucrose) from the diet.

SELECTED READING

Bhagvan, N.V. – *Medical Biochemistry*. Jones and Bartlett Publishers, London, 1992.

Marshall, W.J. – *Clinical Chemistry*, 3rd ed. Gower Medical Publishing, 1995.

Murray, R.K., Granner, D.K., Mayer, P.A., and Rodwell, V.W. (eds.) – *Harper's Biochemistry*, 23rd ed. Appleton and Lange, California, 1993.

Stryer, L. – *Biochemistry*, 4thed. W.H. Freeman and Co., N.Y.,1995.

Watkins, P.J., Drury, P.L. and Taylor, K.W. – *Diabetes and its Management*, 4th ed. Blackwell Scientific Publications, London, 1990.

Whitby, L.G., Smith, A.F., Beckett, G.J. and Walker, S.W. – *Lecture Notes in Clinical Biochemistry*, 5th ed. Blackwell Scientific Publications, London, 1993.

7

LIPIDS

Objectives
To understand:

- The chemistry of lipids
- The biomedical importance of lipids

Lipids are a heterogeneous group of organic biomolecules soluble in non-polar solvents such as ether and benzene. Although certain lipids contain ionised groups (e.g. phosphate or choline), the bulk of any lipid molecule is non-polar. Polar lipids that possess both hydrophilic and hydrophobic regions in the same molecule (e.g. fatty acids, cholesterol and phospholipids) are said to be *amphipathic*.

FATTY ACIDS

All fatty acids are weak acids that have a single carboxyl (-COOH) group at the end of a hydrocarbon chain (Figure 7.1).

Carbon atoms in the fatty acids are numbered from the carboxyl carbon (C1). The end methyl carbon is known as the ω-carbon. The hydrocarbon chain of fatty acids represented by RCOO$^-$ can be either *saturated* (i.e. lacking carbon-carbon double bonds), or *unsaturated* (contains double bonds). The major fatty acids in the human body are shown in Table 7.1.

$$C_n H_{2n+1} COOH$$

Figure 7.1 – General formula of saturated fatty acids.

IMPORTANCE OF UNSATURATED FATTY ACIDS

- the unsaturated fatty acids are required for the *synthesis of glycerophospholipids and sphingophospholipids* that have many important functions in the body

- a high ratio of polyunsaturated fatty acids to saturated fatty acids in the diet has been shown to result in a *lowering of plasma cholesterol level*, and hence, considered to be beneficial in preventing coronary heart disease

- prostaglandins and thromboxanes are synthesised from polyunsaturated fatty acids and can act as local hormones modulating many physiological actions

TRIACYLGLYCEROLS (Triglycerides)

Triacylglycerols are esters of fatty acids and the trihydroxy sugar alcohol glycerol (Figure 7.2). They are also called *neutral fats* because the carboxyl groups of the fatty acids are bound in ester linkage and can no longer function as acids.

If only one or two of the hydroxyl groups of glycerol

MAJOR FATTY ACIDS IN THE HUMAN BODY		
Common Name	Systematic Name	Structural Formula
Saturated		
Palmitic (C16)	n-Hexadecanoic	$CH_3(CH_2)_{14}COOH$
Stearic (C18)	n-Octadecanoic	$CH_3(CH_2)_{16}COOH$
Monounsaturated		
Palmitoleic (C16)	cis-Δ^9-Hexadecenoic	$CH_3(CH_2)_5CH=CH(CH_2)_7COOH$
Oleic (C18)	cis-Δ^9-Octadecenoic	$CH_3(CH_2)_7CH=CH(CH_2)_7COOH$
Polyunsaturated		
Linoleic (C18)	cis-$\Delta^{9,12}$–Octadecadienoic	$CH_3(CH_2)_4(CH=CHCH_2)_2(CH_2)_6COOH$
Linolenic (C18)	all-cis-$\Delta^{9,12,15}$–Octadecatrienoic	$CH_3CH_2(CH=CHCH_2)_3(CH_2)_6COOH$
Arachidonic (C20)	all-cis-$\Delta^{5,8,11,14}$–Eicosatetraenoic	$CH_3(CH_2)_4(CH=CHCH_2)_4(CH_2)_2COOH$

Table 7.1

are esterified with fatty acids, the fat is known as a *mono-* or *diacylglycerol* respectively. When the three fatty acids esterified with glycerol are identical, the triacylglycerol is described as a *pure triglyceride* (e.g. tristearin), but when the fatty acids are not identical, it is described as a *mixed triglyceride* (e.g. oleodistearin). Naturally occurring triacylglycerols are usually mixtures of pure and mixed triacylglycerol.

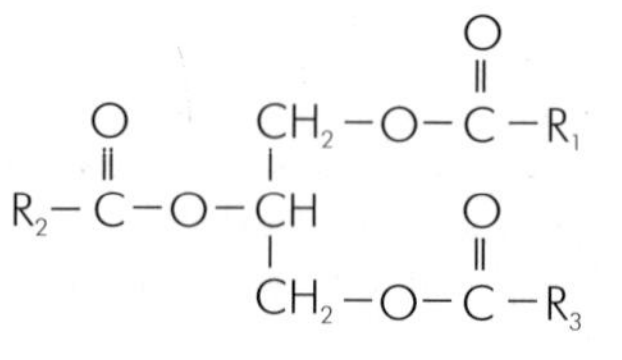

Figure 7.2 – Triacylglycerol.

ENERGY STORAGE BY TRIACYLGLYCEROL

The main function of triacylglycerol is to act as an energy store. Triacylglycerols can store a large amount of energy because they are highly *reduced* and *anhydrous* (because of their non-polar nature). Carbohydrates and proteins are polar and therefore more highly hydrated. One gram of mainly anhydrous fat stores more than six times as much as one gram of hydrated glycogen, which is why triacylglycerol, and not glycogen, serves as the major energy store in the body. It is also economical in terms of bulk, since fatty acids have flexible hydrocarbon chains, and can be stored in a more compact manner than rigid molecules of glycogen. In mammals, triacylglycerols are stored mainly in the cytoplasm of *adipose cells* (*fat cells*).

GLYCEROPHOSPHOLIPIDS (PHOSPHATIDES)

The glycerophospholipids are important biological amphiphiles, since they usually represent up to 50% of the lipids in biological membranes. They may be viewed as being derivatives of **phosphatidic acid** (a glycerol 3-phosphate backbone esterified to two fatty acids). A glycerophospholipid is generally formed by the esterification of a nitrogenous base (*choline, ethanolamine,* or *serine*) to the phosphatidic acid backbone, *phosphatidyl inositol* being an exception.

Plasmalogens are glycerophospholipids in which the 1 (or 2) position has an alkenyl residue containing the vinyl ether aldehydogenic linkage ($-CH_2-O-CH=CH-R^1$) instead of an ester-linked fatty acyl chain. The plasmalogens are an important fraction of the membrane phospholipids in many tissues, especially in nervous tissue. The 1-alkyl-2-acetyl-*sn*-glycerol 3-phosphocholine plasmalogen synthesised from the corresponding 3-phosphocholine derivative is known as the **platelet activating factor** (PAF), because it causes platelet degranulation and aggregates platelets at concentrations as low as 10^{-11} mol/L; it also has hypotensive properties.

MAJOR FUNCTIONS OF GLYCEROPHOSPHOLIPIDS

The main functions performed in the body by glycerophospholipids are shown in Table 7.2.

SPHINGOPHOSPHOLIPIDS

These lipids do not contain glycerol, but are characterised by the presence in their structure of a long-chain aliphatic base, *sphingosine* (Figure 7.3). There are three major classes of sphingophospholipids – *ceramides, sphingomyelin,* and *glycosphingolipids*.

CERAMIDES

A ceramide (Figure 7.3) is formed by the binding of a fatty acid to a sphingosine. The various ceramides differ in their constituent fatty acids. In humans, ceramides function principally as intermediates in the synthesis of other sphingolipids. Ceramides are also thought to be important in cell signalling. Current studies indicate that ceramides may play an important role in the regulation of cell functions such as cell growth, differentiation and apoptosis.

SPHINGOMYELINS

Sphingomyelins are generated by joining choline phosphate or ethanolamine phosphate to ceramides (Figure 7.3). The sphingomyelins are found primarily in nervous tissue, where with the glycolipids, they form important constituents of the myelin sheath surrounding nerve fibres.

GLYCOSPHINGOLIPIDS (Glycolipids)

Glycolipids are formed by the addition of one or more monosaccharide units by a glycosidic linkage to a ceramide . They are widely distributed in the body, particularly in nervous tissue. **Cerebrosides** consist of a hexose sugar such as glucose or galactose, bound to a ceramide (Figure 7.3). **Gangliosides** contain additional

FUNCTIONS OF GLYCEROPHOSPHOLIPIDS	
Glycerophospholipid	Function
Phosphatidylcholine (Lecithin)	Metabolic and structural functions in membranes; influences surface tension in lung alveoli (surfactants).
Phosphatidylethanolamine (Cephalin) and Phosphatidylserine	Structural function in membranes.
Phosphatidylinositol	Important cell membrane phospholipid, especially in nervous tissue. On hormonal stimulation, gives rise to *diacylglycerol* and *inositol triphosphate* which can act as second messengers.
Plasmalogens	Structural function in membranes, especially in nervous tissue and mitochondria. Plasmalogen derivative of 3-phosphocholine function as a platelet activating factor and hypotensive agent.
Cardiolipin	Structural and metabolic function in mitochondrial membrane, especially in the inner membrane.

Table 7.2

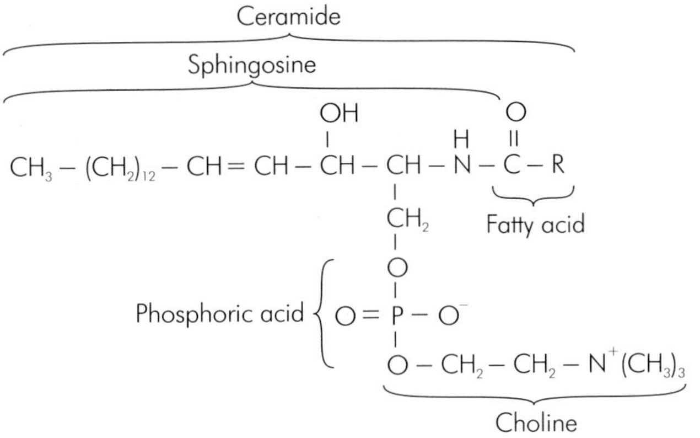

Figure 7.3 – Sphingomyelin, showing its constituent parts.

sugar residues, such as N-acetyl galactosamine and N-acetyl neuraminic acid (sialic acid). Gangliosides appear to have receptor and other functions. A *monosialo-containing ganglioside* named G_{M1} (Figure 7.4) is known to be the receptor in human intestine for cholera toxin. Cells of malignant tumours have unusual gangliosides in their cell membranes. *Sulphatides* are sulphated cerebrosides, or cerebroside-sulphate esters.

Glycerophospholipids and sphingophospholipids in disease

The accumulation or loss of abnormal amounts of glycerophospholipids or sphingophospholipids in tissues, especially in nervous tissue, results in the development of several serious disease conditions.

1. Respiratory distress syndrome

Dipalmitoyl lecithin is an important surfactant pre-venting adherance due to surface tension, of the inner surfaces of lungs. Respiratory distress syndrome of the new born, which is common in premature infants, results from a lack of this surfactant in the lung.

2. Nervous system disorders

Multiple sclerosis is characterised by demyelination due to a loss of glycerophospholipids (particularly,

Ceramide — Glucose — Galactose — N-Acetylgalactosamine — Galactose
   (Acyl- |
 sphingosine)   NeuAc

Figure 7.4 – Structure of G_{M1}

ethanolamine plasmalogen) and of sphingophospho-lipids from white matter. The composition of the white matter then resembles that of grey matter. *Sphingolipidoses* – are a group of inherited diseases, often manifested in childhood. These lipid storage diseases are mainly due to defects in lysosomal enzymes involved in the breakdown of sphingomyelin and gly-colipids. Examples include, *Gaucher's disease* in which glucosyl ceramide accumulates due to a deficiency of β-glucosidase, *Niemann-Pick disease* in which sphin-gomyelin accumulates due to a deficiency of sphin-gomyelinase, and *Tay-Sach's disease,* characterized by the accumulation of GM_2-ganglioside due to a deficiency of hexosaminidase A.

STEROIDS

The steroids include the *sterols* (cholesterol and other steroid alcohols), *steroid hormones* (sex hormones and adrenocortical hormones), and *bile acids*. Structurally, they all contain the same basic nucleus consisting of three fused, cyclohexane rings (A,B and C in Figure 7.5) joined to a cyclopentane ring (D in Figure 7.5). There are a total of 17 carbon atoms in this basic ring structure.

Except for the oestrogens, steroids do not contain aromatic rings. Carbons 3 and 17 always have side groups. The various classes of steroids differ from one another in the number of carbon atoms in the ring structure and the side chains attached to the nucleus.

CHOLESTEROL

Cholesterol is the most abundant representative of sterols in animal tissues, and is the best known steroid because of its association with *atherosclerosis*. Biochemically it is very important because it is the pre-

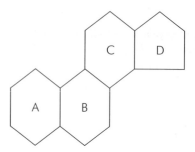

Figure 7.5 – The basic steroid nucleus.

cursor of many other important steroids including the bile acids, adrenocortical hormones, sex hormones, and vitamin D. It is widely distributed in the body, and is often found combined with fatty acids as cholesteryl esters. It is a major constituent of the plasma membrane and of plasma lipoproteins. Cholesterol is predominantly hydrophobic in nature, but the hydroxyl group on C3 of the ring structure confers amphipathic properties that are vital to its role in cell membranes.

In the skin, *vitamin D_3* is synthesised from *7-dehydroc-holesterol* by a UV mediated non-enzymatic photolytic reaction.

SELECTED READING

Vance, D.E. and Vance, J.E. (eds.) – *Biochemistry of Lipids, Lipoproteins and Membranes*. Elsevier, 1991.

Stryer, L. – *Biochemistry*, 4th ed. W.H. Freeman and Co. N.Y., 1995

Murray, R.K., Granner, D.K., Mayer, P.A. and Rodwell, V.W. (eds.) – *Harper's Biochemistry*, 24th ed. Appleton and Lange, California, 1996.

Lehninger, A.L. – *Biochemistry: The molecular basis of cell structure and function*, 3rd ed. Worth Publishers Inc., N.Y., 1993.

8

LIPID METABOLISM AND RELATED DISORDERS

Objectives

To understand:

- The biochemistry of lipoproteins
- Pathways of lipid metabolism
- Disorders of lipid metabolism

Triacylglycerols, fatty acids, cholesterol, cholesteryl esters and phospholipids are the major lipid components of the body. Many cells have the capacity to synthesise them and also possess the mechanisms for the degradation of these lipids to produce energy or convert them to other biologically important compounds.

BLOOD LIPIDS

In addition to the major body lipids, a small amount of non-esterified fatty acids (free fatty acids) are also present in blood. Sources of blood lipids include dietary lipids being transported from the intestine to other tissues, lipids synthesised by the liver being transported to adipose tissue for storage and fatty acids (derived from adipose tissue triacylglycerols) being transported to other tissues to serve as a source of energy (e.g. in fasting or starvation).

FREE FATTY ACID TRANSPORT IN BLOOD

Free fatty acids in the form of sodium salts are transported bound to the plasma protein, albumin, which prevents them from exerting disruptive detergent effects on the circulating proteins and cell membranes. The fatty acid-albumin complex undergoes a dissociation at the plasma membrane, and the free fatty acids are co-transported into the cells with Na^+ by a membrane fatty acid-binding protein. Within cells, the fatty acids bind to other proteins with a high affinity for them (e.g. Z-protein).

TRANSPORT OF OTHER LIPIDS IN BLOOD

The relatively insoluble triacylglycerols, cholesterol and phospholipids, are transported in the plasma as *lipoprotein particles*.

PLASMA LIPOPROTEINS

The plasma lipoproteins are comprised of a hydrophobic core of triacylglycerols or cholesteryl esters, or both, surrounded by an outer layer containing amphipathic lipids such as free cholesterol and phospholipids and a variety of polypeptides known as *apoproteins (apolipoproteins)*. All these lipids are arranged so that their polar portions are exposed on the surface of the lipoprotein, thereby making the particle soluble in aqueous solution.

APOPROTEINS

Ten principal apoproteins have been isolated and characterised. They vary greatly in their molecular characteristics and function in three major ways:

- they provide the structural element to the lipoprotein particles and therefore help in maintaining stability
- they act as ligands for specific receptors
- they act as activators or inhibitors of enzymes involved in lipoprotein metabolism

The apoproteins may be grouped into five major families (A-E), on the basis of their structure and function (Table 8.1). Within each family, several subgroups of apoproteins may be recognised.

PROPERTIES OF THE MAJOR HUMAN APOPROTEINS		
Apolipoprotein	Site of synthesis	Possible function
A-I	I, L	Activation of LCAT Ligand for HDL receptor
A-II	I, L	? Inhibition of LCAT
A-IV	I, L	Structural
B-100	L	Ligand for LDL receptor
B-48	I	Structural
C-I	L	?Activator of LCAT
C-II	L	Activator of LPL
C-III	L	Inhibition of LPL
D	?	? Lipid transfer protein
E	L	Ligand for chylomicron remnant/LDL receptors
I intestine, L liver		

Table 8.1

TYPES OF LIPOPROTEINS

According to their *density* (as determined by their rate of sedimentation on ultracentrifugation), five types of lipoproteins may be recognized, in increasing density, *chylomicrons; very low density lipoproteins (VLDL); intermediate density lipoproteins (IDL); low density lipoproteins (LDL)* and *high density lipoproteins (HDL)*. Of these lipoproteins, the highest triacylglycerol (TG) concentrations are found in chylomicrons and VLDL (85% and 60% of the total composition respectively) and a much lower TG concentration is in LD and HDL (about 15% of total). On the other hand, HDL contains the highest proportion of protein (45% of total composition) while chylomicrons and VLDL contain the lowest amounts of protein. The highest cholesterol concentration is found in LDL (50% of the total composition).

The larger lipoprotein particles (chylomicrons, VLDL) scatter light, and if present in high concentrations (e.g. in uncontrolled diabetes mellitus), they can cause the plasma to appear turbid.

According to their *electrophoretic mobility*, four types of lipoproteins, α, *pre-β, β* and *chylomicrons* may be recognised.

Apolipoprotein (a) is a large, glycated protein of variable size. In a subpopulation of LDL particles, apo (a) can link up with B-100 via disulphide bridges to form a distinct lipoprotein class called lipoprotein (a). This lipoprotein, when present in large quantities in the plasma, has been suggested to increase the risk of coronary heart disease, particularly in individuals with familial hypercholesteraemia. Apo (a) has a strong homology with plasminogen, the precursor of a blood protease whose target is fibrin and may interfere with fibrinolysis and slow down the breakdown of blood clots, important in the aetiology of myocardial infarction.

Lipoprotein X is an abnormal lipoprotein present in plasma of patients with cholestasis and in those with familial lecithin cholesterol acyl transferase (LCAT) deficiency. Phospholipids and free cholesterol are the lipid components of lipoprotein X, the major protein is albumin, but a small amount of apo D is also present.

LIPOPROTEIN METABOLISM

Enzymes involved in lipoprotein metabolism

Four major enzymes are involved in lipoprotein metabolism:

- *lipoprotein lipase (LPL)* – hydrolyses triacylglycerols in chylomicrons and VLDL to produce glycerol and free fatty acids. It is an extracellular enzyme attached by heparan sulphate (a glycosaminoglycan) to capillary endothelial cells, and is present in large amounts in the capillaries of muscle and adipose tissue. Its activity increases after a meal. LPL requires the presence of apo C-II (present on the surface of triacylglycerol-bearing lipoproteins) and phospholipids for full activity

- *lecithin cholesterol acyltransferase (LCAT)* – synthesised by the liver and catalyses the esterification of free cholesterol on the surface of discoidal HDL particles within the circulation. This reaction is stimulated by apo A-I

- *cholesteryl ester transfer protein* – catalyses transfer of cholesteryl esters from HDL to VLDL in an exchange reaction that concomitantly transfers triacylglycerol or phospholipid from VLDL to the HDL

- *hepatic triacylglycerol lipase (HTGL)* – acts on endothelial surface of hepatic capillaries removing triacylglycerol from HDL_2 and HDL_3. It may also act on IDL to generate LDL

Lipoprotein metabolic pathways

Lipoprotein metabolism can be considered to occur in two interconnected cycles, *exogenous* (Figure 8.1) and *endogenous* (Figure 8.2), both centred on the liver.

The **exogenous cycle** is concerned with the metabolism of *chylomicrons* formed from dietary lipids. Long chain fatty acids (C12 and higher) derived from dietary lipids are absorbed in the small intestine and converted to triacylglycerols in the smooth endoplasmic reticulum of the intestinal mucosal cell. These are then complexed with dietary cholesterol, cholesterol esters, phospholipids and apoproteins B-48, A-1 and A-IV synthesized in the mucosal cells, to form *chylomicrons* which are secreted into the lymphatics and reach the blood stream via the thoracic duct. In the circulation, there is a rapid transfer of apo C (C-II and C-III) and apo E together with some phospholipids and cholesterol from HDL to the nascent chylomicron. Triacylglycerol is gradually removed from these lipoproteins by the action of *lipoprotein lipase* (LPL) present in the capillaries of a number of tissues, predominantly adipose tissue and skeletal muscle. LPL requires apo C-II and phospholipids on circulating lipoprotein particles as cofactors. As chylomicrons lose triacylglycerol, excess surface components, phospho-

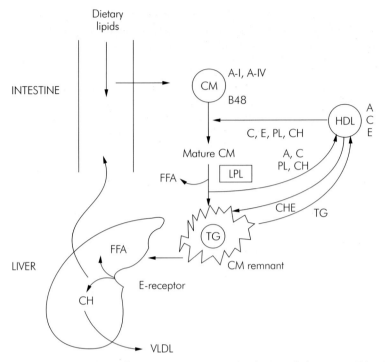

Figure 8.1 – Metabolism of lipoproteins – Exogenous cycle. CM-chylomicrons, TG–triacylglycerol, CH – Cholesterol, CHE – Cholesterol ester, PL – phospholipid, LPL – lipoprotein lipase; A, B, C, D, E, – apoproteins, VLDL – very low density lipoprotein; FFA – free fatty acids, HDL – high density lipoproteins.

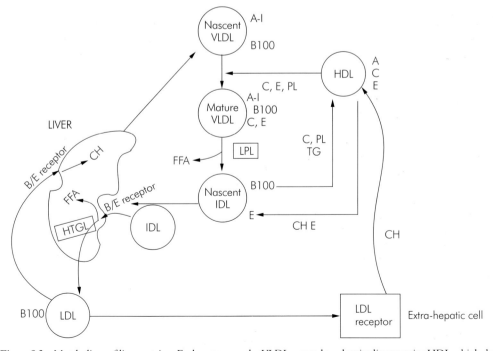

Figure 8.2 – Metabolism of lipoproteins: Endogenous cycle; VLDL – very low density lipoprotein; HDL – high density lipoprotein; LDL – low density lipoprotein; IDL – intermediate density lipoprotein; FFA – free fatty acids; TG – triacylglycerol; CH – cholesterol; CHE – cholesteryl ester; PL – phospholipid; LPL- lipoprotein lipase; HTGL – hepatic triacylglycerol lipase; A,B,C,E – apoproteins A,B,C and E respectively.

lipids, free cholesterol and the C-apoproteins are also returned to HDL and they become smaller *chylomicron remnants* which are removed from circulation by the liver; uptake appears to be mediated by a receptor specific for apo-E present on hepatocyte membranes. The cholesterol from these remnants may be utilised by the liver to form cell membrane components or bile salts, or may be excreted in bile.

The **endogenous cycle** is concerned with the metabolism of VLDL, LDL and HDL.

VLDL, synthesised in the liver, are released from this organ as *nascent* VLDL particles containing apo B-100 and apo A-I. They obtain apo C-II and apo E from circulating HDL to become *mature* VLDL particles which undergo the same form of delipidation as chylomicrons, by the action of LPL resulting in the formation of an *intermediate density lipoprotein (IDL)*. The surface components including the C and E apoproteins are transferred back to HDL. The IDL is subsequently taken up by tissues or converted to LDL by the transfer of cholesteryl esters from HDL to IDL in an exchange reaction that concomitantly transfers triacylglycerol or phospholipid from IDL to HDL. This exchange is accomplished by the *cholesteryl ester transfer protein* (CETP). CETP may be a pro-atherogenic factor as CETP-deficient subjects have high HDL concentrations and appear to be resistant to atherosclerosis.

LDL functions primarily to provide cholesterol for peripheral tissues. Most of the LDL enters cells by binding to specific cell surface *LDL receptors*. LDL may be metabolised slowly by uptake in most tissues through the LDL specific B/E receptors and also by non-specific mechanisms known as *scavenger pathways*.

The LDL receptor is concentrated in special membrane depressions called coated pits. After it binds to the receptor, the LDL-receptor complex is internalized within the cell where it undergoes lysosomal degradation. Its apo B is hydrolysed to its constituent amino acids and its cholesteryl ester is hydrolysed to free cholesterol which acts as a signal by which the cellular cholesterol content is precisely regulated by three co-ordinated reactions. First, the enzyme, which is rate-limiting for cholesterol biosynthesis (3-hydroxy 3-methyl glutaryl CoA reductase, HMGCoA reductase) is repressed, thus effectively centralising cholesterol biosynthesis to organs such as the liver and gut. Second, the synthesis of the LDL receptor itself is suppressed. Third, acyl CoA: cholesterol O-acyl transferase (ACAT) is activated so that any excess cholesterol is converted to cholesteryl ester, which

because of its hydrophobic nature forms into droplets within the cytoplasm and is stored. A similar mechanism is used for the cellular uptake and degradation of chylomicron remnants and HDLs by the liver. Chemically modified (by acetylation or oxidation) LDL can be 'scavenged' by receptors on macrophages. This process can be inhibited by antioxidants such as vitamin E. The modified LDL taken up by macrophages does not regulate intracellular cholesterol levels and cholesterol accumulates in these cells transforming them into 'foam cells' that participate in formation of atheromatous plaques.

The other quantitatively important mechanism for entry of LDL into cells is by a non-receptor-mediated pathway. LDL binds to cell membranes at sites other than those where LDL receptors are located and some of it passes through the membrane by pinocytosis. Unlike receptor-mediated entry, non-receptor-mediated LDL uptake is not saturable and continues to increase with increasing extracellular LDL concentrations. This pathway assumes greater quantitative importance than entry via LDL receptors when there is a relatively high LDL concentration (e.g. in individuals consuming high fat diets).

HDL particles are derived mainly from the liver, although a small amount can be synthesised by the intestine. Newly secreted HDL particles are disc-shaped, containing predominantly unesterified cholesterol, phospholipids and apoproteins A,C and E. In the circulation, lecithin-cholesterol acyltransferase (LCAT) helps to esterify cholesterol from peripheral tissues taken up by HDL.

LCAT is activated by apo A-1 of the HDL. With the accumulation of cholesteryl ester, the nascent HDL particles become spherical (HDL_3). Formation of the cholesteryl ester increases the capacity of the surface of the HDL particles for free cholesterol, which is acquired from cell membranes, possibly after interaction with specific HDL receptors. Along with the accumulation of cholesterol, apoproteins C-I, C-II, C-III and E, and phospholipids are also acquired from VLDL and chylomicrons, and the HDL is converted to lipid enriched particles of lower density HDL_2. In moderate consumers of ethanol, HDL_3 cholesterol concentrations may be increased, while HDL_2 cholesterol concentrations remain unchanged. However, it is not certain whether this can reduce the risk of coronary heart disease.

The HDL_2 is taken up directly by the liver, or indirectly by being transferred to other circulating lipoproteins which then return it to the liver. HDL particles can also act as donors of cholesteryl ester to chylomicron and VLDL remnants to be transported to and internalised by the liver. These processes are thought to be anti-atherogenic, and an elevated HDL cholesterol level has been shown to confer a decreased risk of coronary heart disease. HDL enters the hepatocyte via the apo B/E receptor for which the E interaction appears to be the major component.

FATTY ACID BIOSYNTHESIS

Fatty acid biosynthesis occurs by *de novo* biosynthesis, chain elongation, or, in the case of unsaturated fatty acids, by desaturation.

DE NOVO FATTY ACID BIOSYNTHESIS

De novo fatty acid biosynthesis occurs in the soluble cell cytoplasm of primarily, the liver and lactating mammary gland, and to a lesser extent in adipose, kidney, brain and lung tissue. This process involves the incorporation of carbon atoms from several units of acetyl CoA, utilising ATP and reduced nicotinamide adenine dinucleotide phosphate (NADPH).

Source of acetyl CoA for fatty acid biosynthesis

Glucose is the main source of acetyl CoA for fatty acid synthesis. The pyruvate formed from glucose during glycolysis is converted to acetyl CoA in the mitochondria. Pyruvate formed during the metabolism of certain amino acids (e.g. alanine, serine glycine and threonine) may also be converted to acetyl CoA.

Transfer of acetyl CoA into the cytosol

The first step in the fatty acid biosynthetic process (Figure 8.3) involves the transfer of acetate from mitochondrial acetyl CoA to the cytosol to from cytosolic acetyl CoA. Since the CoA portion of acetyl CoA cannot cross the mitochondrial membrane, acetate units are transferred to the cytosol in the form of citrate. The efflux of citrate is mediated by a specific transporter in the inner mitochondrial membrane called *citrate-malate antiporter* because it exchanges citrate for malate. On translocation of citrate from the mitochondrion into the cytosol, it is cleaved by *citrate lyase* to produce cytosolic acetyl CoA and oxaloacetate. Malate returns to the mitochondria via the malate

shuttle, enters the citric acid cycle and helps to maintain the flux of intermediates around the cycle.

Incorporation of acetyl CoA units into fatty acids

Once acetyl CoA enters the biosynthetic pathway directly the remainder must be converted to malonyl CoA before they enter the pathway (Figure 8.4). The carboxylation of acetyl CoA to produce malonyl CoA is the rate-limiting reaction in the fatty acid biosynthetic pathway. The reaction is catalysed by *acetyl CoA carboxylase,* that requires *biotin* as a coenzyme. Bicarbonate supplies the CO_2 required in this reaction. All further reactions in the fatty acid biosynthetic pathway are catalysed by the *fatty acid synthase complex*. In eukaryotes, this enzyme complex exists as a dimer (Figure 8.4), each monomer of which has seven distinct enzyme activities plus a domain that covalently binds a molecule of *4-phosphopantetheine*. In prokaryotes, this portion known as *acyl carrier protein* (ACP) is a separate protein.

As shown in Figure 8.3, the synthesis of fatty acids begins with the attachment of one molecule of acetate (transferred from its CoA derivatives) to the ACP region of the fatty acyl synthase through the phosphopantetheine group in a reaction catalysed by *acetyl CoA-ACP transacylase*. This is followed by the transfer of a three-carbon malonate unit from malonyl CoA to the ACP with help from *malonyl CoA-ACP transacylase*. Carbon chain elongation begins with the condensation of these acetyl and malonyl groups, and the elimination of CO_2 from the malonyl group. The product *β-ketoacyl-ACP* then undergoes reduction and dehydration, resulting in the generation of a four-carbon compound whose three terminal carbons are fully saturated, and that remains attached to the ACP. This cycle of reactions is repeated six more times, each time incorporating a two-carbon unit (derived from malonyl CoA) into the growing fatty acid chain until a fully saturated molecule of *palmitic acid* (C16) is formed.

CONTROL OF DE NOVO BIOSYNTHESIS OF FATTY ACIDS

Control of fatty acid biosynthesis may involve short- or long-term control mechanisms.

Short-term control involves the *regulation of the activity of acetyl CoA carboxylase*, a key enzyme of the fatty acid biosynthetic pathway. The inactive form of this enzyme consists of a protein made of four subunits. Citrate activates acetyl CoA carboxylase by causing

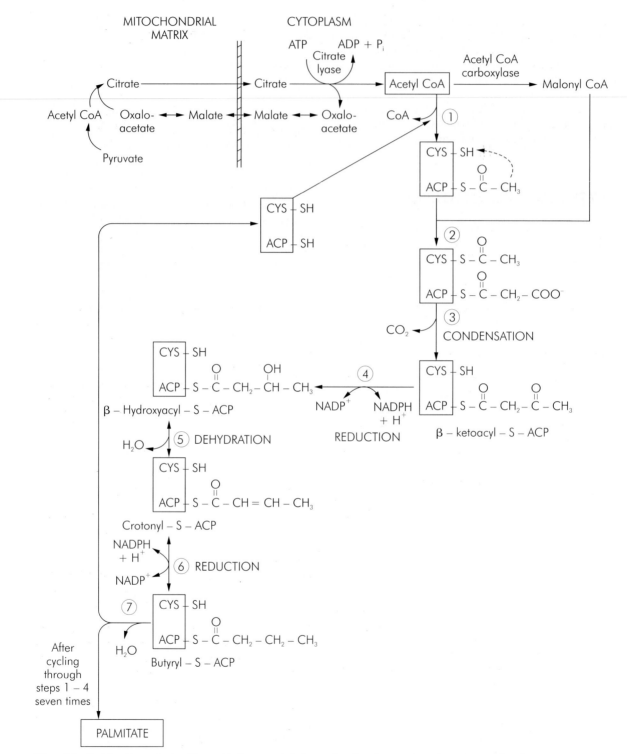

Figure 8.3 – *De Novo* biosynthesis of fatty acids from acetyl CoA transferred to the cytoplasm from the mitochondria via citrate:
① – AcetylCoA ACP transacylase; ② – MalonylCoA ACP transacylase; ③ – β-ketoacyl ACP synthase; ④ – β-ketoacyl ACP reductase;
⑤ – β-hydroxyacyl ACP dehydratase; ⑥ – 2,3-trans-enoyl ACP reductase; ⑦ – Palmitoyl thioesterase.

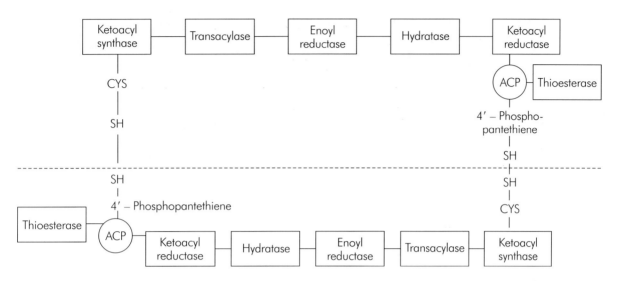

Figure 8.4 – Fatty acid synthase multienzyme complex.

aggregation of the enzyme subunits (*feed forward activation*). Palmityl CoA (and also malonyl CoA) inactivates the enzyme by maintaining the four subunits in the depolymerised form (*feedback inhibition*).

Short-term control of acetyl CoA carboxylase may also be achieved by reversible phosphorylation of the enzyme. Adrenaline causes phosphorylation of the enzyme (analogous to the mechanism of inactivation of glycogen synthase) while insulin activates the enzyme by dephosphorylation through the activation of a protein phosphatase. Insulin can also increase fatty acid biosynthesis by converting pyruvate dehydrogenase complex to the active form in the adipose tissue (but not in the liver). In diabetes mellitus, there will be a decrease in fatty acid biosynthesis due to insulin deficiency. The effects of these short-term measures manifest themselves very rapidly because they involve modulation of the activity of an already existing enzyme.

Long-term control involves *changes in the content of fatty acid biosynthesising enzymes* within the cell. Prolonged consumption of high carbohydrate or fat free diets causes an increase in enzyme synthesis. Conversely, enzyme content is decreased by prolonged feeding of a high fat diet or fasting.

ELONGATION OF FATTY ACYL CHAINS

Of all fatty acids in humans, 60% have chain lengths of ≥ 18 carbon atoms (C20, C22, and C24 fatty acids are the most common). Lengthening of fatty acyl chains occurs mainly in the endoplasmic reticulum, catalysed by a *microsomal elongase enzyme system*. The process is very similar to that producing short-chain fatty acids in that malonyl CoA donates the two-carbon units and the same four reaction sequence, as shown in Figure 8.3, occurs. The major difference is that palmitate participates as a CoA rather than an ACP derivative. Fatty acid elongation also occurs to a limited extent in mitochondria by a slightly different reaction sequence.

DESATURATION OF FATTY ACIDS

Introduction of double bonds into fatty acids also occurs in the endoplasmic reticulum and involves *cytochrome b_5, cytochrome b_5 reductase* and a specific *desaturase*. Humans lack the ability to introduce double bonds beyond carbons 9–10, and therefore must have the polyunsaturated fatty acids linoleic (18: 2 *cis*-$\Delta^{9,12}$) and linolenic (18: 3 *cis*-$\Delta^{9,12,15}$) acids provided in the diet; these fatty acids are therefore *essential fatty acids*. Arachidonic acid (20: 4 *cis*-$\Delta^{5,8,11,14}$) becomes essential if its precursor, linoleic acid, is missing in the diet.

Desaturation is regulated according to the needs of the body. Carbohydrate feeding increases activity of desaturases, and starvation or feeding unsaturated fat decreases the activity of the enzymes.

BIOSYNTHESIS OF TRIACYLGLYCEROLS

Triacylglycerols (TG) can be synthesized by two pathways. The first is the *general pathway* (Figure 8.5) that is

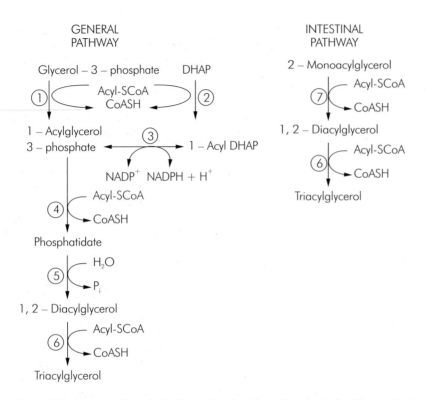

Figure 8.5 – General and intestinal pathways for triacylglycerol synthesis: ① – Glycerol-3-phosphate acyltransferase; ② – Dihydroxyacetone phosphate acyltransferase; ③ – 1-Acyl dihydroxyacetone phosphate reductase; ④ – 1-Acyl-3-phosphate acyltransferase; ⑤ – Phosphatase; ⑥ – 1,2- Diacylglycerol transferase; ⑦ – 2-Monoacylglycerol acyltransferase.

operational in the liver and other organs where fatty acid biosynthesis occurs. Phosphatidate, which is a precursor of triacylglycerols, may be derived from dihydroxyacetone phosphate (a glycolytic intermediate) or from glycerol-3-phosphate. The second is the *intestinal pathway* that is responsible for the resynthesis of triacylglycerols in the intestinal epithelium from 2-monoacylglycerols formed during the intestinal digestion of triacylglycerols.

MOBILISATION OF STORED FATS AND OXIDATION OF FATTY ACIDS

The fatty acids stored in the adipose tissue as triacylglycerols serve as the major fuel store of the body. The complete oxidation of fatty acids to CO_2 and H_2O yields 9 kcal/g as compared with 4 kcal/g of carbohydrate or protein. The triacylglycerol stores in the adipose tissue are continuously undergoing lipolysis and re-esterification. These two processes occur by separate pathways involving different reactants and

enzymes. The balance between these processes determines the rate of release of free fatty acids (FFA) from adipose tissue.

MOBILISATION OF STORED FATS

The hydrolytic release of fatty acids and glycerol from triacylglycerol initiates the mobilisation of stored fat. This process begins by the removal of a fatty acid from C1 or C3 of a triacylglycerol by a *hormone-sensitive lipase* located in adipose tissue cells. Additional lipases specific for diacylglycerol or monoacylglycerol remove the remaining fatty acids.

REGULATION OF THE ACTIVITY OF THE HORMONE-SENSITIVE LIPASE

Hormone-sensitive lipase is activated when phosphorylated by a *3′, 5′- cAMP-dependent protein kinase*. Several hormones such as *adrenaline, noradrenaline, glucagon, adrenocorticotrophic hormone (ACTH)*, and *growth hormone* (primarily adrenaline), promote lipolysis through activation of the hormone-sensitive lipase.

Processes that destroy cAMP inhibit lipolysis. *Cyclic 3,5-nucleotide phosphodiesterase* degrades cAMP to 5'-AMP. It is inhibited by methylxanthines such as *caffeine* and *theophylline. Insulin*, on the other hand, decreases lipolysis by inhibiting the hormone-sensitive lipase activity, thus reducing the release not only of FFAs but also of glycerol. *Insulin, nicotinic acid*, and *prostaglandin E* inhibit the synthesis of cAMP at the adenylate cyclase site, acting through a G-protein. Insulin also stimulates the phosphodiesterase that destroys cAMP, and the lipase phosphatase that inactivates hormone-sensitive lipase.

FATE OF GLYCEROL RELEASED FROM TRIACYLGLYCEROL

Further metabolism of glycerol cannot occur in adipocytes because they lack *glycerol kinase*. The glycerol is therefore transported into the liver where it is phosphorylated to glycerol phosphate which can be converted to triacylglycerol in the liver, or be converted to dihydroxyacetone phosphate that can enter the glycolytic or gluconeogenic pathways.

THE OXIDATION OF SATURATED FATTY ACIDS

Saturated fatty acids are chiefly oxidised by the mitochondrial *β-oxidation pathway* in which two-carbon fragments are successively removed from the carboxyl end of the fatty acyl CoA, producing acetyl CoA (Figure 8.6). The acetyl CoA formed undergoes further oxidation via the citric acid cycle.

ENTRY OF FATTY ACIDS INTO MITOCHONDRIA

Fatty acids cannot pass easily through the inner mitochondrial membrane. The fatty acids in the cytosol are therefore first activated to an acyl CoA derivative at the outer mitochondrial membrane by *fatty acyl CoA synthetase (thiokinase)*.

Since bulky molecules such as CoA cannot traverse easily across the inner mitochondrial membrane, the acyl group from the cytosol is carried into the matrix (Figure 8.6), by the specialized carrier molecule *carnitine* via the *carnitine shuttle*. This process involves the

participation of *carnitine acyl transferase I*, located on the outer surface of the inner mitochondrial membrane, and *carnitine acyl transferase II*, located on the inner surface of the inner mitochondrial membrane. Malonyl CoA inhibits carnitine acyl transferase I. Therefore, when fatty acid synthesis occurs in the cytosol (as indicated by high levels of malonyl CoA) the newly formed fatty acids cannot be transferred to the mitochondria for oxidation.

Genetic defects in the enzymes of the carnitine shuttle in skeletal muscle, or low concentrations of carnitine due to defective synthesis, result in an inability to use long chain fatty acids to produce energy and causes myoglobinaemia and weakness following exercise.

THE β-OXIDATION SCHEME

As shown in Figure 8.6, the acyl CoA molecule in the mitochondrial matrix is degraded by a recurring sequence of four reactions: oxidation linked to flavin adenine dinucleotide (FAD); hydration; oxidation linked to nicotinamide adenine dinucleotide (NAD^+); and a thiolysis by CoA. At the end of these reactions, the fatty acyl CoA is shortened by two carbon atoms, and $FADH_2$, NADH, and acyl CoA are generated. This sequence will be repeated until a 4C acetoacetyl CoA remains.

The individual reactions involved in the β-oxidation of short- and medium-chain fatty acids are catalysed by separate enzymes. There are three *fatty acyl CoA dehydrogenase* (Figure 8.6) species in mitochondria that have specificities for short-, medium-, and long-chain fatty acids. Medium-chain length acylCoA dehydrogenase deficiency is found in approximately 1:10,000 births; in this condition there is a decrease in fatty acid oxidation and severe hypoglycaemia and in a few cases is thought to be a cause of *sudden infant death syndrome (SIDS)*.

Energy produced by fatty acid oxidation through the β-oxidation scheme

A large amount of ATP is produced by the β-oxidation of fatty acids. For example, palmitic acid (16C) will produce eight molecules of acetyl CoA. Each acetyl CoA will yield 12 ATP on its passage through the citric acid cycle; the total from the eight acetyl CoA molecules would therefore be 96 ATP. Transport in the respiratory chain of electrons from reduced FAD and NAD formed will also lead to the synthesis of 5ATP for each of the first seven acetyl CoA molecule formed by the β-oxidation of palmitate (total 35 ATP).

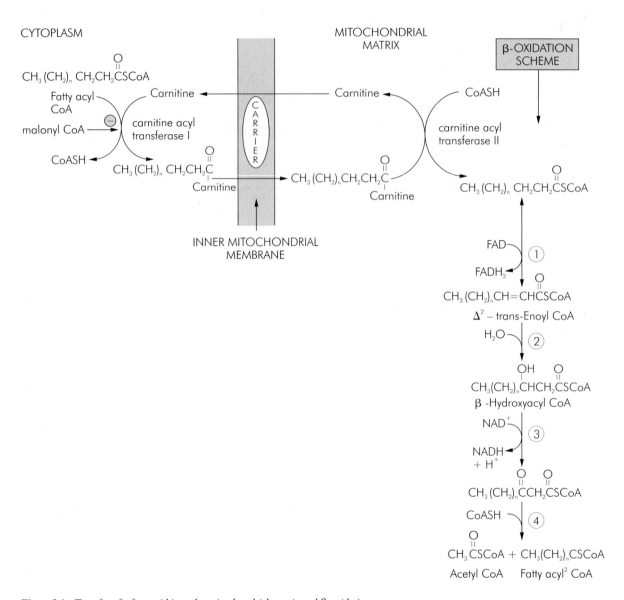

Figure 8.6 – Transfer of a fatty acid into the mitochondrial matrix and β-oxidation :
① – Acyl CoA dehydrogenase; ② – EnoylCoA dehydratase; ③ – β-Hydroxyacyl CoA dehydrogenase; ④ – AcylCoA acyl transferase (thiolase).

Therefore on subtracting the 2ATP used for the initial activation of the fatty acid from the total ATP formed during its oxidation (131–2), the oxidation of one molecule of palmitate will yield a net gain of 129 molecules of ATP.

PEROXISOMAL OXIDATION OF FATTY ACIDS

Very long chain fatty acids (e.g. C20, C22) can also undergo oxidation in peroxisomes by a modified form

of β-oxidation; end products are acetyl CoA and hydrogen peroxide. The peroxisome is required for the initial stages of oxidation of acyl groups > 18 carbons, as mitochondria can oxidise only fatty acids of 18 carbons or less. This system is not linked directly to phosphorylation and the generation of ATP, and is induced by high fat diets and hypolipidaemic drugs such as *clofibrate*. That this peroxisomal pathway is physiologically important is illustrated by a rare group of hereditary peroxisomal disorders typified by

Zellweger syndrome; in individuals with these disorders (due to a defect in peroxisome biosynthesis), long-chain fatty acids accumulate in the blood.

α AND ω-OXIDATION OF FATTY ACIDS

A specialised pathway that does not require CoA intermediates exists in the brain for the α-oxidation (removal of one carbon at a time from the carboxyl end of the molecule) of fatty acids. α-Oxidation, which occurs in peroxisomes, involves molecular oxygen, cytochromes, free fatty acids, an *α-hydroxylase*, and an *α-oxidase*. The metabolism of *phytanate*, a degradation product of chlorophyll, requires the α-oxidation pathway for metabolism because the presence of a methyl group on the β-carbon of phytanate prevents it being oxidised by the β-oxidation pathway. The β-oxidation step, helps to generate a substrate for the β-oxidation pathway. *Refsum's disease (phytanate storage disease),* is a rare inborn error of lipid metabolism resulting from a defect in the α-hydroxylase step of α-oxidation and is characterized by retinitis pigmentosa, peripheral neuropathy, nerve deafness and cerebellar ataxia. Treatment consists of a diet low in phytanate.

ω-Oxidation is a very minor pathway that occurs in the endoplasmic reticulum.

OXIDATION OF FATTY ACIDS WITH AN ODD NUMBER OF CARBON ATOMS

The β-oxidation of a saturated fatty acid with an odd number of carbon atoms proceeds until the final three carbon atoms are reached. The *propionyl CoA* so formed undergoes carboxylation by an ATP dependent reaction to D-methyl malonyl CoA; which in turn undergoes isomerisation to the L-form. This L-methyl malonyl CoA is finally converted to succinyl CoA by the B_{12}-dependent enzyme, methyl malonyl CoA isomerase.

OXIDATION OF UNSATURATED FATTY ACIDS

Fatty acids with one or more double bonds require modification to convert them into intermediates of the β-oxidation pathway. The acyl CoA derivatives of monounsaturated fatty acids (e.g. oleate) are also degraded by the same enzymes involved in the oxidation of saturated fatty acids (Figure 8.7), until an inter-mediate with a *cis*-double bond between C3 and C4 is formed. This prevents the normal dehydrogenation reaction in the β-oxidation scheme which involves formation of a *trans*-double bond between C2 and C3. The conversion of *cis*-Δ^3 bond to a *trans*-Δ^2 bond is carried out by a specific *enoyl CoA isomerase*. In the case of polyunsaturated fatty acids such as linoleic acid, the enoyl CoA isomerase plus additional enzymes are used to convert the *cis*-double-bonded intermediate to the *trans*-Δ^2 form that can eventually enter the β-oxidation scheme for complete oxidation.

KETONE BODY METABOLISM

In the liver, acetyl CoA in excess of the amount that can be metabolised by the citric acid cycle is converted to the ketone bodies *acetoacetate* and *3-hydroxybutyrate (β-hydroxybutyrate)* (Figure 8.7). Acetoacetate may spontaneously decarboxylate to produce *acetone* which is volatile, and may be exhaled. Acetone may be detected in the breath of patients with severe and untreated diabetes.

Ketone body synthesis occurs within the mitochondria. High ratios of NADH to NAD^+ inhibit the citric acid cycle and divert acetyl CoA into the synthesis of ketone bodies. The ketone bodies move out of the mitochondria through an inner membrane transporter in exchange for pyruvate.

PHYSIOLOGICAL SIGNIFICANCE OF KETONE BODIES

Ketone bodies are very important for the provision of energy to peripheral tissues (especially during starvation) for the following reasons:

- they are water-soluble, so do not need to be incorporated into lipoproteins or bound to albumin for transport in the blood

- they are produced in the liver when the amount of acetyl CoA present exceeds the oxidative capacity of the liver

- extrahepatic tissues such as heart, skeletal muscle and renal cortex use ketone bodies in proportion to their concentration in the blood; heart muscle and renal cortex use ketone bodies in preference to glucose. The brain adapts to the utilization of ketone bodies in hypoglycaemic conditions and during starvation in an attempt to conserve glucose. This also helps to conserve muscle by reducing the

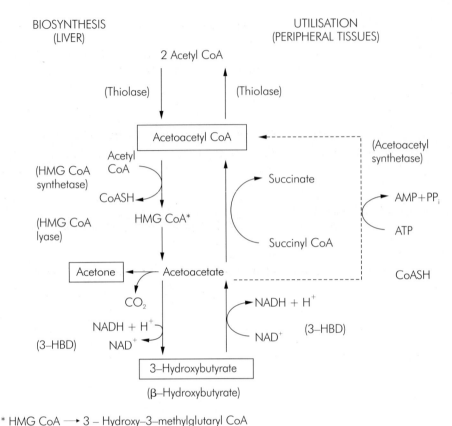

BIOSYNTHESIS
(LIVER)

UTILISATION
(PERIPHERAL TISSUES)

* HMG CoA ⟶ 3 – Hydroxy–3–methylglutaryl CoA
3-HBD – 3 – Hydroxybutyrate dehydrogenase

Figure 8.7 – Ketone body metabolism.

need for protein catabolism for gluconeogenesis. In prolonged starvation, 75% of the fuel needs of the brain are met by acetoacetate

Although the liver produces ketone bodies, it lacks *β-ketoacyl transferase* and therefore cannot reconvert acetoacetate to acetoacetyl CoA, and cannot itself use them as fuels.

Utilization of ketone bodies by peripheral tissues

Ketone bodies synthesised in the liver are converted to acetyl CoA in peripheral tissues.

CHOLESTEROL METABOLISM

BIOSYNTHESIS

Cholesterol is present in the diet and is also synthesised in most tissues of the body (in the liver, intestine

and skin) from acetyl CoA; the brain actively synthesises cholesterol during myelination. Cholesterol synthesis occurs in the microsomal and cytosolic fractions of the cell. The biosynthesis of cholesterol occurs in five stages:

Stage 1 – Acetyl CoA is converted to the 6C compound *mevalonate*. Two molecules of acetyl CoA react to form a molecule of acetoacetyl CoA which, with a further acetyl group (from acetyl CoA) generates 3-hydroxy, 3-methylglutaryl CoA (HMG CoA). The HMG CoA so formed undergoes an NADPH-dependent reduction to mevalonate. The *HMG CoA reductase* step is the rate-limiting step in cholesterol biosynthesis. In the liver, the activity of the reductase is decreased by glucagon and increased by insulin. Enzyme activity is also inhibited by cholesterol (or its metabolites). In the intestine, this reaction is inhibited by bile acids.

Stage 2 – The formation of a 5C compound *isopentenyl pyrophosphate* from mevalonate. This process involves several phosphorylated intermediates and a decarboxylation reaction. This 5C compound is the building unit not only of steroids, but also of other compounds such as vitamins D, E, K and ubiquinone.

Stage 3 – Three units of isopentenyl pyrophosphate condense to form a 15C alcohol *farnesyl pyrophosphate*.

Stage 4 – Two units of farnesyl pyrophosphate condense to form the 30C unsaturated hydrocarbon *squalene*.

Stage 5 – Cyclisation of squalene occurs with oxidation and methyl transfer reactions leading to the production of *cholesterol* via an intermediate cyclic compound *lanosterol*.

CHOLESTEROL DEGRADATION

The ring structure of cholesterol is eliminated from the body by:

- conversion to bile acids which are excreted in the faeces; 80% of cholesterol is excreted in this manner. Part of the bile acids may be reabsorbed during fat absorption and later re-excreted

- secretion of unesterified cholesterol into the bile for transport into the intestine for elimination

Conversion of cholesterol to bile acids

In the liver, cholesterol is converted first to the *primary bile acids cholic acid* and *chenodeoxycholic acid* (Figure 8.8). The rate-limiting step in the synthesis of bile acids is catalyzed by microsomal *7α-hydroxylase*. A high cholesterol diet stimulates the activity of this enzyme while the bile acids (especially cholic acid) can inhibit the enzyme activity by a feedback mechanism.

Conversion of bile acids to bile salts

Before the bile acids are excreted from the liver they

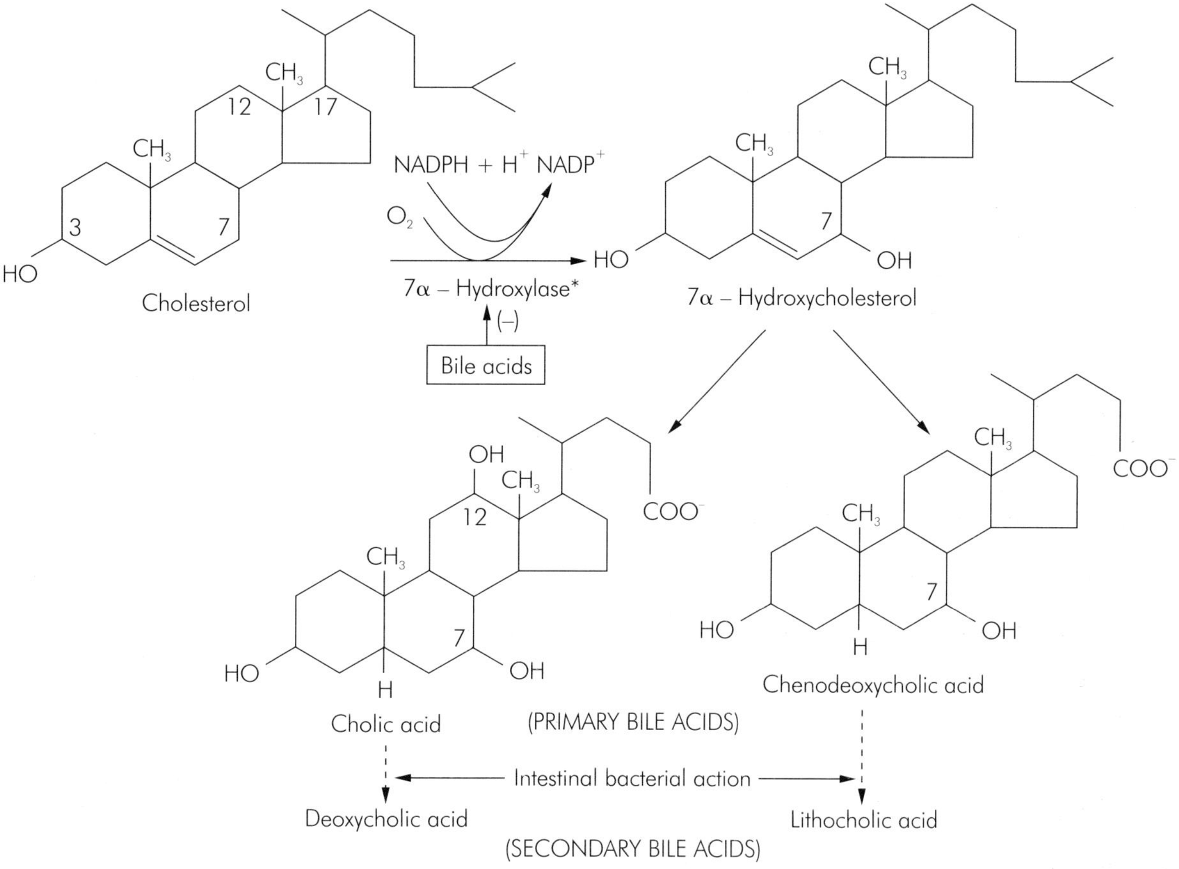

Figure 8.8 – Conversion of cholesterol to bile acids.

are conjugated to either glycine or taurine (an end-product of cysteine metabolism) to form *glycocholic* or *taurocholic acid* respectively. Since bile contains significant amounts of Na^+ and K^+ and is alkaline, these amino acid conjugates usually exist in the salt forms referred to as *bile salts*. Bile salts and free cholesterol enter the gall bladder and are secreted into the intestine where bacterial action helps to remove glycine and taurine from bile salts. A portion of the primary bile acids derived from the bile salts can also be converted by intestinal bacterial action to the *secondary bile acids, deoxycholic acid,* and *lithocholic acid* (Figure 8.8).

Biliary cholesterol represents one of the major excretory pathways for sterol elimination from the body and plays a central role in *cholesterol gallstone* formation. One of the major events in this is the secretion by hepatocytes of more cholesterol than can be effectively solubilised in phospholipid unilamellar vesicles and bile acid-phospholipid mixed micelles. A significant proportion of patients with cholesterol gallstones present with high rates of biliary cholesterol secretion associated with normal secretory concentrations of bile acids and phospholipids. The mechanisms that cause abnormal cholesterol secretion are not clear. It may be possible that some high cholesterol secretory states as those associated with obesity or gallstone disease could be mediated by the over expression of a specific carrier protein (similar to the sterol carrier protein, SPC-2, in rat) involved in transport of newly synthesised biliary cholesterol.

Enterohepatic circulation of bile salts

When bile empties into the intestine, nearly 60% of the bile salts, together with some primary and secondary bile acids, get reabsorbed into the ileum by a process of active transport and reach the liver parenchymal cells via portal blood. The primary and secondary bile acids are reconverted in the liver to bile salts which are again secreted into the bile. The continuous process of secretion of bile salts into the intestine, where some are converted into bile acids, and their subsequent return to the liver as a mixture of bile acids and salts is referred to as the *enterohepatic circulation*.

PLASMA CHOLESTEROL CONCENTRATION

Plasma cholesterol concentration is influenced by age, race, sex and other genetic factors. Its concentration is very low at birth (total cholesterol < 2.6 mmol/L) and increases rapidly in the first year of life, but remains < 4.1 mmol/L in childhood; early adult concentration starts to increase further (by about 0.2 mmol/L per decade). Plasma cholesterol is affected by diet. In general, an intake of saturated fats with a low polyunsaturated: saturated fatty acid (P:S) ratio raises the plasma cholesterol concentration whereas an intake of mono- and polyunsaturated fats cause a fall in plasma cholesterol.

METABOLISM OF PHOSPHOLIPIDS

DEGRADATION OF GLYCEROPHOSPHOLIPIDS

The degradation of glycerophospholipids is carried out by three types of *phospholipases*.

Phospholipase A_1 removes the fatty acid at the C1 position of the phospholipid (Figure 8.9).

Phospholipas A_2 hydrolyses the ester bond in position 2 of the phospholipid molecule to form a free fatty acid and a *lysophospholipid*.

Phospholipase C attacks the ester bond in position 3 of the phospholipid molecule liberating 1,2-diacylglycerol plus a phosphoryl base. Membrane bound phospholipase C plays an important role in producing second messengers.

DEGRADATION OF SPHINGOMYELIN

Sphingomyelin is degraded by the combined action of lysosomal *sphingomyelinase* and *ceramidase* to form sphingosine and a free fatty acid. An inherited deficiency of sphingomyelinase results in *Niemann-Pick disease*.

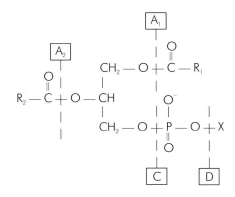

Figure 8.9 – Phospholipase action on a glycerophospholipid: A_1-Phospholipase A_1; A_2- Phospholipase A_2 ; C-Phospholipase C; D-Phospholipase D.

DISORDERS OF LIPID METABOLISM

Disorders of lipid metabolism may be broadly categorised into two groups:

- those resulting in an alteration in the blood lipid concentration – *hyperlipidaemias* and *hypolipidaemias*
- those causing an accumulation of an abnormal amount of lipid in a specific tissue or organ – *deposition disorders*

HYPERLIPIDAEMIAS

Primary hyperlipidaemias are due to a genetically determined defect affecting one or more stages in the course of lipoprotein formation, transport, or destruction. *Secondary hyperlipidaemias,* which are more common, may result from excessive dietary intake of lipid or carbohydrate, or as a manifestation of some other disease or drug effect (Table 8.2). In most cases it is impossible to distinguish primary from secondary hyperlipidaemias on the basis of the lipoprotein abnormality, and indeed some of the pathogenetic mechanisms may be common to both types of disorders. In addition, systemic disorders may alter the expression of the primary hyperlipidaemias, often greatly increasing their severity.

CLASSIFICATION OF PRIMARY HYPERLIPIDAEMIAS

Hyperlipidaemias have been classified in several ways. The WHO classification is essentially a phenotypic classification based on the type of lipoprotein involved. This classification does not differentiate primary from secondary causes of any particular phenotype and does not give any indication of the genetic basis of the manifested lipoprotein disorder, or a guide to its management. Furthermore, this classification is concerned only with the apo-B-containing lipoproteins and takes no account of HDL cholesterol. The following description of hyperlipidaemias is based on the genetic classification that is replacing that of the WHO.

Familial chylomicronaemia

This is a rare, autosomal-recessive disorder causing hypertriacylglycerolaemia and chylomicronaemia. The plasma is very turbid because of the accumulation of chylomicrons. The primary defect is deficiency of either lipoprotein lipase or its activator, apo CII, or the presence of an inhibitor. Presentation of this condition is usually in childhood, with eruptive xanthomata, abdominal pain due to pancreatitis, and sometimes splenomegaly. The major complication of the chylomicronaemic syndromes is recurrent pancreatitis.

Chylomicronaemia may also be seen when a genetic predisposition for hypertriacylglycerolaemia is exacerbated by other conditions such as obesity, diabetes mellitus or alcohol ingestion. Management involves a reduction in fat intake, with substitution of some fat by triacylglycerols based on medium-chain fatty acids (these do not produce chylomicrons because they are absorbed from the gut directly into the bloodstream).

Familial hypercholesteraemia (FH)

In individuals with FH, there is a specific genetic defect in the production or nature of high-affinity tissue apo-B100 receptors. This condition is inherited as an autosomal-dominant characteristic with a frequency in the population of 1:500. FH is characterised by high plasma cholesterol concentrations (increased LDL fraction) from early childhood. Many heterozygotes have tendon xanthomata and symptoms of coronary heart disease appear in about 50% of heterozygotes by the fourth or fifth decade; in homozygotes, symptoms of heart disease appear much earlier (in childhood or in the second decade).

THE MORE COMMON CAUSES OF SECONDARY HYPERLIPOPROTEINAEMIAS	
Cause	Examples
Endocrine	Diabetes mellitus, thyroid disease, pregnancy
Nutritional	Obesity, alcohol excess, anorexia nervosa
Renal disease	Nephrotic syndrome, chronic renal failure
Drugs	Some β-adrenoreceptor blockers, thiazide diuretics, oestrogen therapy or oral contraceptives, retinoic acid derivatives
Hepatic disease	Cholestasis, hepatocellular dysfunction

Table 8.2

Polygenic (common) hypercholesterolaemia

In about 95% of patients with primary hypercholesterolaemia, the abnormality is due to a combination of dietary and genetic factors. Plasma cholesterol is not as high as in FH.

Familial dysbetalipoproteinaemia

This is also known as *remnant hypercholesterolaemia* or *broad-β disease* (increased IDL and chylomicron remnant fractions) and is an uncommon disorder, characterised clinically by lipid deposition in the palmar creases, tuberous xanthomata (over bony prominences) and a high risk of premature ischaemic heart disease. Patients are also at risk of developing peripheral and cerebral vascular disease.

Patients with broad-β disease have only the E_2 form of apoprotein E which cannot react with the hepatic E receptor and therefore have impaired IDL uptake by the liver.

Familial hypertriacylglycerolaemia

This is due to hepatic triacylglycerol (TG) production with increased VLDL secretion from the liver. It is transmitted as an autosomal dominant trait, usually becoming apparent only after the fourth decade of life. It may be associated with obesity, glucose intolerance and hyperuricaemia. Management should include calorie restriction to achieve ideal weight and avoidance of diets rich in carbohydrates (particularly with sucrose or fructose) and alcohol. In severe cases, there is a risk of pancreatitis; it is not certain whether these patients have an increased risk of coronary heart disease.

Familial combined hyperlipidaemia

This is inherited as an autosomal-dominant characteristic with a frequency in the population of 1:300. The condition is due to excessive hepatic production of apo B, leading to increased VLDL secretion and increased production of LDL from VLDL. The lipid abnormalities only become apparent after the third decade. These patients may have eruptive xanthomata and have a high risk of developing coronary heart disease.

Familial hyperalphalipoproteinaemia

This is an abnormality that gives rise to increased plasma HDL concentrations. Coronary heart disease risk is decreased and no treatment is required.

RELATIONSHIP OF HYPERLIPIDAEMIA TO ATHEROSCLEROSIS

Atherosclerosis is a serious consequence of hyperlipidaemia, characterised by the deposition of plaques (*atheroma*) containing cholesterol and cholesteryl esters of lipoproteins containing apo-B100 in the connective tissue of arterial walls. Such atheromatous plaques may eventually lead to the development of *ischaemic heart disease* or *cerebral vascular disease* due to narrowing of blood vessels.

Although cholesterol is often singled out as being chiefly responsible for the development of atheroma, patients with arterial disease can have any one of the following abnormalities: elevated VLDL (TG) with normal LDL (cholesterol) concentration; elevated VLDL (TG) and LDL (cholesterol); and elevated LDL (cholesterol) with normal VLDL (TG). Diseases in which prolonged elevated concentrations of VLDL, IDL or LDL may occur in blood (e.g. diabetes mellitus, hypothyroidism, lipid nephrosis) are often accompanied by premature or more severe atherosclerosis. Evidence also suggests a strong predictive relationship between the LDL:HDL cholesterol ratio and coronary heart disease (CHD). An inverse relationship between CHD and blood HDL (HDL_2) concentration has been found. This relationship is explainable because of the roles of LDL in transporting cholesterol to the tissues and of HDL acting as a scavenger of cholesterol in reverse cholesterol transport.

Total triacylglycerol and cholesterol concentrations can easily be measured in the laboratory. HDL cholesterol can be determined after first using a simple precipitation technique to separate HDL from LDL. The following formula can then be used to calculate LDL concentration:

$$\text{LDL cholesterol} = \text{Total cholesterol} - (\text{HDL cholesterol} + \text{TG}/2.2),$$

where all quantities are expressed in mmol/L. This formula assumes that the total TG/2.2 approximates the value for VLDL cholesterol. This formula should not be used if the triacylglycerol concentration exceeds 4.5 mmol/L (>400 mg/dL) or in the presence of either chylomicrons or the TG-rich lipoproteins (VLDL remnants, IDL) seen in dysbetalipoproteinaemia.

MANAGEMENT OF HYPERLIPIDAEMIA

The management of secondary hyperlipidaemias requires treatment of the underlying cause. The most commonly used methods for management of primary hyperlipidaemia are *dietary control* and *treatment with lipid lowering drugs*. Individuals with concentrations of total cholesterol >6.5 μmol/L LDL cholesterol >5.0 mmol/L, HDL cholesterol <0.9 mmol/L or triacylglycerols >2.5 mmol/L are considered to be at high risk of developing coronary heart disease.

Dietary control

It is recommended that red meat and dairy product consumption is reduced while that of vegetables, fruits, pulses and fish is increased. The ω-3 fatty acids in oily fish such as mackerel are also beneficial because they give rise to certain prostanoids that help to prevent platelet aggregation. Dietary alterations to reduce fat intake should focus on decreasing saturated fat to < 10% of dietary energy intake and substituting it with a mixture of unrefined carbohydrates and monounsaturated and polyunsaturated fats. Fibre is also thought to be beneficial as a part of a cholesterol lowering diet.

Drug therapy

A number of lipid lowering drugs are currently available. Some e.g. cholestyramine, lorastatin help to reduce only plasma cholesterol while others e.g. fibrates and nicotinic acid help to reduce both plasma cholesterol and triacylglycerol.

In homozygous familial hypercholesteraemia, *plasma exchange* at intervals or a *liver transplant* may be the only effective treatment.

HYPOLIPIDAEMIAS

Hypolipidaemia is rare and often genetic. A *betalipoteinaemia* is a defect in apo-B synthesis. Triacylglycerol (TG) accumulates in the liver and intestine and malabsorption of fat soluble vitamins occurs, resulting in an autonomic neuropathy.

DEPOSITION DISORDERS

FATTY LIVER

Lipids (mainly as triacylglycerol) can accumulate in the liver for many reasons. Chronic accumulation of fat in the liver may result in fibrotic changes in liver cells progressing to *impaired liver function*. In some alcoholic patients, fatty liver may progress to *cirrhosis*.

Fatty liver develops in conditions where the rate of triacylglycerol (TG) synthesis is not balanced by the rate of TG efflux from the liver. This imbalance can occur:

- in conditions resulting in an elevation of the plasma fatty acid concentration (e.g. chronic alcoholism, uncontrolled diabetes mellitus, starvation, high fat diets); uptake of fatty acids by the liver increases resulting in increased triacylglycerol synthesis

- in conditions where the liver produces normal amounts of TG, but there is a metabolic block in either the synthesis of VLDL or its excretion from the liver (e.g. kwashiorkor, toxic liver injury)

THE LIPIDOSES

Certain rare inborn errors of metabolism are associated with abnormalities in the synthesis or disposal of intracellular lipid, while the levels of circulating lipids are within the normal range. These lipidoses (e.g. *Niemann-Pick disease, Tay-Sach's disease, Gaucher's disease, Fabry's disease*) are characterised by the accumulation of ceramide containing complex lipids (e.g. sphingomyelin, gangliosides) in various tissues due to specific enzyme defects in lysosomes. Most of these lipidoses are autosomal recessive disorders and most patients die in the first years of life.

SELECTED READING

Feher, M. and Richmond, W. – *Lipids and Lipid Disorders*. Gower Medical Publishing, London, 1991.

Hunningshake, D.B. (ed.) – Lipid Disorders. *The Medical Clinics of North America* 1994; **78**: 1–266.

Marshall, W.J. *Clinical Chemistry*, 3rd ed. Mosby, London, 1995.

Murray, R.K., Granner, D.K., Mayes, P.A. and Rodwell, V.W. (eds.) – *Harper's Biochemistry*, 24th ed. Prentice Hall International (UK) Ltd., London, 1996.

Puglielli, L., Rigotti, A., Amigo, L., Nunez, L., Greco, A.V., Santos, M.J. and Nervi, F. - Modulation of intrahepatic cholesterol trafficking: evidence by *in-vivo* antisense treatment for the involvement of sterol carrier protein-2 in newly synthesized cholesterol transport into rat bile. *Biochemical Journal* 1996; **317**: 681–687.

Strasberg, S.M. and Harvey, P.R.C. - Biliary cholesterol transport and precipitation. *Hepatology* 1990; **12**: 1S – 5S.

Stryer, L. – *Biochemistry*, 4th ed. W.H. Freeman and Co., N.Y., 1995.

9

PROTEINS AND PROTEINS AS FUNCTIONAL UNITS

Objectives
To understand:

- The biochemistry of amino acids

- Protein structure

- Enzyme action and the importance of enzymes and isoenzymes in clinical diagnosis

PROTEINS

Proteins are complex *polymers of amino acids* that are produced by all living cells. Each protein is composed of only 20 amino acids in varying numbers and sequences. The sequence of amino acids which ultimately determines the characteristics of a protein, is determined by genetic information contained in the cell nucleus. All proteins contain C,H,O, and N (about 16%) ; some contain S. The presence of N differentiates proteins from carbohydrates and lipids.

CLASSIFICATION OF PROTEINS

Proteins may be broadly classified as *simple proteins* that contain only amino acids and *complex proteins* that have non-protein components as integral parts of their molecules. Examples of complex proteins include the *metalloproteins* such as haemoglobin and cytochromes, the *glycoproteins* containing carbohydrates, and the *lipoproteins* responsible for lipid trans· ·t in the plasma.

BIOLOGICAL FUNCTIONS OF PROTEINS

Proteins perform different, very important functions in the body. Each of these functions is performed by a specific type of protein (Table 9.1).

Proteins have a definite life span, and eventually get degraded to their constituent amino acids, to be replaced by newly synthesised protein.

AMINO ACIDS

Amino acids are carboxylic acids which also contain an amino ($-NH_2$) group, and have the general formula shown in Figure 9.1.

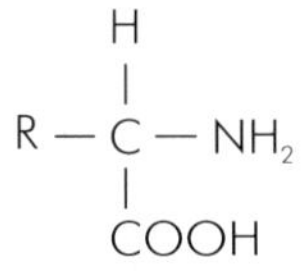

$$R - \overset{\overset{\displaystyle H}{|}}{\underset{\underset{\displaystyle COOH}{|}}{C}} - NH_2$$

Figure 9.1 – General formula of an amino acid.

R represents the side chain attached to the central carbon atom known as the α-carbon atom.

ISOMERIC FORMS OF AMINO ACIDS

With the exception of glycine, in which R=H, the α-carbon atom of amino acids is joined to four different groups, and is thus *asymmetric*. Amino acids other than glycine can therefore exist in two different isomeric

FUNCTIONS OF PROTEINS	
Function	Example
Regulation of cellular activities	Enzymes, Receptors, Repressors, Hormones (e.g.*insulin, growth hormone*) and Growth factor proteins
Transport and storage of small molecules and ions	Haemoglobin, Albumin, Globulins, Myoglobin and Lipoproteins
Co-ordination of motion	Actin, Myosin
Provision of mechanical support	Structural proteins (eg *collagen, keratin, muscle proteins*)
Defence against foreign substances	Antibodies, Complement, Cytokines

Table 9.1

forms, the *D* - and *L – forms*, according to their relationship to the structures of D- and L-glyceraldehyde.

Only *L-amino acids* are used in the synthesis of proteins. *D-amino acids* are less common in nature, and can be found in some fungal polypeptide antibiotics (e.g. polymyxin contains D-leucine), and as components of the muropeptide of the cell wall of gram positive bacteria. *Proline*, which is commonly considered to be an amino acid, is strictly speaking, an *imino acid*.

CLASSIFICATION OF AMINO ACIDS

Amino acids can be conveniently grouped into two different classes – *hydrophilic (polar)* and *hydrophobic (non-*

polar), depending on the nature of their side chains or R-groups (Figure 9.2 and 9.3).

The polar amino acids may be *neutral, acidic,* or *basic*, depending on the charges carried by the R-group.

Amino acids can also be classified as *aliphatic, aromatic*, or *heterocyclic* according to the type of ring structure found in the molecule.

AMINO ACIDS NOT FOUND IN PROTEINS

Some amino acids that are found in cells do not take part in protein synthesis. However, they, perform some essential functions in the cell (Table 9.2).

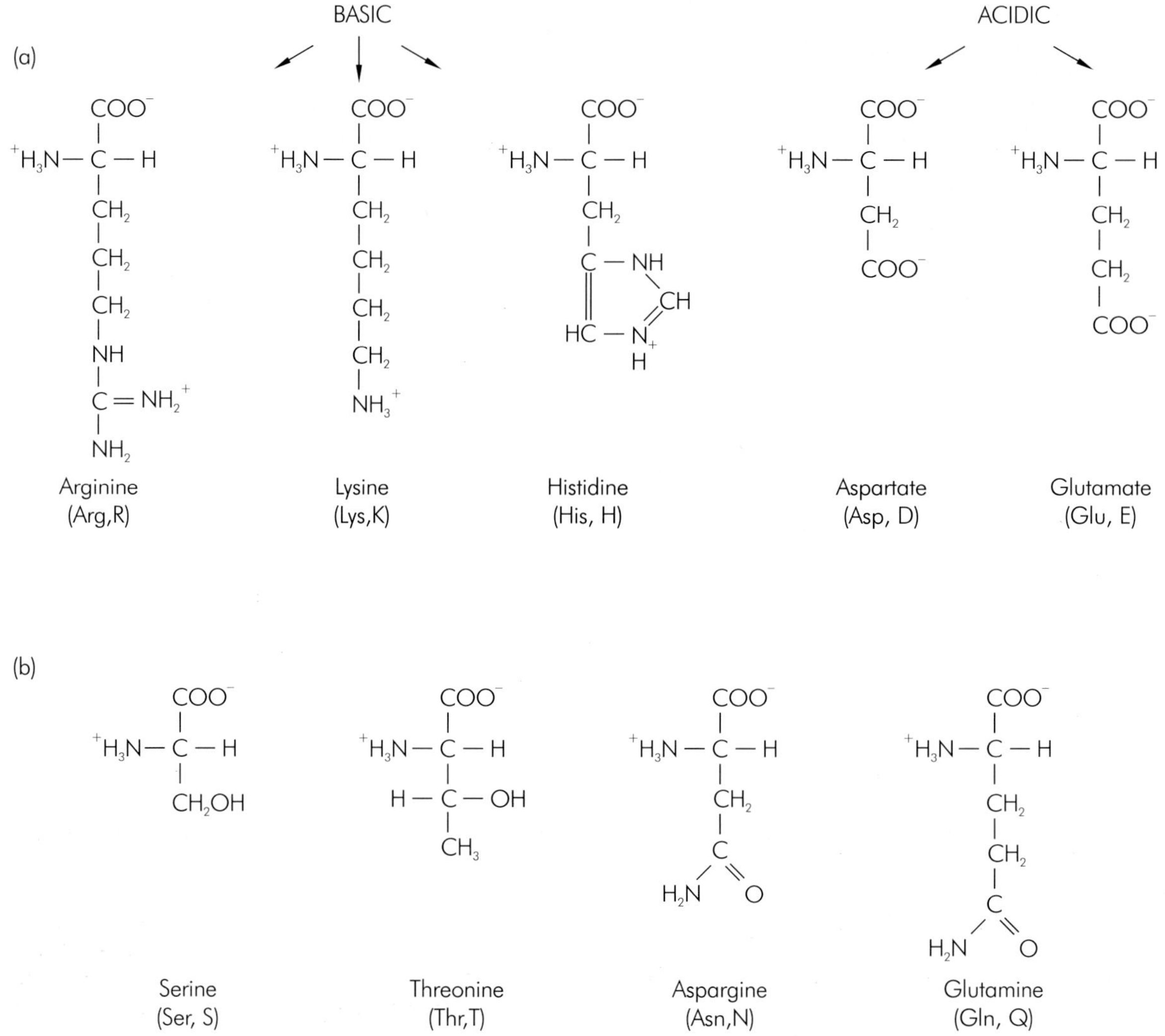

Figure 9.2 – Hydrophilic (Polar) amino acids that participate in protein synthesis, (a) polar charged R-groups, (b) polar, uncharged R-groups.

(a)

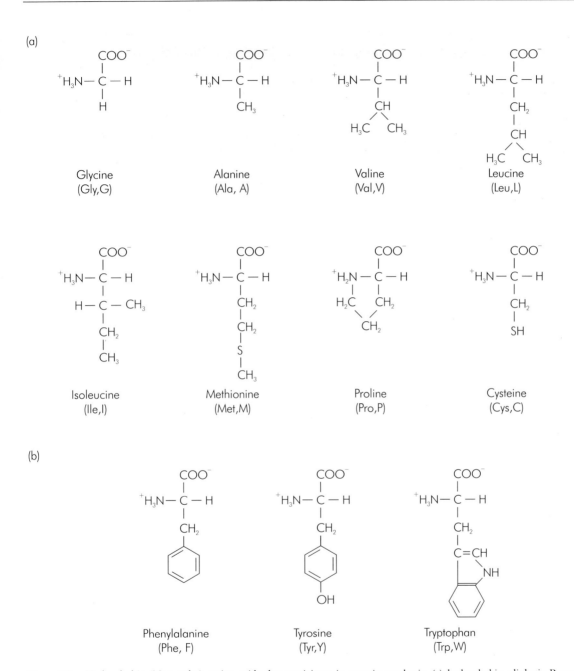

Figure 9.3 – Hydrophobic (Non-polar) amino acids that participate in protein synthesis. (a) hydrophobic, aliphatic R-groups, (b) hydrophobic aromatic R-groups.

IONIC STATES OF AMINO ACIDS

Amino acids are *amphoteric compounds*. They contain acidic (-COOH) and basic (-NH$_2$) groups in the same molecule. In solution, the -NH$_2$ group can accept a proton and exist as -NH$_3^+$, resulting in the amino acid containing two weakly acidic groups (-COOH and -

NH$_3^+$). Both the -NH$_3^+$ and -COOH groups of amino acids ionise in aqueous solutions (-COOH ionises before NH$_3^+$). The extent to which either group is ionized depends on the pH of the solution. At physiological pHs (pH between 6.9–7.4), most common amino acids exist as dipolar ions or *zwitterions*. The COO$^-$ group can act as a proton acceptor,

PHYSIOLOGICALLY IMPORTANT AMINO ACIDS NOT FOUND IN PROTEINS	
Amino acid	Importance
α-amino acid	
Homocysteine	Intermediate in biosynthesis of cysteine from methionine
Ornithine	Intermediate in urea biosynthesis
Citrulline	Intermediate in urea biosynthesis
Dihydroxyphenyl-alanine (DOPA)	Precursor of melanin
Mono (or di)-iodo tyrosine	Precursor of thyroid hormones
Non-α-amino acid	
β-Alanine	Part of coenzyme A and the vitamin pantotheine
Taurine	In bile, combined with bile acids
γ-Aminobutyric acid (GABA)	Inhibitory neurotransmitter in central nervous system
δ-Aminolaevulinic acid (δ-ALA)	Intermediate in haem biosynthesis

Table 9.2

while the NH_3^+ can act as a proton donor. *The zwitterion has a net zero charge.*

The pH at which the zwitterion form may predominate together with minute, but equal amounts of the cationic and anionic forms, is called the *isoelectric pH* or *pI*. At this pH, the predominant ionic form has a net zero charge. The pI is the pH at the midpoint between the pK values on either side of the zwitterion species.

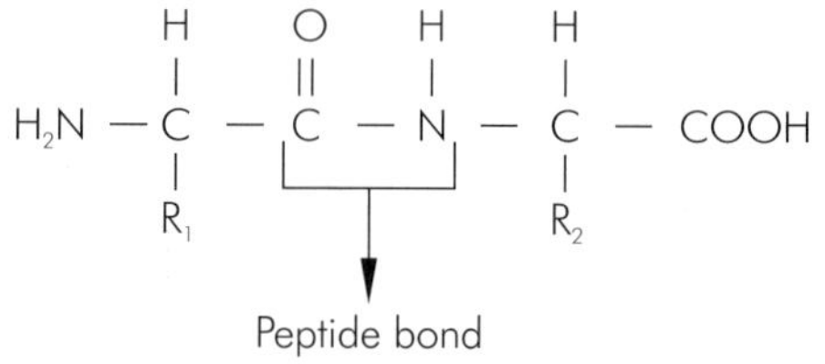

PEPTIDE BOND FORMATION

The covalent binding of an α-amino group of one amino acid with the carboxyl group of a second amino acid with the elimination of water, results in the formation of a *peptide bond* (Figure 9.4); polymers of amino acids formed in this way are known as *peptides*.

A *dipeptide* contains two amino acid residues; a *tripeptide* contains three. An amino acid chain with less than 25 amino acid residues is called an *oligopeptide* while a *polypeptide* has more than 25 amino acids. A *protein* may consist of a long polypeptide or several polypeptide

Figure 9.4 – Formation of a peptide bond.

subunits. Normally, the amino acid residues found in peptides are named in the order starting from the N-terminal end.

PHYSIOLOGICALLY IMPORTANT OLIGOPEPTIDES

A variety of low molecular weight polypeptides of physiological interest are formed by specific cleavage from larger peptides, or synthesised independently. Examples include the following :

Glutathione – is a tripeptide (*γ-glutamyl cysteinyl glycine*),

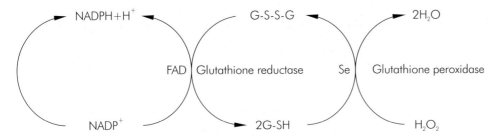

Figure 9.5 – The reversible oxidation of glutathione.

which is ubiquitous in mammalian cells. Within cells, the sulphydryl (-SH) group of the cysteine is about 95% reduced *(GSH)*. The sulphydryl groups of two molecules of glutathione can undergo simultaneous oxidation to form a disulphide 'bridge' (-S-S-) between the two molecules. The resulting compound is referred to as *oxidised glutathione (GSSG)*. This oxidation can be reversed by *glutathione reductase* (Figure 9.5).

Functions of glutathione include the following:

- *preventing peroxide and free radical mediated cell injury*

- *transporting amino acids across membranes in kidney*

- *functioning as an intracellular reducing agent.* Due to its ability to undergo reversible oxidation, glutathione helps to maintain the -SH groups of amino acids in various proteins in a reduced, active state

- *detoxication of foreign compounds* (e.g. drugs), by forming water-soluble glutathione conjugates

Oxytocin and Vasopressin (antidiuretic hormone, ADH)
These are hormones secreted by the posterior pituitary gland. *Oxytocin* stimulates contraction of the uterus. *Vasopressin* decreases water excretion by the kidney.

Angiotensin - the *renin-angiotensin system* plays a pivotal role in sodium metabolism, and regulation of arterial blood pressure.

THERAPEUTICALLY USEFUL PEPTIDES AND AMINO ACID DERIVATIVES

PEPTIDES

Peptide hormones and vaccines
Many hormones in the body (e.g. *insulin, growth hormone*), are polypeptides. These hormones are frequently given to patients to correct corresponding deficiency states (e.g. administration of insulin to patients suffering from *diabetes mellitus*). Improved molecular biological techniques have enabled the rapid chemical synthesis of these hormones as well as the synthesis of certain viral peptides and proteins for use as *vaccines.*

Antibiotics and Antitumour agents

Valinomycin and *Gramicidin* are two examples of peptide antibiotics. *Bleomycin* is an example of a peptide used as an antitumour agent.

AMINO ACID DERIVATIVES

N-Acetylcysteine
N-Acetylcysteine (NAC), is a synthetic derivative of cysteine, and a precursor of reduced glutathione. It is used to replenish hepatic levels of glutathione and prevent hepatotoxicity due to overdosage with paracetamol. It has also become a promising cancer chemotherapeutic agent. NAC is also used as a mucolytic agent (e.g. in *cystic fibrosis*) because it cleaves disulphide linkages of mucoproteins.

S-Adenosylmethionine

S-Adenosylmethionine (SAMe) is a naturally occurring amino acid derivative. Due to its prominent role in transmethylation reactions, and as a precursor of sulphur-containing compounds (e.g. glutathione), SAMe is currently being used as a novel therapeutic agent to restore normal hepatic function in the presence of various chronic liver diseases, and to reverse hepatotoxicity due to drugs or chemicals such as alcohol, paracetamol, steroids, and lead.

PROTEIN STRUCTURE

In proteins that consist of a single polypeptide chain,

there are three levels of organisation – **primary, secondary**, and **tertiary**. For proteins that contain two or more polypeptide chains, each chain is a subunit, and there is a **quaternary** level of structure.

PRIMARY STRUCTURE

The primary structure describes the type and sequence of covalently linked amino acids in a polypeptide chain. The primary structure is unique to each polypeptide, and determines which higher structure it assumes. Further, the biological, chemical, and physical properties of a polypeptide depends on its primary structure. For example, *sickle cell haemoglobin* (HbS) differs from normal haemoglobin (HbA) only by one amino acid, but the replacement of a negatively charged glutamic acid residue in the sixth position of the β-globin chain by an uncharged valine changes the properties of the haemoglobin drastically.

SECONDARY STRUCTURE

The secondary structure describes the manner in which certain lengths of polypeptides interact through the formation of *intermolecular* or *intramolecular* hydrogen bonds between -C=O and -NH groups of the peptide bonds in the polypeptide backbone. This type of folding enables the protein to attain a stable *conformation* (a 3-dimensional arrangement of groups of atoms that can be altered without breaking any covalent bonds). Common types of secondary structure include the right handed α-*helix*, parallel and antiparallel β-*pleated sheets,* the *triple helix* peculiar to collagen, and β-*turns*.

α-Helix

An α-helix is formed by *intrachain hydrogen bonding* (Figure 9.6) usually between the -C=O and -NH within the same polypeptide chain. These bonds are parallel to the axis of the helix.

Most α-helixes contain between 4 and 50 amino acid residues, most commonly about 12, with 3–6 residues per turn. Certain amino acids tend to disrupt the α-helix. For example, proline and hydroxyproline cause termination of the α-helix, while glycine and amino acids with charged, or bulky R-groups (e.g. arginine, aspartate, isoleucine, glutamate) electrostatically or physically interfere with helix formation.

β-pleated sheet

The β-pleated sheet structure is formed by *interchain*

hydrogen bonding between -C=O and -NH groups of adjacent polypeptide chains. A preponderance of certain amino acids (e.g. glycine and alanine) in the polypeptide chains promotes the formation of β-pleated sheets. In this structure the peptide chain is almost fully extended, and hydrogen bonding is perpendicular to the axis of the chain. Depending on whether hydrogen bonding occurs between chains aligned in the same direction with respect to the N-terminal and C-terminal regions, or in opposite directions, a *parallel sheet structure* or an *antiparallel sheet structure* will be formed.

Clinical importance of β-pleated sheets

The β-pleated structure occurs as a principal secondary structure in proteins found in a certain types of disease known as *amyloidosis*. Since the aggregates of twisted β-pleated sheet fibrils found in amyloidosis are insoluble and resist proteolysis, they accumulate and crowd out normal tissue. The amyloid deposit, which occurs in several different tissues, is produced in certain *chronic inflammatory diseases, in some cancers,* and in the brain *in some neurodegenerative diseases* (e.g. *Alzheimer's disease*). The amyloid fibrils found in amyloid deposits in the brain in Alzheimer's disease have been shown to be composed of antiparallel β-sheets.

The triple helix

The triple helix is formed by three polypeptide chains coiling around one another. Carbon-carbon double bonds and hydrogen bonds hold these chains together. This type of secondary structure is peculiar to *collagen.*

Collagen - is the most abundant structural protein in the body, especially in the organic matrix of bones and tendons. It usually occurs as a glycoprotein. More than 15 different types of collagen have been found in mammalian tissues. In collagen, each chain of the triple helix is coiled in a left handed manner due to the presence of a large amount of glycine. The three chains coil around one another in a right handed manner to form a *tropocollagen* molecule. The mature collagen consists of many tropocollagen molecules joined end to end, and parallel to one another. The staggered positions of the ends of the tropocollagen molecules create the striations in collagen seen under the electron microscope.

The 3 polypeptide chains in the triple helix may be identical ($3\alpha_1$), or may consist of two identical chains and one dissimilar chain ($2\alpha_1 + \alpha_2$). In addition to the presence of large amounts of glycine, each chain of the triple helix characteristically contains much proline, hydroxyproline, and fair amounts of lysine and

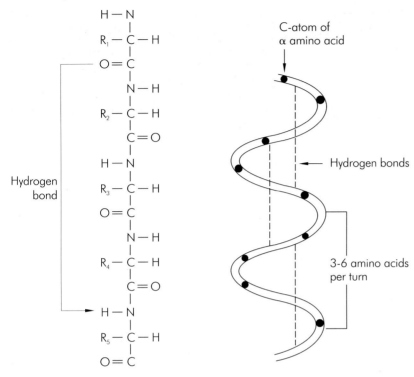

Figure 9.6 – Diagrammatic representation of an α-helix.

hydroxylysine (formed by the hydroxylation of some lysine residues by the enzyme *lysyl hydroxylase*). The three chains are joined by interchain hydrogen bonds and cross-links between lysyl and hydroxylysyl residues. Cross-linking is carried out by the enzyme *lysyl oxidase*. Carbohydrate residues are usually attached to the hydroxylysine residues in the chains.

COLLAGEN AND CONNECTIVE TISSUE DISORDERS

Inherited defects of collagen synthesis result in the development of various disease conditions the clinical features of which depend on the type of collagen affected. Examples include osteogenesis imperfecta, characterised by bone fragility, epidermolysis bullosa in which skin breakage and blistering occurs after minimal trauma and Alport's syndrome in which renal damage occurs.

β-Turns

β-Turns are formed by a reversal in the direction of a polypeptide chain. This configuration involves the formation of a loop in which a -C=O group forms a hydrogen bond with the -NH group of the amino acid residue 3 positions further along the polypeptide chain. β-Turns cause polypeptide chains to be compact molecules (e.g. *globular proteins* with spherical or ellipsoidal shapes).

Regions of protein that are not identifiably organised as helical or pleated sheets are described as being in *random coil* formation. A protein may possess predominantly one kind of secondary structure (e.g. α-keratin of hair, and silk fibroin contain mostly α-helix and β-pleated structure respectively), or may have more than one kind (e.g. globular proteins such as haemoglobin).

TERTIARY STRUCTURE

The tertiary structure of a protein describes how the chains with secondary structure further interact through the R-groups of amino acid residues to give a 3-dimensional shape. In general, proteins may have either of two tertiary forms – *globular* or *fibrous*. Bonds that help to maintain the stability of the tertiary structure include:

- *hydrophobic bonds* formed between amino acids with hydrophobic R-groups (e.g. alanine, leucine, isoleucine, phenylalanine and tryptophan)

- *hydrogen bonding* between amino acid side chains

- *ionic* (or *electrostatic*) *bonds* between amino acids containing oppositely charged side chains

- *covalent bonds*; the most common type is the disulphide bond of cystine between cysteine residues

In general, *fibrous proteins* (e.g. collagen, α-keratin) are elongated and water insoluble, while *globular proteins* are spherical and water soluble, and they consist mainly of random coils with occasional stretches of α-helices.

QUATERNARY STRUCTURE

The arrangement of polypeptide chains in relation to one another in a multiple-chained protein is called the *quaternary structure*. Insulin, haemoglobin, collagen, and many enzymes are examples of proteins where several subunits interact non-covalently to form the active protein molecule. The interacting subunits may be of the same type (e.g. *heart lactate dehydrogenase*), or of different types (e.g. *haemoglobin, insulin*).

PROTEIN DENATURATION

Denaturation can conveniently be defined as the loss of biological activity due to alterations in the proper 3-dimensional structure of a protein. During this process, the polypeptide chain unfolds due to alterations in the secondary, tertiary, and quaternary structures.

Denaturing agents include:

- *heat* that causes disruption of weak forces such as hydrogen bonds that maintain protein structure

- *extremes of pH* that cause disruption of hydrogen bonds and alters the charge on proteins

- *organic solvents* which alter the aqueous environment and prevent formation of hydrophobic bonds, or interactions with water molecules

- *strong detergents* which perturb hydrophobic interactions

PROTEINS AS FUNCTIONAL UNITS

Proteins perform three major functions in the body: **structural, binding** and **catalytic**.

STRUCTURAL PROTEINS

Structural proteins may be located extracellularly (*e.g. keratin*, found in skin and hair, and *collagen* in connective tissue), or intracellularly (e.g. the muscle proteins *actin* and *myosin*). Many structural proteins are synthesised as soluble precursors that are subsequently converted to the mature (insoluble) structural proteins by post-translational modifications. Structural proteins usually have regions of regular secondary structure (e.g. β-pleated structure of β-keratin or triple helix of collagen), and are stabilised by disulphide bond formation.

BINDING PROTEINS

Binding proteins include soluble and membrane bound globular proteins, folded in such a manner that areas on their exposed surfaces can act as highly specific sites for ligand binding. Ligand binding occurs at specific binding sites and is maintained by weak interactions such as hydrogen or hydrophobic bonds. Some proteins (e.g. haemoglobin) will bind only one type of ligand, while others can bind two or more different ligands at different sites. Binding of ligands may result in a local conformational change that is transmitted to a second binding site (e.g. the catalytic binding site of an enzyme or oxygen binding site of haemoglobin) and alters the activity of the second site. The ligand is then said to act in an *allosteric* manner.

CATALYTIC PROTEINS – ENZYMES

Enzymes are highly specialised protein catalysts that speed up biological reactions without themselves undergoing any chemical change. *Substrates* are molecules acted on by enzymes; *products* are formed as a result of an enzyme-substrate interaction:

$$\text{S} \quad + \quad \text{E} \quad \rightarrow \quad \text{P} \quad + \quad \text{E}$$
$$\text{substrate} \quad \text{enzyme} \quad \text{product} \quad \text{enzyme}$$

HOW ENZYMES ACT AS CATALYSTS

The conversion of any substrate to its product/s depends on the number of substrate molecules that are in an energised or activated state; only molecules in the activated state can react. *Free energy of activation* refers to the energy required to bring all the molecules in one mole of a substrate to the activated state at any given temperature. The rate of a reaction can be increased by either increasing the number of activated molecules (e.g. by increasing the temperature) or by lowering the energy of activation. *An enzyme increases the rate of a reaction by lowering the energy of activation.* Enzymes are thought to lower the energy of activation by forming a stable enzyme-substrate (ES) complex intermediate:

$$E \quad + \quad S \quad \rightarrow \quad ES \quad \rightarrow \quad P \quad + \quad E$$

| enzyme | substrate | enzyme-
substrate
complex | product | enzyme |

By lowering the energy of activation, an enzyme increases the rate of the reaction by a factor of $10^8 - 10^{20}$.

ROLE OF THE ACTIVE SITE IN FORMATION OF THE ENZYME-SUBSTRATE COMPLEX

The binding of the substrate to the enzyme is not random, but occurs at a specific *active* (or *catalytic*) *site*. Here, various chemical groupings important in substrate binding are brought together in a spatial arrangement conferring specificity.

CLASSES OF ENZYMES

Enzymes may be classified according to composition of the active enzyme or the type of reactions they catalyse:

According to the composition, enzymes can be classified as:

- *Simple* – protein structure alone is sufficient for catalytic activity (e.g. *trypsin, chymotrypsin, elastase*)
- *Complex* – enzyme requires additional non-protein cofactors for full catalytic activity. A complete catalytically active enzyme together with its cofactor is known as a *holoenzyme*. Cofactors may be organic in nature (*coenzymes*) or metal ions (Table 9.3), and are involved in group transfer reactions. Cofactors are not destroyed by heat, whereas the apoenzyme (being a protein) is denatured by heat. Most cofactors are linked to enzymes by non-covalent bonds. A cofactor that is bound by covalent bonds to the enzyme (e.g. pyridoxal phosphate), is referred to as a *prosthetic group*

COFACTORS AND THEIR FUNCTIONS		
Type of cofactor	Function	
Organic cofactors *(Coenzymes)*	*Transfer of hydrogen*	*Transfer of groups* *other than hydrogen*
	NAD$^+$, NADP$^+$, FMN, FAD, Lipoic acid, Coenzyme Q, Biopterin	Coenzyme A – acyl groups Thiamine pyrophosphate -aldehyde groups Biotin -CO_2 Cobamide (B_{12}) – alkyl groups Pyridoxal phosphate – amino groups Folate coenzyme – methyl, methylene or formyl groups
Metal ions	*Assist enzyme activity by* *forming part of the* *catalytic group* Fe^{2+}/Fe^{3+} in cytochrome oxidase, catalase, peroxidase	*Assist substrate binding without* *being an integral part of the enzyme* Mg^{2+} in enzymes involved with phosphate group transfer(e.g. hexo- kinase, glucose 6-phosphatase)
	Cu^{2+}in superoxide dismutase Zn^{2+}in superoxide dismutase, DNA poly- merase, carbonic anhydrase, alcohol dehydrogenase	Mn^{2+} in arginase K$^+$ and Mg^{2+} in pyruvate kinase

Table 9.3

According to the type of reaction catalysed, enzymes are grouped into six major classes. Within each of these classes, there are several sub-groups of enzymes. Table 9.4.

ENZYME SPECIFICITY

Enzymes interact with one or a few specific substrates, and catalyse only one type of chemical reaction. Some enzymes show absolute specificity. For example, *pyruvate kinase* catalyses the transfer of a phosphate group only from phosphoenol pyruvate to ADP during glycolysis. *L-Amino acid oxidase* that acts on only L-amino acids and not D-amino acids shows *stereospecificity.* Many enzymes show *group specificity.* For example, *hexokinase* transfers phosphate groups from ATP to several sugars (e.g. D-glucose, D-fructose, D-mannose).

ENZYME ACTIVITY

The activity of an enzyme is usually expressed in *units.* One international unit (IU) is the quantity of enzyme that will catalyse the reaction of one μmol of substrate per minute.

A *katal (kat)* is the catalytic amount of an enzyme that catalyses a reaction rate of one mole/second (mol/s) and is the SI unit of enzyme activity.

FACTORS AFFECTING THE RATE OF AN ENZYME CATALYSED REACTION

Substrate concentration

When all other factors (e.g. enzyme concentration, pH, temperature and electrolyte composition in solution) are kept constant, the rate of an enzyme catalysed increases until a maximum velocity (V_{max}) is reached (*a hyperbolic curve* – Figure 9.7).

The *Michaelis constant* (K_m) is defined as the substrate concentration at which the enzyme reaction proceeds at half its maximum velocity under specified reaction conditions. A low K_m indicates that the enzyme has a high affinity for the substrate, and vice versa. The K_m

CLASSIFICATION OF ENZYMES ACCORDING TO THE TYPES OF REACTIONS THEY CATALYZE	
Major Classes	**Reaction type catalyzed**
Oxidoreductases	Oxidation-reduction reactions (transfer of hydrogen between substrates) – e.g. *lactate dehydrogenase.*
Transferases	Transfer of functional groups containing C, N or P – e.g. *aminotransferases.*
Hydrolases	Cleavage of bonds by addition of water – e.g. *acetyl-cholinesterase.*
Lyases	Cleavage of C-C, C-O, or C-N bonds other than by hydrolysis or by oxidation-reductions – e.g. *pyruvate decarboxylase.*
Isomerases	Conversion between *cis-* and *trans-* isomers, D- and L-isomers, or aldoses and ketoses – e.g. *phospho-glucose isomerase* and *triosephosphate isomerase.*
Ligases	ATP-dependent condensation reactions – e.g. *pyruvate carboxylase.*
Selected sub-classes	
Epimerases	Conversion between molecules that differ in configuration around on specific carbon bond – e.g. *UDP-hexose 4-epimeraxse.*
Hydratases	Addition of water between carbon-carbon double bonds without bond breakage, or remove water to create a double bond – e.g. *serine dehydratase.*
Kinases	Transfer of a phosphate group from a high energy phosphate compound (e.g. ATP) to a substrate – e.g. *hexokinase.*
Mutases	Shifts the position of a group intramolecularly – e.g. *phosphoglycerate mutase.*

Table 9.4

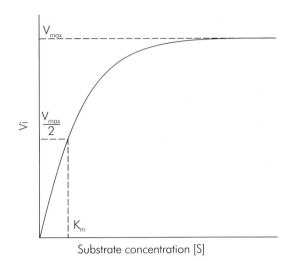

Figure 9.7 – Effect of substrate concentration on rate of an enzyme-catalyzed reaction.

and V_{max} of a reaction can be established by plotting the reciprocals of the initial velocity (V_i) versus the reciprocal of the substrate concentration ([S]) (see Figure 9.8 – the *Lineweaver-Burk plot*).

pH

Each enzyme has an optimal operating pH. This is usually close to the pH of the tissue that contains the enzyme (e.g. pepsin in the stomach has an optimal pH of about 2). Changes in pH alter the charge distribution along the entire length of the enzyme molecule and change its conformation, thereby affecting its catalytic activity.

Temperature

Increasing the temperature speeds up the reaction rate (provided the higher temperature does not denature the enzyme) because there is an increase in the kinetic energy of the molecules in solution, and hence more frequent collisions between enzyme and substrate molecules.

Inhibitors

There are two main types of enzyme inhibitors: irreversible and reversible.

Irreversible inhibitors bind covalently to enzymes and dissociate very slowly. They bear no structural resemblance to the substrate and generally inactivate the enzyme permanently. This type of inhibition is non-specific and many enzymes can be inhibited by the same inhibitor. The inhibition of cyclooxygenase by *aspirin* is an example of an irreversible enzyme inhibition.

Reversible inibitors bind non-covalently to enzymes through hydrogen bonds or ionic bonds. These inhibitors may be *competitive* or *non-competitive*.

Competitive inhibitors are usually chemical analogues of the true substrate which bind to the active site and, compete with the substrate for enzyme binding. Inhibition can be overcome by increasing the substrate concentration. As shown in Figure 9.8(b), in competitive inhibition, V_{max} remains unchanged while apparent K_m is increased in the presence of the inhibitor.

Non-competitive inhibitors do not resemble the substrate and bind to enzymes in areas other than the active site. Increasing [S] will not overcome the inhibition; the degree of inhibition depends on the concentration of the inhibitor. Therefore, in contrast to competitive inhibition, V_{max} decreases while the K_m usually remains unchanged (Figure 9.8(c)). The non-competitive inhibitor binds to either the free enzyme or the ES complex, and slows down the reaction. *Heavy metals* such as Hg^{2+} and Pb^{2+} bind to the -SH groups of enzymes and inhibit non-competitively.

APPLICATIONS OF COMPETITIVE INHIBITION IN MEDICINE

Some examples of the clinical applications of competitive inhibition are:

Inhibition of acetylcholinesterase by neostigmine

Neostigmine is a structural analogue of acetylcholine and is administered when prolongation of the action of acetylcholine is desired, for example, in the treatment of *myasthenia gravis* (a chronic disease characterised by progressive muscular weakness due to failure of neuromuscular transmission).

The use of sulpha drugs as antibacterial agents

Sulphanilamides competitively inhibit the enzyme that converts p-aminobenzoic acid (PABA) to folic acid, interfering with bacterial cell division, therefore functioning as antibacterial agents.

The use of ethanol for the prevention of methanol toxicity

Methanol is converted, by the actions of alcohol

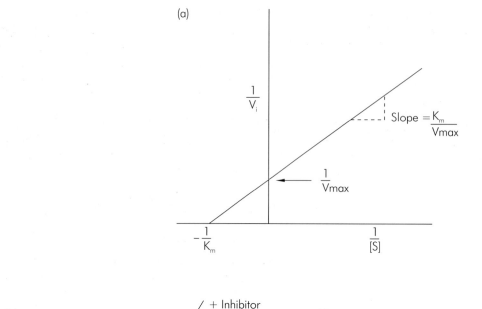

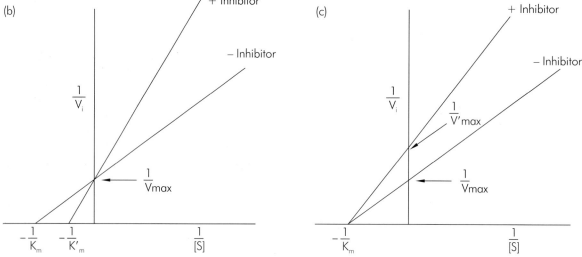

Figure 9.8 – Lineweaver–Burk plots of enzyme reactions.
(a) – Double reciprocal plot ($1/V_0$ vs $1/$[S] in a reaction to evaluate K_m and V_{max}.
(b) and (c) – Double reciprocal plots of classic competitive inhibition, and reversible non-competitive inhibition respectively.

dehydrogenase in the liver and kidney, to formaldehyde (that can cause retinal cell damage), and formic acid. Toxic effects of methanol can be reduced by the administration of the structural analogue ethanol that can competitively inhibit the activity of alcohol dehydrogenase.

ALLOSTERIC ENZYMES

An *allosteric enzyme's* activity can be altered in a positive or negative manner by the binding of a modulator molecule (usually non-covalently) to a regulatory site *(allosteric site)*. Binding of the allosteric effector causes a conformational change in the quaternary structure of the enzyme molecule making it more, or less active. An *allosteric activator* enhances substrate binding (e.g. activation of isocitrate dehydrogenase by ADP). An *allosteric inhibitor* decreases or inhibits enzyme activity (e.g. inhibition of phosphofructokinase by ATP).

Allosteric enzymes are often found strategically placed at the first step in a long metabolic pathway so that the whole pathway can be activated or slowed down by alterations in the activity of the first enzyme. The inhibition of the pathway by a final product is known as *feedback inhibition*.

When the initial velocity of a reaction catalysed by an allosteric enzyme is plotted against [S], a sigmoidal curve is obtained, indicating that binding of one substrate molecule, facilitates the binding of additional substrate molecules (*cooperative effect*) to other active sites. This resembles what is observed during the binding of oxygen molecules to the subunits of haemoglobin.

ISOENZYMES

Enzymes can exist in more than one molecular form in the same tissue or even in the same cell. Different molecular forms that catalyse the same reaction, are known as *isoenzymes*. *Creatine kinase, alkaline phosphatase* and *lactate dehydrogenase* are examples of enzymes that exist as isoenzymes. The pattern of isoenzymes detectable in plasma reflects their origin and can be useful in the diagnosis of disease (Table 9.5).

NUCLEIC ACIDS AND NUCLEOTIDES

The nucleic acids (DNA and RNA) are formed by the polymerisation of a large number of *nucleotide units*.

NUCLEOTIDES

A *nucleotide* is a compound that contains a nitrogenous heterocyclic base (a purine or a pyrimidine) connected to a phosphorylated pentose sugar unit (deoxyribose or ribose). A nucleotide minus the phosphate group (base connected to a sugar unit) is referred to as a *nucleoside*.

The bases in nucleosides and nucleotides

The principal *purine bases* found in the body (Figure 9.9) are *adenine* (A), and *guanine* (G). Other purine bases include *xanthine* and *hypoxanthine*.

Pyrimidine bases in the body are *cytosine* (C), *uracil* (U), and *thymine* (T).

Nucleoside and nucleotide nomenclature

Both nucleosides and nucleotides are named after the bases from which they are derived). The *nucleosides of ribose* with adenine, guanine, cytosine, thymine and uracil are called *adenosine, guanosine, cytidine, thymidine,* and *uridine* respectively.

The corresponding *nucleotides* are called *adenylic acid* or *adenosine monophosphate* (AMP), *guanylic acid* or *guanosine monophosphate* (GMP), *cytidylic acid* (CMP), *uridylic acid* (UMP) and *thymidylic acid* (TMP). If deoxyribose is present rather than ribose, the prefix *deoxy* is used, as in *deoxyuridine* (dU) or *deoxyuridylic acid* (dUMP).

Linkage of the base and sugar units

In both nucleosides and nucleotides, the purine or

SERUM ENZYMES USEFUL IN CLINICAL DIAGNOSIS	
Enzyme	Major diagnostic use
Alkaline phosphatase	Bone disorders; Liver disease.
Alanine aminotransferase (ALT)	Liver disease
Aspartate aminotransferase (AST)	Myocardial infarction; Liver disease.
Amylase	Acute pancreatitis
Creatine kinase	Myocardial infarction (MB isoenzyme); Muscle disorders (MM isoenzyme)
γ-Glutamyl transpeptidase	Liver disease (mainly cholestatic liver disease)
Lactate dehydrogenase (especially LD_1 and LD_2 isoenzymes)	Myocardial infarction
Pancreatic lipase	Acute pancreatitis

Table 9.5

Base Formula	Base (X = H)	Nucleoside (X = ribose or deoxyribose)	Nucleotide (X = ribose phosphate)
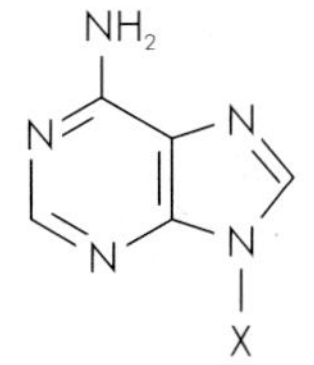	Adenine (A)	Adenosine	Adenosine monophosphate (AMP)
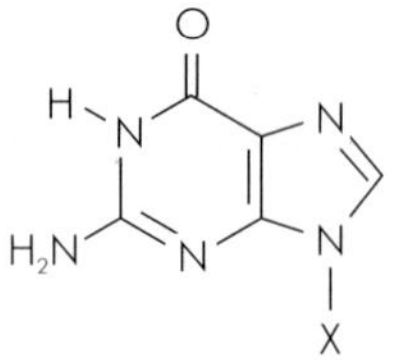	Guanine (G)	Guanosine	Guanosine monophosphate (GMP)
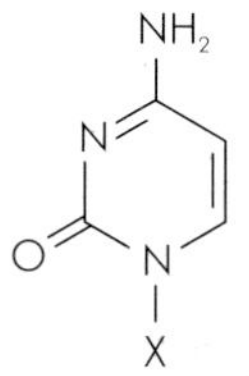	Cytosine (C)	Cytidine	Cytidine monophosphate (CMP)
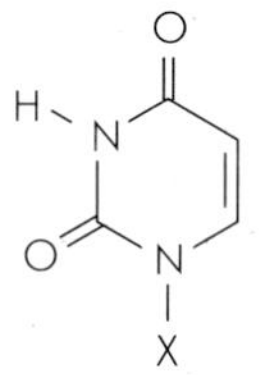	Uracil (U)	Uridine	Uridine monophosphate (UMP)
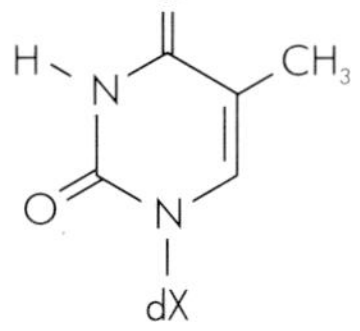	Thymine (T)	Thymidine	Thymidine monophosphate (TMP)

Figure 9.9 – The nomenclature of nucleosides and nucleotides.

pyrimidine base is linked to the pentose sugar by a glycosidic linkage. The C-1 of the pentose is linked to the N-1 of the pyrimidine ring, or N-9 of the purine ring. The atoms in the sugar unit are numbered with a prime to distinguish them from atoms in the bases. It is important to indicate the position at which esterification of the sugar has occurred (e.g. *adenosine 3′-monophosphate*, or *adenosine 5′-monophosphate*). Unless otherwise stated, reference to, for example, an adenine nucleotide in the text implies that it is a 5′-ester.

Polynucleotides

Several nucleotides can link with one another to form *polynucleotide chains* (e.g. DNA and RNA). The nucleotides in a polynucleotide chain are linked to one another by *phosphodiester bonds* formed between the 5′-

phosphate of one nucleotide and the 3'-OH group of the adjacent nucleotide.

IMPORTANT BIOLOGICAL FUNCTIONS OF NUCLEOTIDES

Nucleotides have a number of important functions:

- *precursor units for the synthesis of the nucleic acids DNA and RNA*

- *linkage of energy yielding reactions to those which require energy* – adenosine 5'-diphosphate (ADP) and adenosine 5'-triphosphate (ATP) play a central role in this function. The 5'-diphosphates and 5'-triphosphates of guanosine, inosine, uridine and cytidine can also function in this manner

- *activated intermediates in many biosynthetic processes* – for example, UDP-glucose and CDP-diacylglycerol are precursors of glycogen and glycerophospholipids respectively. S-Adenosyl methionine serves as a form of 'active' methionine and acts as a methyl donor in many diverse reactions, and as a source of propylamines for the synthesis of polyamines

- *synthesis of important coenzymes* – adenine nucleotides are important in the synthesis of NAD$^+$ (nicotinamide adenine dinucleotide), FAD (flavin adenine dinucleotide), and coenzyme A, which takes part in many cellular metabolic reactions

- *metabolic regulation* – cyclic AMP (cAMP), adenosine 3',5'-monophosphate and cyclic GMP (cGMP) act as important second messengers that mediate the actions of many hormones. Some nucleotides can also regulate certain metabolic pathways by allosteric or covalent modulation of key enzymes (e.g. regulation of glycolysis by the actions of ATP and AMP on key enzymes

MEDICAL APPLICATIONS OF NUCLEOBASES, NUCLEOSIDES AND NUCLEOTIDES

Synthetic analogues of naturally occurring nucleobases, nucleosides or nucleotides that can act as enzyme inhibitors or replace naturally occurring nucleotides in nucleic acids are increasingly being used in the chemotherapy of cancer and certain other clinical conditions.

CANCER CHEMOTHERAPY

Examples of synthetic analogues used in cancer chemotherapy include *5'-fluorouracil, 6-mercaptopurine,* and *cytosine arabinoside.*

ANTIFUNGAL AGENTS

Flucytosine (5-fluorocytosine) acts as an antifungal agent through conversion to 5-fluorouracil in the fungal cells.

ANTIVIRAL AGENTS

Idoxuridine (iododeoxyuridine) is effectively used in the treatment of corneal infections by herpes virus. It acts as a competitive inhibitor (via phosphorylated derivatives) of the incorporation of thymidylic acid into DNA.

Azathymidine, or *3'-azido-3'-deoxythymidine* (AZT) which converts to the corresponding 5'-triphosphate inhibits viral reverse transcriptase and is used in the treatment of AIDS.

TREATMENT OF HYPERURICAEMIA AND GOUT

Allopurinol (4-hydroxypyrazolopyrimidine), a structural analogue of hypoxanthine is widely used as an inhibitor of *de novo* purine biosynthesis, and of *xanthine oxidase.*

Selected reading

Gething, M.J. and Sambrook, J. – Protein folding in the cell. *Nature* 1992; **355**: 33–45.

Lehninger, A.L. – *Biochemistry: The molecular basis of cell structure and function,* 3rd ed. Worth Publishers Inc., N.Y., 1993.

Murray, R.K., Granner, D.K., Mayes, P.A. and Rodwell, V.W. (eds) – *Harper's Biochemistry,* 24th ed. Appleton and Lange, California, 1996.

Stryer, L. - *Biochemistry,* 4th ed., W.H. Freeman and Co., N.Y., 1995.

10

METABOLISM OF PROTEINS AND AMINO ACIDS

Nitrogen metabolism regulates body nitrogen and ensures its use in the synthesis of important nitrogenous compounds. Most nitrogen in the body is in proteins. Other important nitrogenous compounds include nucleic acids, nucleotides, hormones, neurotransmitters and the porphyrin components of proteins such as cytochromes and haemoglobin. This chapter will consider in detail only the metabolism of proteins and nucleotides as the metabolism of nitrogen-containing hormones, neurotransmitters and porphyrin containing compounds are discussed in other chapters in the text.

PROTEIN METABOLISM

FATE OF DIETARY PROTEIN

Dietary proteins are hydrolysed to amino acids by enzymes in the gastrointestinal tract, and are absorbed by various active transport processes. Amino acids are transferred to the liver where some are used for the biosynthesis of plasma proteins (e.g. albumin, prothrombin) and others are passed to extrahepatic tissues for use in protein synthesis. Excess amino acids are degraded in the liver and the nitrogen used for the synthesis of urea and several physiologically active nitrogenous compounds (Figure 10.1). The carbon skeletons are used for the synthesis of various intermediates encountered in the metabolism of carbohydrates and lipids.

DYNAMIC STATE OF BODY PROTEINS

Most proteins in the body undergo continual synthesis, along with degradation (*protein turnover*). The rate of protein turnover varies widely for individual proteins. For example, digestive enzymes and plasma proteins have half-lives measured in hours or days while structural proteins such as collagen have half-lives measured in months or years. It is thought that the rate of protein degradation is influenced by some structural aspect of the protein. For example, proteins rich in sequences containing proline, glutamate, serine and threonine (PEST sequences) are rapidly degraded. Chemically altered proteins (e.g. due to oxidation) are also preferentially degraded.

Although protein turnover includes both synthesis and degradation, this chapter will consider in detail only the catabolism of proteins (and amino acids).

PROTEIN DEGRADATION

The degradation of proteins results in the formation of *free amino acids*. Within cells, various intracellular *proteases* hydrolyse proteins to peptides which are then degraded to free amino acids by *peptidases*. *Endopeptidases* cleave internal bonds forming shorter peptides. Amino acids from the N- and C-termini of these peptides are then removed by *aminopeptidases* and *carboxypeptidases* respectively.

In eukaryotes, extracellular, membrane-associated proteins are degraded in *lysosomes* by an *ATP-independent process*, while abnormal and other short-lived proteins are degraded by *cytosolic, ATP-dependent proteases* located in *proteosomes*. The proteases will not be active unless signalled by specific molecules (the best known is *ubiquitin*) attached to the proteins that require degradation. Ubiquitin is a small protein present in all eukaryotic cells, and is covalently attached (via specific enzymes) to proteins to be degraded.

Proteins in circulation become targets for destruction when they lose a sialic acid moiety from the non-reducing ends of their oligosaccharide chains. These asialoglycoproteins are recognised and internalised by liver cell *asialoglycoprotein receptors* for degradation by lysosomal proteases termed *cathepsins*.

CATABOLISM OF AMINO ACIDS

Amino acids are catabolised mainly in the liver. The first step in the catabolism of all amino acids involves

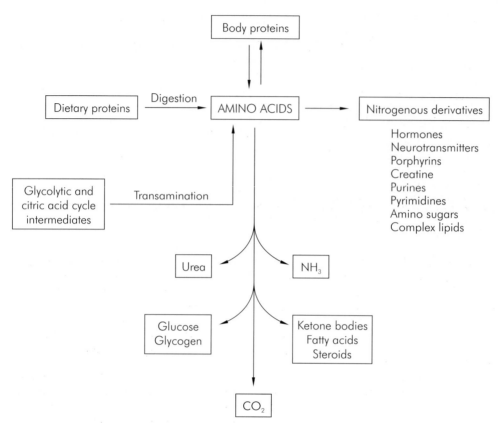

Figure 10.1 – Sources of amino acids and their fate in the body.

the removal of the α-amino groups leaving α-keto acids. The amino group may be released as ammonia or be transferred to other compounds.

REMOVAL OF THE AMINO ACID NITROGEN

The α-amino group in an amino acid is removed by a process of *transamination* or *deamination*.

Transamination is the process by which the amino group of one amino acid is transferred to an α-keto acid (mainly α-ketoglutaric acid) by a *transaminase* or *amino-transferase*. It requires *pyridoxal phosphate*, a member of the vitamin B_6 group, as a coenzyme, the latter acting as the carrier of the -NH_2 group by forming pyridoxamine phosphate (Figure 10.2).

Transaminases are widely distributed in the body, being found in cytosol as well as mitochondria. Only L-amino acids can undergo transamination. Lysine, proline, hydroxyproline, and threonine cannot undergo transamination.

Physiological importance of transaminases

- synthesis of non-essential amino acids from intermediates generated during the metabolism of carbohydrates for example, *alanine* can be synthesised from *pyruvate; aspartate* from *oxaloacetate; glutamate* from α-*ketoglutarate*. The *glutamate* can be converted to *proline, glutamine,* and *arginine*.

  Glycine can be generated from *serine,* which in turn can be synthesised from *3-phospho-glycerate* via the intermediates 3-phosphohydroxypyruvate and phosphoserine.

- synthesis of glucose from glucogenic amino acids.

- the carbon skeleton can be used as a source of energy.

Clinical importance of transaminases

The presence of elevated plasma aminotransferase activity generally indicates cellular damage (e.g. due to physical trauma or disease). Two aminotransferases of

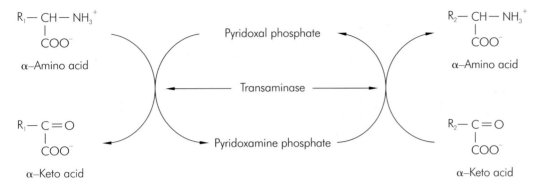

Figure 10.2 – Removal of the α-amino group in an amino acid by transamination.

particular diagnostic importance are *aspartate amino-transferase* (AST) and *alanine aminotransferase* (ALT). The actions of AST and ALT are shown in Figure 10.3. ALT is located in the cell cytosol while AST has two major isoenzymes, one cytoplasmic, the other mitochondrial.

Plasma AST and ALT may be elevated in liver disease, especially in conditions that cause extensive cell necrosis. Aminotransferases may also be elevated in non-hepatic disease such as myocardial infarction and muscle disorders.

Deamination

In this process the α-amino group, instead of being transferred to a keto acid, is liberated as ammonia. Deamination can be *oxidative* or *non-oxidative*. These reactions occur primarily in the liver and kidney.

Oxidative deamination

The chief enzyme utilised for oxidative deamination is *L-glutamate dehydrogenase* which is a mitochondrial enzyme requiring NAD^+ or $NADP^+$ as a coenzyme. The amino groups of most amino acids eventually get funnelled to glutamate by means of transamination with α-ketoglutarate. The reaction is reversible, and functions both in amino acid catabolism and biosynthesis. The combined sequences of transamination and deamination by glutamate dehydrogenase (Figure 10.4) provides a pathway where the amino groups of most amino acids are released as ammonia.

Amino acid oxidases can oxidatively deaminate α-amino acids, requiring FMN or FAD as cofactors. Liver and kidney contain amino acid oxidases that can remove amino groups from D- or L- amino acids (Figure 10.5).

Non-oxidative deamination is the main route for removing the α-amino groups from asparagine, cysteine, glutamine, histidine and serine. The reaction starts with the elimination of water or H_2S (from cysteine) by a *dehydrase* followed by a deamination reaction (Figure 10.6).

Decarboxylation of amino acids plays only a minor role in the catabolism of amino acids, resulting in the synthesis of a number of biomedically important amines (Table 10.1).

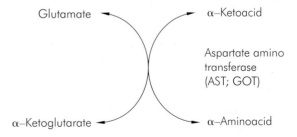

Figure 10.3 – Actions of alanine aminotransferase, and aspartate aminotransferase.

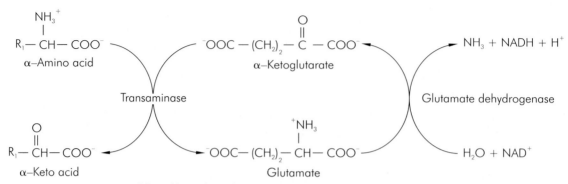

Figure 10.4 – Transamination followed by oxidative deamination by glutamate dehydrogenase.

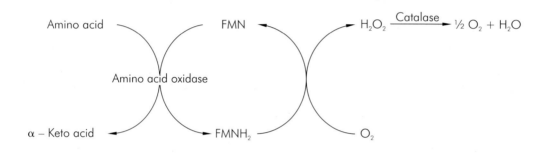

Figure 10.5 – Deamination by an amino acid oxidase.

AMMONIA METABOLISM

SOURCES OF BODY AMMONIA

Ammonia in the body can be derived from three major sources:

- *deamination of amino acids*, especially in the liver and kidney

- *hydrolytic deamination of glutamine* (mainly in the kidney) by *glutaminase* (Figure 10.7). Some glutamine obtained from the blood or from the digestion of dietary protein can also be hydrolyzed by an intestinal glutaminase

- *intestinal bacterial action on dietary protein* and / or urea present in fluids secreted into the gastrointestinal tract. Cleavage of urea to $CO_2 + NH_3$ occurs by the action of the bacterial *urease*. Ammonia is absorbed from the intestine by way of the portal vein and transported to the liver

Smaller amounts of ammonia are generated during the *action of amine oxidase* on dietary amines or monoamines that serve as hormones or neurotransmitters and the *catabolism of purines and pyrimidines*.

BLOOD AMMONIA CONCENTRATION

The normal concentration of ammonia in human plasma is 5–50 μmol/L (10–80 mg/dL). Ammonium ions are toxic to the central nervous system (see below).

REMOVAL OF EXCESS AMMONIA FROM CIRCULATION

Excess ammonia in circulation is usually removed by the following methods:

- *conversion to urea for excretion in the urine.* This is the most important pathway in the liver for the disposal

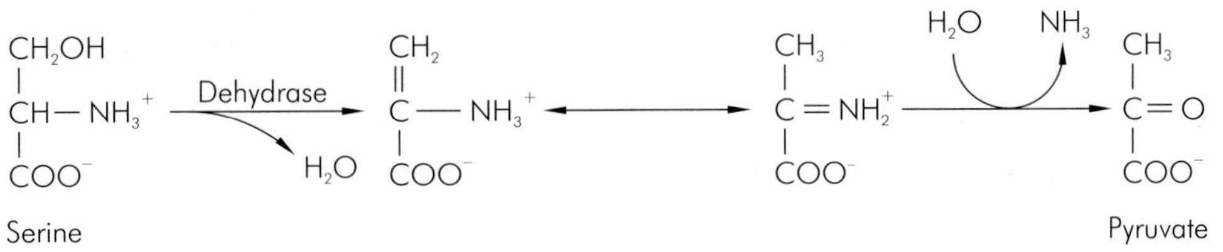

$$\begin{array}{ccc} CH_2OH & & CH_2 \\ | & \xrightarrow{\text{Dehydrase}} & \| \\ CH-NH_3^+ & & C-NH_3^+ \\ | & H_2O & | \\ COO^- & & COO^- \end{array} \longleftrightarrow \begin{array}{c} CH_3 \\ | \\ C=NH_2^+ \\ | \\ COO^- \end{array} \xrightarrow{H_2O \quad NH_3} \begin{array}{c} CH_3 \\ | \\ C=O \\ | \\ COO^- \end{array}$$

Serine   Pyruvate

Figure 10.6 – Non-oxidative deamination.

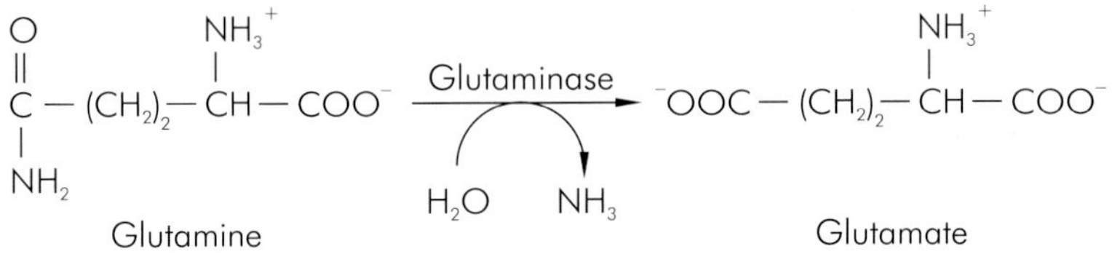

$$\begin{array}{c} O \quad\quad NH_3^+ \\ \| \quad\quad\quad | \\ C-(CH_2)_2-CH-COO^- \\ | \\ NH_2 \end{array} \xrightarrow[\;H_2O\quad NH_3\;]{\text{Glutaminase}} {}^-OOC-(CH_2)_2-\overset{\overset{\displaystyle NH_3^+}{|}}{C}H-COO^-$$

Glutamine   Glutamate

Figure 10.7 – Deamination of glutamine by glutaminase.

BIOMEDICALLY IMPORTANT AMINES GENERATED BY DECARBOXYLATION OF AMINO ACIDS.		
Amino acid	**Product**	**Biomedical importance of product**
Aspartate	β-Alanine	Component of pantothenic acid, and therefore of coenzyme A
Glutamate	γ-Aminobutyric acid (GABA)	Inhibitory neurotransmitter
Histidine	Histamine	Causes peripheral vasodilatation, bronchiolar constriction. Local release, especially in allergic reactions, causes fluid leakage into tissues resulting in oedema and urticaria
Serine	Ethanolamine	Component of phospholipid
Tryptophan	5-Hydroxytryptamine (5-HT, serotonin)	In muscle – causes vasoconstriction. In brain – involved in several psychiatric disorders. Decreased concentration implicated in development of endogenous depression
		Deamination of serotonin followed by oxidation yields 5-hydroxyindoleacetic acid (5-HIAA). The urinary excretion of 5-HIAA is elevated in the *carcinoid syndrome*

Table 10.1

of ammonia and is the major pathway for disposal of most circulating ammonia (see below)

* *used in amidation of glutamate to glutamine* by the action of *glutamine synthetase* found in the mitochondria of liver, kidney, brain, muscle and some other tissues (Figure 10.8)

* *the formation of glutamine* occurs primarily in muscle

and liver, but is also the major mechanism by which ammonia is detoxified in the brain

* *increased renal excretion*

* *synthesis of non-essential amino acids* by amination of α-keto acids arising from carbohydrate metabolism

* *used for the biosynthesis of pyrimidine bases*

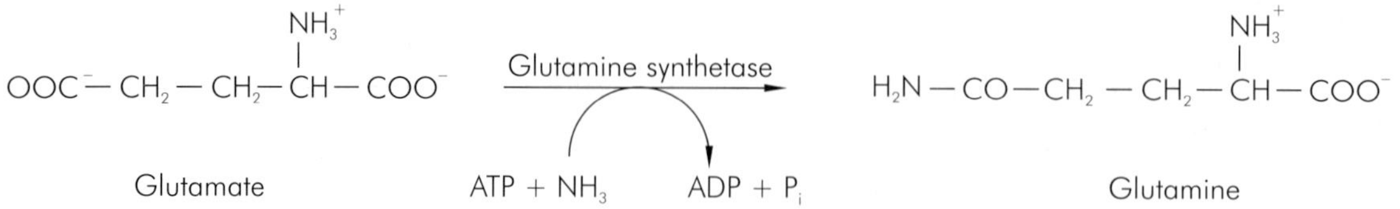

$$OOC - CH_2 - CH_2 - \overset{\overset{\displaystyle NH_3^+}{|}}{CH} - COO^- \quad \xrightarrow[\text{ATP} + NH_3 \qquad \text{ADP} + P_i]{\text{Glutamine synthetase}} \quad H_2N - CO - CH_2 - CH_2 - \overset{\overset{\displaystyle NH_3^+}{|}}{CH} - COO^-$$

Glutamate   Glutamine

Figure 10.8 – Amidation of glutamate to glutamine by the action of glutamine synthetase.

UREA CYCLE

Urea is a relatively non-toxic, water-soluble base accounting for about 90% of the nitrogen-containing components of urine. Other nitrogenous constituents in urine include small amounts of ammonia, amino acids, urate, creatinine and some other identified and non-identified nitrogenous compounds. Urea produced by the liver via *the urea cycle* is excreted in the urine. In a healthy adult, the plasma urea concentration is about 3.3–6.6 mmol/L (20–40 mg/dL).

Reactions of the urea cycle

The reactions of the urea cycle are shown in Figure 10.9. The first two reactions in the cycle, the *carbamoylphosphate synthetase* and *ornithine transcarbamoylase* reactions occur in the mitochondria while the remaining reactions occur in the cytosol.

A high protein diet increases the rate of synthesis of arginase in the liver. The urea cycle is regulated by the intrahepatic concentration of *N-acetylglutamate*, an essential activator for carbamoylphosphate synthetase I, which is the rate-limiting step in the urea cycle.

Urea production in acidosis

Normally, the proportion of ammonia nitrogen diverted for urea formation in the liver is much greater than that used for the synthesis of glutamine. With increasing acidosis, however, a greater proportion of nitrogen is diverted for glutamine synthesis in the liver, with a concurrent fall in the rate of urea production. Glutamine so formed is transported from the liver by the blood to the kidney where it is acted on by the renal glutaminase to release ammonia and glutamate. The ammonia so produced helps to bind H^+ in the tubular lumen and excrete it in the urine as NH_4^+.

HYPERAMMONAEMIA

Elevated levels of ammonia in blood cause symptoms of *ammonia intoxication* such as flapping tremor, slurring

of speech, blurring of vision, and in severe cases coma and death.

Acquired hyperammonaemia

Impaired liver function is one of the major causes of acquired hyperammonaemia. Other causes include urinary tract infections and leukaemia. When the liver cannot function normally (e.g. in cirrhosis), or is bypassed by the establishment of a porto-caval shunt, ammonia in the blood cannot be efficiently converted to urea or glutamine in the liver, and there can be a marked rise in the circulating concentration of ammonia. Hyperammonaemia is thought to be a contributory factor for the development of *hepatic encephalopathy* in some patients with liver disease.

Hereditary hyperammonaemia

Genetic defects in each of the five urea cycle enzymes have been reported. In each case, during the first few weeks after birth, hyperammonaemia results due to a failure to synthesize urea from ammonia.

AMINO ACID BIOSYNTHESIS

ESSENTIAL AND NON-ESSENTIAL AMINO ACIDS

In humans certain *essential* amino acids cannot be synthesised and must be provided in the diet. Amino acids which can adequately be synthesised in the body are *non-essential* and the absence of one of these in the diet does not impair protein synthesis. In man, eight of the ten essential amino acids (*leucine, isoleucine, valine, methionine, threonine, tryptophan, phenylalanine and lysine*) are essential at all times, whereas *arginine* and *histidine* are required only during periods of rapid tissue growth characteristic of childhood or recovery from illness.

Cysteine and *tyrosine* are synthesised from essential amino acids. For example, when cysteine is absent from the diet, methionine requirement increases by

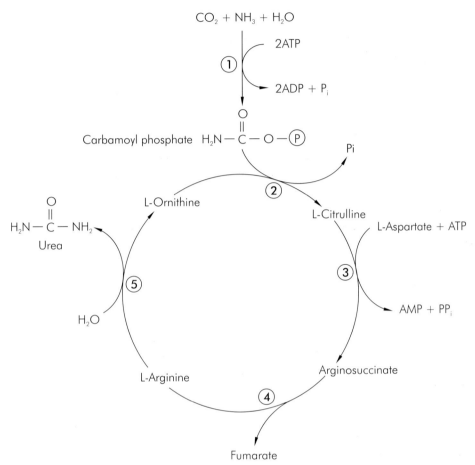

Figure 10.9 – The urea cycle. À – Carbamoyl phosphate synthetase I; Á – Ornithine transcarbamoylase; Â – Arginosuccinate synthetase; Ã – Arginosuccinate lyase; Ä – Arginase.

about 30% because cysteine is synthesised from methionine (Figure 10.10). When sufficient cysteine is present in the diet, the requirement for dietary methionine will be decreased.

The absence of tyrosine increases the phenylalanine requirement because phenylalanine is irreversibly converted to tyrosine (Figure 10.11). The presence of sufficient tyrosine in the diet has a 'sparing effect' on phenylalanine.

Free amino acid pool

Both essential and non-essential amino acids are found in body fluids and tissues as the *free amino acid pool* in the body. Over 50% of the total free amino acid pool is in skeletal muscle, with only a very small proportion found in plasma (0.2–0.6% for individual amino acids). The addition of amino acids to the pool takes place by

absorption from the gut, degradation of cellular proteins and synthesis of non-essential amino acids.

General principles governing synthesis of amino acids

- the synthesis of most amino acids occurs by transamination of the corresponding keto acids; glutamate generally supplies the amino group.

- the enzymes for the synthesis of the carbon chains of non-essential amino acids are contained in the liver.

- the rates of amino acid synthesis can be controlled in one of two ways: *allosteric inhibition* of enzymes in the biosynthetic pathway – generally, the first reaction in the biosynthetic sequence is inhibited by the product of the pathway so that it operates only if there is a deficiency of the product; and increasing

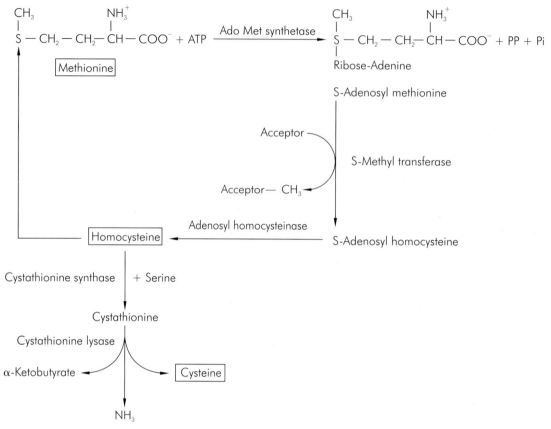

Figure 10.10 – Synthesis of cysteine from methionine.

METHIONINE AND CYSTEINE METABOLISM

Methyl groups liberated from methionine are used for the synthesis of many other important compounds such as phosphatidylcholine, adrenaline, creatine, acetylcholine and methylated bases used in nucleic acid synthesis. Rare inherited defects in *cystathionine synthase* or *cystathionine lyase* (Figure 10.10), will result in the conditions of *homocystinuria* and *cystathioninuria* respectively. Both homocystinuria and cystathioninuria are autosomal recessive disorders. In homocystinuria, due to a defect in cystathionine synthase, associated clinical findings include the occurrence of thromboses, osteoporosis, dislocated lenses in the eyes and developmental delay. Mild to moderate hyperhomocystinaemia (mainly due to a defect in an enzyme involved in the reconversion of homocysteine to methionine) has also been implicated in the pathogenesis of various types of

cardiovascular disorders. The clinical course of cystathioninuria is benign; pyridoxine treatment often leads to a reduction in the quantity of cystathionine in the urine. Some individuals with homocystinuria also respond to pyridoxine treatment. Both homocystinuria and cystathioninuria respond to dietary methionine restriction and cysteine supplementation.

Cysteine is catabolised in mammals via a direct oxidative or transamination pathway to pyruvate with the liberation of sulphate. Urinary sulphate arises almost entirely from oxidation of L-cysteine. Cysteine also serves as a precursor of the thioethanolamine portion of coenzyme A and of taurine that conjugates with bile acids, forming taurocholic acid and other products.

PHENYLALANINE AND TYROSINE METABOLISM

The metabolism of phenylalanine and tyrosine is summarised in Figure 10.11. Phenylalanine is converted to tyrosine by the action of the enzyme *phenylalanine hydroxylase*. *Tetrahydrobiopterin* (BH_4), a pteridine com-

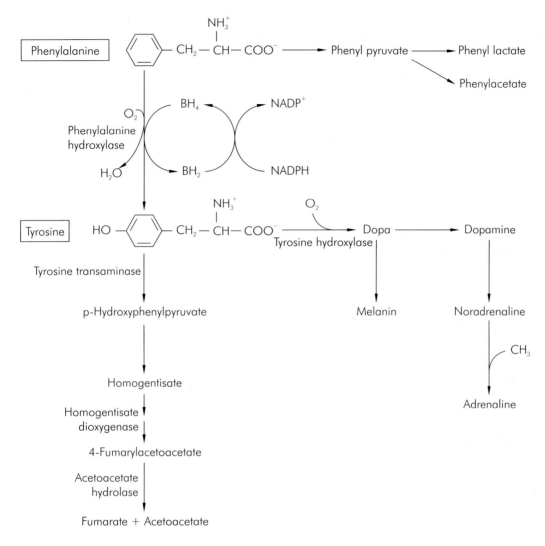

Figure 10.11 – Phenylalanine and tyrosine metabolism. Only the enzymes of clinical importance have been named. BH_2 – dihydro-biopterin; BH_4 – tetrahydrobiopterin; Dopa – 3,4-dihydroxy phenylalanine.

pound resembling folic acid is an essential coenzyme in the phenylalanine hydroxylase reaction. During this reaction, BH_4 gets oxidized to *dihydrobiopterin* (BH_2). NADPH regenerates BH_4 from BH_2.

The major pathway by which tyrosine is metabolised involves a transamination of tyrosine to *p*-hydrox-yphenylpyruvate, which in turn is oxidised to homogentisate by an enzyme using ascorbate as a coenzyme. The homogentisate is ultimately converted to fumarate and acetoacetate. Alternatively, tyrosine can be hydroxylated to dihydroxyphenylalanine (Dopa) which in turn can be metabolised to melanin or the neurotransmitter noradrenaline. Methylation of the noradrenaline by S-adenosylmethionine results in the synthesis of adrenaline.

DISORDERS ARISING FROM DEFECTS IN PHENYLALANINE AND TYROSINE METABOLISM

Phenylketonuria (PKU) is an autosomal recessively inherited disorder with a frequency of about 1: 10,000 live births. *Classical PKU* is caused by a *deficiency of phenylalanine hydroxylase* (Figure 10.11). Hyperphenylalaninaemia may also be caused by deficiencies in the enzymes that synthesise BH_4 (*dihydrobiopterin reductase*) or convert it to BH_2 (*dihydrobiopterin synthetase*). It is important to distinguish among these different forms of hyperphenylalaninaemia because clinical management is different (see below).

Biochemical features include elevated phenylalanine concentrations in tissues, blood and urine, and increased concentration in the blood and urine of minor metabolites such as phenylpyruvate (a phenylketone, hence the name of the condition), phenyllactate and phenylacetate; much of the phenylacetate is excreted as phenylacetylglutamine.

In the first few weeks of life PKU may present with irritability and vomiting. Both microcephaly and epilepsy are common. Developmental delay occurs and is thought to be due to the effect of excess phenylalanine on brain development. Additional clinical signs include *eczema, psychoses,* and a *'mousy odour'* (the origin of which is probably phenylacetic acid). There is usually a *tendency for decreased melanin synthesis* because phenylalanine competetively inhibits the activity of tyrosine hydroxylase, the first step in the synthesis of melanin (Figure 10.11).

Management of PKU is by dietary restriction of phenylalanine. Abnormalities of dihydrobiopterin reductase and dihydrobiopterin synthetase require, in addition, treatment with BH_4. The diet of women with PKU planning pregnancy must also be strictly controlled because maternal hyperphenylalaninaemia can affect the fetus and cause microcephaly and congenital heart disease.

All new-born infants in the UK are screened for PKU, within 5–10 days of life, using capillary blood obtained from a heel prick. The delay after birth allows the establishment of protein intake because high blood levels of phenylalanine may not occur until this time.

Albinism includes a spectrum of clinical disorders characterised by *hypomelanosis* due to heritable defects in eye and skin melanocytes. Albinism inherited in an autosomal recessive manner and may occur due to a lack of, or defective, *tyrosine hydroxylase* (Figure 10.11). Reduced pigmentation in the eye causes photosensitivity, and decreased skin pigmentation associated with an increased risk of skin cancer. Catecholamine production is normal in albino individuals because the tyrosine hydroxylase (*tyrosinase*) involved in catecholamine

synthesis is a different isoenzyme, controlled by a different gene.

Alkaptonuria is a relatively harmless condition (inherited in an autosomal recessive manner) arising as a result of an absence of *homogentisate dioxygenase* required for the further metabolism of homogentisate derived from tyrosine (Figure 10.11). Homogentisate accumulates and is excreted in the urine, which turns dark on standing due to the oxidation of homogentisate to a melanin-like substance. Oxidation occurs more rapidly at alkaline pH. Individuals with alkaptonuria develop pigmentation of the connective tissue called *ochronosis* and develop arthritis.

Tyrosinaemia Type I is an autosomal recessive condition due to a deficiency of *fumarylacetoacetate hydrolase* (Figure 10.11). This condition usually presents between 2–6 months of age with vomiting, diarrhoea, oedema, ascites, hepatosplenomegaly, hypoglycaemia and failure to thrive. Other characteristic features include renal tubular damage leading to hypophosphataemic rickets; bleeding diathesis may occur due to prothrombin deficiency. If untreated, death may occur from hepatic failure during the first year of life or from primary liver cancer in the cirrhotic liver, usually in the first two decades.

Restricted intake of tyrosine and phenylalanine may reduce the excretion of the precursors of fumarylacetoacetate, and produce regression of the renal tubular defects. A metabolic inhibitor blocking the pathway before homogentisic acid, 2-nitro-4-trifluoromethyl benzoyl-1,3 cyclohexanedione, NTBC, reduces the production of toxic metabolites and can be used in treatment.

Tyrosinaemia Type II *(Richner Hanhaart syndrome)* is an inherited metabolic defect thought to be due to abnormality of *tyrosine transaminase* (Figure 10.11). Clinical findings include eye and skin lesions and moderate impairment of mental development. The pathology is considered to be secondary to the deposition of tyrosine crystals in cells, precipitating an inflammatory response. Treatment includes use of a low tyrosine and phenylalanine diet.

Neonatal tyrosinaemia is an inherited disorder thought to result from a relative deficiency of *p-hydroxyphenylpyruvate hydroxylase* (Figure 10.11). Blood levels of tyrosine and phenylalanine are elevated, as are urinary concentrations of tyrosine, p-hydroxyphenylacetate, N-acetyltyrosine and tyramine. Therapy consists of a diet low in protein.

BRANCHED-CHAIN AMINO ACID METABOLISM

The three branched-chain amino acids, *leucine, isoleucine* and *valine* are degraded by transamination to α-keto acids which are oxidised and decarboxylated to acyl CoA thioesters by mitochondrial α-keto acid dehydrogenases. The ultimate end product of valine and isoleucine catabolism is *propionyl CoA* which undergoes carboxylation to *methylmalonyl CoA* and is then converted to succinyl CoA by the *vitamin B_{12}*-dependent enzyme *methylmalonyl CoA isomerase*.

Maple syrup urine disease (MSUD) is an autosomal recessive disorder arising due to inherited *defects in the branched-chain keto acid dehydrogenase*. There is an increased excretion of the branched-chain amino acids and their α-keto acids in urine, giving rise to the characteristic 'maple syrup' odour. Common features include vomiting, acidosis, dehydration and ketosis. The dinitrophenylhydrazine test for keto acids can be used for rapid diagnosis, with measurement of the defective enzyme activity providing confirmation. Rapid treatment is essential because the condition may progress to coma and apnoea. Mortality is high and survivors may show dystonia, psychomotor impairment and other neurological abnormalities. Dietary protein restriction is part of treatment.

ROLE OF TETRAHYDROFOLATE IN AMINO ACID METABOLISM

Tetrahydrofolate (FH_4) is the biologically active form of the B-vitamin folic acid. It is produced in the body by a two-step reduction of folate by *dihydrofolate reductase* (Figure 10.12).

FH_4 plays an important role in the transfer of one-carbon groups produced during metabolism (mainly amino acid catabolism). One-carbon groups transferred by FH_4 are methyl ($-CH_3$), methylene ($-CH_2$), hydroxymethyl ($-CH_2OH$), and formimino ($-CH=NH$) groups (Figure 10.12). Transfer of one carbon groups by FH_4 plays a very important role in the biosynthesis of purines and pyrimidines, and therefore in cell division. Dietary deficiency of folic acid (and therefore FH_4) results in megaloblastic anaemia, due to the inability of red blood cells to divide. Vitamin B_{12} deficiency can also cause symptoms of this disorder because vitamin B_{12} is required for the conversion of methyl FH_4 to FH_4 (Figure 10.12).

METABOLISM OF NUCLEOTIDES

Mammals are capable of synthesizing purine and pyrimidine nucleotides *de novo*, and are thus not dependent upon exogenous sources of these important compounds.

PURINE NUCLEOTIDES

BIOSYNTHESIS

In man purine nucleotides are synthesised for the monomeric precursors of nucleic acids and for other functions. The reactions involved in the *de novo* biosynthesis of purine nucleotides are outlined in Figure 10.13. Phosphoribosyl pyrophosphate (PRPP) is the initial substrate from which purines are synthesised. It is generated by pyrophosphorylating ribose-5-phosphate with ATP. The enzyme catalysing this reaction, *phosphoribosyl pyrophosphate synthetase* is allosterically inhibited by ADP and GDP:

$$\text{Ribose-5-phosphate + ATP} \xrightarrow{\text{PRPP synthetase}} \text{PRPP + AMP}$$

Phosphoribosyl pyrophosphate amidotransferase then catalyses the replacement of the pyrophosphate group of PRPP with the amide amino group of glutamine, forming the amino sugar phosphate 5-phosphoribosylamine. An entire molecule of glycine is next incorporated into phosphoribosylamine to form phosphoribosyl glycinamide. This compound undergoes several complex reactions before being converted to inosine monophosphate (IMP) which can be considered to be the parent compound from which all purine nucleotides are derived. The synthesis of AMP and GMP from IMP is shown in Figure 10.13.

Important points about the purine biosynthetic pathway include:

- *tetrahydrofolate* (FH_4) a folic acid derivative, is essential for two of the reactions in the pathway. Two of the ring carbons (C2 and C8) are added from N^{10}-formyl-tetrahydrofolate. Any condition that reduces the concentration of the vitamin folic acid in the body can therefore affect the level of purines, and hence the nucleic acid synthesis

- the first step in the biosynthetic pathway (the *phosphoribosylamidotransferase* reaction) is the rate controlling step. It is subject to feedback inhibition by its products AMP and GMP. Other allosteric inhibitors of this enzyme are GTP, ADP and ATP

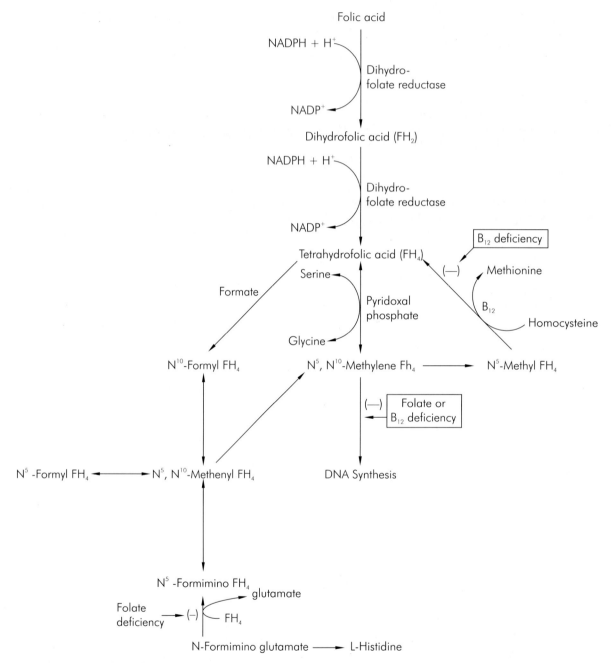

Figure 10.12 – Biosynthesis of tetrahydrofolate from folic acid and the interconversions of one carbon units attached to tetrahydrofolate.

•. the rate of the pathway is also dependent on the intracellular concentration of PRPP and the availability of energy. Four molecules of ATP are consumed in the reactions converting PRPP to IMP

GENERATION OF PURINE NUCLEOTIDES BY THE SALVAGE PATHWAYS

AMP and GMP can be regenerated from adenine and guanine derived from the catabolism of nucleic acids by the action of two salvage pathways. As shown in

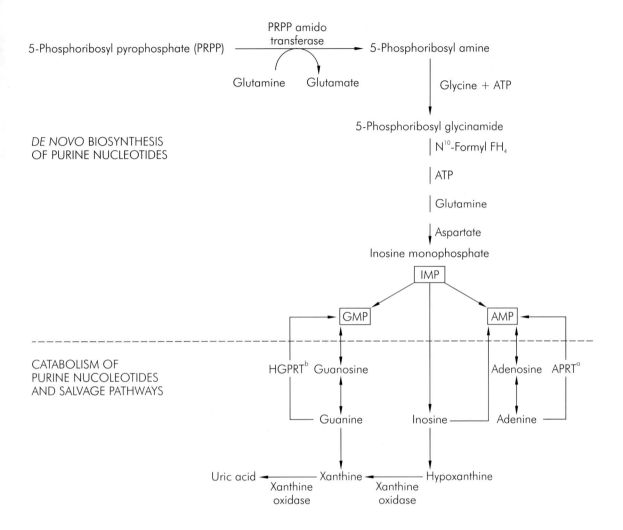

Figure 10.13 – An outline of purine biosynthesis and catabolism.
a – Adenine phosphoribosyl transferase; b- Hypoxanthine-guanine phosphoribosyl transferase.

Figure 10.13, *adenine phosphoribosyl transferase* helps to add ribose phosphate from PRPP to adenine to regenerate AMP. The analogous reaction with guanine or hypoxanthine is catalyzed by hypoxanthine- guanine phosphoribosyl transferase (*HGPRTase*).

In the second pathway for purine salvage, ribose-1-phosphate is added to adenine and guanine to generate adenosine and guanosine respectively, which are phosphorylated with ATP to yield AMP and GMP.

CATABOLISM

The ultimate catabolite of purines is *uric acid*. (Figure 10.13). Adenosine undergoes deamination and deribosylation to form hypoxanthine which is then converted by *xanthine oxidase* (containing molybdenum and iron) to xanthine. Guanosine also undergoes a deribosylation followed by a deamination to form xanthine. The xanthine so formed is converted to uric acid by the xanthine oxidase.

Uric acid can exist as a mixture of relatively insoluble uric acid and a highly soluble sodium urate. At pH < 5.75, the predominant form in body fluids is uric acid while at pH > 5.75 sodium urate will predominate in solution.

PYRIMIDINE NUCLEOTIDES

BIOSYNTHESIS

The synthesis of the pyrimidine ring commences with the formation of carbamoyl phosphate from glutamine,

ATP and CO_2 in a reaction catalyzed by *carbamoylphosphate synthetase II* (CPSII) located in the cell cytosol (Figure 10.14). In animal cells, the cytosolic CPSII is part of a multienzyme complex catalysing the three steps from carbamoyl phosphate to dihydroorotic acid. The other two enzymes in this complex are *aspartate transcarbamoylase* and *dihydroorotase*. *Uridine monophosphate* (UMP) is the primary end poduct of the pyrimidine biosynthetic pathway. A second enzyme complex, *UMP synthetase*, catalyzes the last two reactions in the synthesis of UMP. In man, CPSII is the rate limiting enzyme in the pyrimidine biosynthetic pathway. This

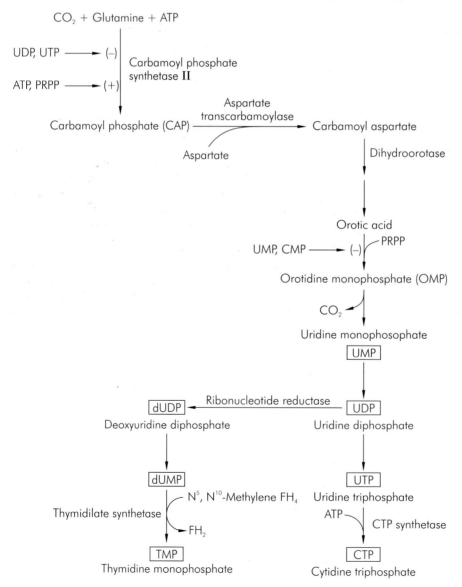

Figure 10.14 – An outline of pyrimidine nucleotide biosynthesis.

enzyme complex is inhibited by the end products of pyrimidine biosynthesis, uridine diphosphate (UDP) and uridine triphosphate (UTP) and is activated by ATP and PRPP.

Although the pyrimidine nucleus is simpler and its synthetic pathway shorter than that of the purine nucleus, several common precursors (phosphoribosyl pyrophosphate, glutamine, CO_2 and aspartate) are used for the synthesis of both purines and pyrimidines.

Tetrahydrofolate (in the form of N^5, N^{10}-FH_4) is also essential for the synthesis of the thymidine nucleotide TMP from UMP (Figure 10.14). *Folic acid antagonists* such as *methotrexate* are used in the treatment of leukemia because they block folate-dependent steps in nucleic acid synthesis such as the thymidylate synthetase reaction. The pyrimidine analogue *5-fluorouracil* (5-FU) used in the treatment of many solid tumours in man, also inhibits thymidylate synthetase. 5-FU gets activated to 5-fluoro-dUMP which competitively inhibits thymidylate synthetase because it resembles dUMP structurally.

CATABOLISM

Pyrimidine catabolism occurs mainly in the liver. It results in the production of a series of highly soluble products (CO_2, NH_3, β-alanine and β-aminoisobutyric acid). This contrasts with the production of sparingly soluble uric acid by purine catabolism.

SYNTHESIS OF DEOXYRIBONUCLEOTIDES

All nucleotides are synthesised initially as ribonucleotides. Deoxyribonucleotides (dNTPs) are derived from cellular ribonucleotides by direct reduction at the 2-carbon in the ribose moiety of the corresponding nucleotide after it has been converted to the respective nucleoside diphosphate. As shown in Figure 10.15, reduction of the ribonucleotide diphosphates to deoxyribonucleotide diphosphates is catalysed by *ribonucleotide reductase* (that requires *thioredoxin*, a protein cofactor), *thioredoxin reductase* (a flavoprotein) and NADPH as a cofactor. The immediate electron donor to the nucleotide is thioredoxin that has been reduced by NADPH.

DISORDERS OF PURINE METABOLISM

HYPERURICAEMIA

The miscible urate pool in the body is reflected by the sodium urate concentration in the serum. At pH 7.4 and 37°C, the solubility of sodium urate in an aqueous medium is 0.57 mmol/L. In plasma, the presence of proteins appears to reduce the solubility of sodium urate. *Hyperuricaemia* is a condition that results when the plasma sodium urate concentration exceeds its solubility limit in the plasma. In the UK, the reference range for plasma urate in males is 0.12–0.42 mmol/L, while in females it is 0.09–0.36 mmol/L, increasing slightly with age. Hyperuricaemia may occur due to overproduction of urate, by decreased renal excretion of urate or a combination of both (Table 10.2). Excessive dietary intake of purine-containing foods or alcohol can exacerbate the hyperuricaemia and should be avoided by individuals with this condition.

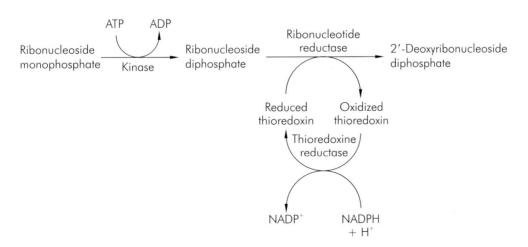

Figure 10.15 – Synthesis of deoxyribonucleoside diphosphates from ribonucleoside diphosphates.

CAUSES OF HYPERURICAEMIA	
Category	Examples of responsible factors or conditions
Overproduction of urate *Increased de novo purine synthesis*	Idiopathic Overactivity of specific enzymes in the purine biosynthetic pathway (e.g. PRPP synthetase or PRPP amidotransferase). Deficiency of specific enzymes in pathways associated with the *de novo* purine biosynthetic pathway (e.g. HGPRT in Lesch-Nyhan syndrome; glucose-6-phosphatase in Von Gierke's disease).
Increased turnover of pre-formed purines	Myeloproliferative disorders (e.g. polycythaemia rubra vera). Lymphoproliferative disorders (e.g. lymphocytic leukaemia, lymphoma). Miscellaneous (e.g. carcinomatosis, secondary polycythaemia, psoriasis).
Defective elimination of urate	Idiopathic Renal disease (e.g. chronic renal failure, lead nephropathy). Drugs (e.g. diuretics, low-dose salicylates) Metabolic acidosis (e.g. lactic acidosis, ketoacidosis).

Table 10.2

GOUT

Gout comprises a group of metabolic disorders whose clinical problems result from tissue deposition of crystals of sodium urate. Gout is classified as *primary (idiopathic)* or *secondary* (when a condition known to cause hyperuricaemia is present). However, gout is uncommon when hyperuricaemia develops secondarily to other conditions. The prevalence of gout is higher in men than in women: in the latter, it is very rare in the pre-menopausal years. Shortly before and during an acute attack of gout, the plasma urate rises to about 0.9 mmol/l. In chronic gout, between acute episodes, plasma urate is usually in the high normal range.

Owing to its low solubility, sodium urate tends to precipitate and the deposition of the crystals in soft tissues and joints form deposits called *tophi* causing an inflammatory reaction. Visualisation under a polarising light microscope of needle-shaped, intensely negatively birefringent crystals of sodium urate in joint fluid is diagnostic of gout.

Precipitation of urate in tissues may be enhanced by local factors such as tissue pH and trauma. Local inflammation due to urate precipitation attracts leucocytes to the area. Production of lactate by the leucocytes which produces an acid environment, hence reducing the solubulity of urate. Damage to leucocyte membranes by urate crystals also results in the release of their lysosomal contents leading to local and systemic manifestations of gout.

A reduction in the renal clearance of uric acid is thought to be the major cause of *primary gout*. In about 10% of patients hyperuricaemia is thought to be the consequence of an inherited metabolic defect resulting in an increased endogenous synthesis of uric acid. Inherited defects in the purine biosynthetic enzymes PRPP synthetase (which synthesizes PRPP) and PRPP amidotransferase (which catalyzes the rate-limiting step in IMP synthesis), which cause them to be overactive, resistant to feed back inhibition or have low affinities for their substrates, are thought to be responsible for the development of primary gout in some individuals.

Secondary gout may develop as a complication of several other disorders that cause a reduced renal clearance of uric acid (e.g. reduced renal perfusion, diuretic therapy, especially thiazides), or an overproduction of uric acid.

TREATMENT OF HYPERURICAEMIA

Acute attacks of gout may be treated with anti-inflammatory drugs such as indomethacin (uricosuric drugs and allopurinol should be avoided at this stage), although they have no effect on the hyperuricaemia. Long-term treatment with the aim of reducing hyperuricaemia includes:

- *dietary measures.* Reduction of purine intake, avoidance of alcohol and drugs known to exacerbate the condition (e.g. diuretics)

- *increasing renal excretion of urates with uricosuric drugs* (e.g. probenecid, salicylates)

- *reducing urate production by drugs.* The most widely used drug is allopurinol (an isomer of hypoxanthine) that competitively inhibits xanthine oxidase, thereby causing a fall in urate concentration in plasma and urine. Urinary xanthine excretion is increased, but xanthine is more water soluble than urate. In patients with a tendency to form urate stones, a high fluid intake and alkalisation of the urine will help to reduce the likelihood of stone formation

INHERITED METABOLIC DISORDERS ASSOCIATED WITH HYPERURICAEMIA

Lesch-Nyhan syndrome is an X-linked disorder. Owing to the lack of the salvage pathway enzyme HGPRT, purines cannot be recycled to form purine nucleotides and urate production from them increases resulting in severe hyperuricaemia. This syndrome is associated with gout, together with a neurological syndrome comprising choreoathetosis, spasticity, a variable degree of developmental delay and a striking behavioural disturbance characterized by self mutilation.

Glucose 6-phosphatase deficiency (*von Gierke's disease*)

In this condition an increased metabolism of glucose-6-phosphate through the pentose phosphate pathway increases forming increased amounts of ribose 5-phosphate, a substrate for purine nucleotide synthesis. In

these patients there is also a marked elevation in the serum lactate concentration. In most patients with glucose-6-phosphatase deficiency, the hyperuricaemia is a consequence of both, an excessive purine synthesis *de novo*, and a decreased urate excretion secondary to competitive inhibition of renal tubular urate secretion by lactate.

HYPOURICAEMIA

This condition is not as common as hyperuricaemia. Hypouricaemia may be caused by either *a decreased production of uric acid* such as occurs with use of xanthine oxidase inhibitors (e.g. allopurinol), in the rare disorder of *xanthinuria* (congenital xanthine oxidase deficiency) or severe liver disease; or *increased urinary urate excretion* due to the excessive use of uricosuric drugs such as probenicid or renal tubular defects (e.g. *Fanconi syndrome*). Some patients with xanthine oxidase deficiency develop xanthine stones in the urinary tract from the increased xanthine (and hypoxanthine) excretion that occurs in this condition, but the condition may be asymptomatic.

DISORDERS OF PYRIMIDINE METABOLISM

As the end-products of pyrimidine metabolism are highly water-soluble, detectable abnormalities due to pyrimidine overproduction are rarely evident. The few pyrimidine related disorders known are due to some defect in the synthesis of pyrimidines (either due to a deficiency of folate or vitamin B_{12} or an enzyme in the synthetic pathway).

The only well recognized disorder of pyrimidine synthesis is the very rare *hereditary orotic aciduria*. This condition results from a deficiency of the protein with the two enzyme activities, orotate phosphoribosyl transferase and orotidine 5-phosphate decarboxylase. Affected children develop megaloblastic anaemia and show developmental delay.

SELECTED READING

Marshall, W and Bangert, S.K. (eds) – *Clinical Biochemistry*. Churchill Livingstone, London, 1995.

Mousseau, D.D. and Butterworth, R.F. – Current theories on the pathogenesis of hepatic encephalopathy (43770). *Proceedings of the Society for Experimental Biology and Medicine* 1994; **vol 26**: 329–344.

Murray, R.K., Granner, D.K., Mayes, P.A. and Rodwell, V.W. (eds). – *Harper's Biochemistry*, 24th ed. Appleton and Lange, California, 1996.

Roskoski, R. – *Biochemistry*. W.B. Saunders and Co., Philadelphia, 1996.

Stryer, L. – *Biochemistry*, 4th ed. W.H. Freeman and Co., N.Y., 1995.

Smith, A.F., Beckett, G.J. and Walker, S.W. – *Lecture Notes on Clinical Biochemistry*, 6th ed. Blackwell Scientific Publications, London, 1998.

Wetherall, D.J., Ledingham, J.G.G. and Warrell, D.A. (eds) – *Oxford Textbook of Medicine*, 3rd ed. Vol 2, Oxford Medical Publications, 1996.

11

COMMUNICATION BETWEEN CELLS AND TISSUES IN THE BODY

Objectives
To understand:

- The nature of cellular communication
- Tissue receptors and mechanisms of signal transduction
- Disorders of signal transduction systems

across a synapse but response to transmitters can be modified by other substances.

Local mediators are signal molecules released from cells and they act locally on nearby target cells. Examples include *growth factors, eicosanoids, nitric oxide, cytokines* and *leukotrienes*. However, it is becoming apparent that the distinction (biochemically or physiologically) between hormones, neurotransmitters and local mediators is not absolute.

The survival of multicellular organisms depends on their ability to integrate and coordinate differentiated cell functions to maintain homeostasis. Small groups of cells can communicate with each other by direct cell-to-cell contact. For example, *gap junctions* permit adjacent cells to exchange small molecules and coordinate metabolic responses. Mechanisms also exist for cells to produce a variety of chemicals called *signal molecules* that generate signals triggering changes in the patterns of activity within the cells.

SUB-DIVISION OF SIGNAL MOLECULES ACCORDING TO THE RELATIONSHIP BETWEEN THE PRODUCTION SITES AND THE TARGET SITES

Signal molecules can be sub-divided into three groups, *autocrine, paracrine,* and *endocrine.*

In *autocrine signalling,* molecules released from certain cells influence the behaviour of the same cells (e.g. *some growth factors, eicosanoids*).

In *paracrine signalling,* the signalling molecules released from certain cells influence the activity of target cells that lie very close to them (e.g. *neurotransmitters* and *neurohormones*).

In *endocrine signalling,* molecules released from the endocrine glands are transported to distant target tissues for activity.

PRINCIPAL TYPES OF SIGNAL MOLECULES UTILIZED FOR COMMUNICATION BETWEEN CELLS AND TISSUES

Hormones, neurotransmitters and local mediators are the principal types of signal molecules that function in communication between cells and tissues.

Hormones are classically defined as chemical messenger molecules secreted by certain cells in minute quantities, and transported in the blood to distant target cells where they regulate metabolism and thereby produce their physiological effects. This definition is not strictly true because certain substances that function as hormones (e.g. eicosanoids) can also have local actions. According to the relationship of hormones generated by endocrine glands to the central nervous system, three levels of hormones can be recognised.

Neurotransmitters are chemical substances secreted by neurons and they convey messages from one neuron to a target cell. At the target cells, the neurotransmitters may alter ion flow (*depolarise* or *hyperpolarise*), or they may alter the cellular metabolism. The transmitter substances carry out the actual passage of a signal

SUB-DIVISION OF SIGNAL MOLECULES ACCORDING TO THEIR CHEMICAL NATURE

Chemically, signal molecules can be grouped into four major classes:

- amino acids or their derivatives (e.g. *catecholamines, thyroid hormones,* and *many neurotransmitters*)

- peptides (e.g. *from the pancreas and gut*

- steroidal compounds (e.g. *sex hormones*)

-        fatty acid derivatives (e.g. *eicosano*

SIGNAL MOLECULE AND RECEPTOR INTERACTION

VARIATION IN THE TYPE OF CELLULAR RESPONSE TO SIGNAL MOLECULE-RECEPTOR INTERACTION

A signal molecule that binds to, or fits into a special binding site on a receptor protein is generally referred to as a *ligand*.

All *receptors* to which signal molecules bind are proteins and have at least two functional domains – one that recognises and binds to the signal molecule, and another that initiates a response (signal transduction). Some cells have more than one receptor type for the same ligand, each inducing a different response. For example, adrenaline can bind to β-adrenergic receptors in the heart and to α-adrenergic receptors in smooth muscle cells. Some ligands can generate different responses in different cell types, via the same receptor type. Acetylcholine slows the rate of contraction in heart muscle cells but, in pancreatic acinar cells, it triggers exocytosis of secretory granules that contain digestive enzymes.

SPEED AND DURATION OF RESPONSES TO RECEPTOR-MEDIATED SIGNALS

The response of a target cell to a signal molecule may last a few milliseconds or be sustained for several hours or days. *Rapid responses* are required for changes in the rates of reactions involved in metabolic regulation (e.g. by hormones) and are generally achieved by an alteration in the activity (e.g. by phosphorylation or dephosphorylation) of a key enzyme. Termination of the rapid response occurs by inactivation of the hormone or its intracellular messenger, or by a reversal of the enzyme modification.

Slow responses occur when a signal molecule acts at the gene level. The concentration of a particular enzyme can be altered by influence of the hormone on the pattern of gene expression. *Thyroid hormones, steroid hormones and some eicosanoids bring about slow and sustained responses* in this manner. Such responses are especially important for the regulation of growth and differentiation of cells.

PLASMA MEMBRANE RECEPTORS, AND THE MECHANISMS BY WHICH LIGANDS THAT BIND TO THESE RECEPTORS MEDIATE CELLULAR RESPONSES

Water-soluble signal molecules (e.g peptide hormones and amino acid derivatives, with the exception of thyroid hormones) bind to receptors on the plasma membrane of target cells. According to the type of response generated by the binding of a signal molecule to the receptor, three principal types of receptors, each of which transduces signals in a different way, can be recognised (Figure 11.1):

- *receptors that function as ion channels* – transmitter-gated ion channels that open or close briefly in response to ligand binding

- *receptors linked to G-proteins* – these indirectly activate or inactivate enzymes bound to the plasma membrane, or ion channels, with assistance from trimeric GTP-binding proteins (G-proteins)

- *catalytic or enzyme-linked receptors* – these act either directly as enzymes, or are associated with enzymes; the enzymes are usually protein kinases that phosphorylate specific proteins in the target cell

RECEPTORS THAT THEMSELVES FUNCTION AS ION CHANNELS

Neurotransmitters are the principal signal molecules that mediate their actions via receptors that can function as ion channels. Most channel-linked receptors are transmembrane proteins or protein complexes that possess a ligand-binding domain on the outer surface of the cell, and a channel-forming domain that traverses the width of the membrane (Figure 11.2). The receptor is therefore an integral part of the ion channel.

Binding of neurotransmitters to channel-linked receptors generally produces changes in electrical activity within the cells by altering the membrane permeability to ions.

Under resting conditions, all cells maintain a negative electromotive force known as the *resting potential*. *Excitatory neurotransmitters* (e.g. *acetylcholine, glutamate, noradrenaline*) bind to receptors linked to cation channels, and promote an increased entry of Na^+ into cells accompanied by a movement of K^+ out of cells, each moving down a concentration gradient. The influx of Na^+ results in a dissipation of the normal resting

RECEPTOR FUNCTIONING AS ION CHANNEL

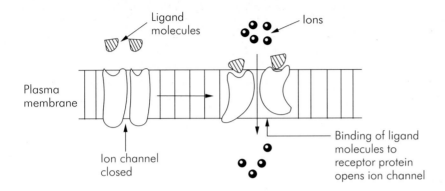

G-PROTEIN LINKED RECEPTOR

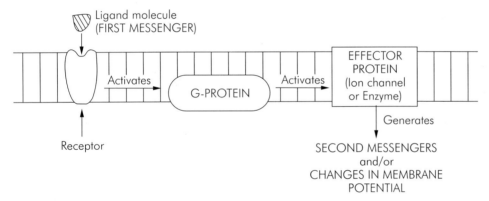

ENZYME-LINKED RECEPTORS

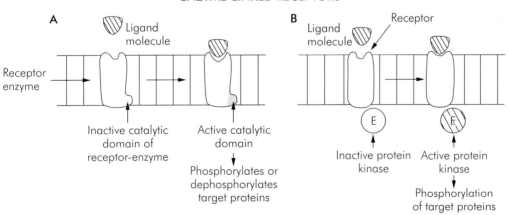

Figure 11.1 – Types of plasma membrane receptors and the mechanisms by which they mediate signal transduction.

potential and a *depolarisation* that triggers a nerve discharge. *Inhibitory neurotransmitters* (e.g. *γ-aminobutyric acid or GABA, glycine*) on the other hand, bind to anion-linked channels and increase the flow of anions (mainly Cl⁻) into cells causing a *hyperpolarisation* (an increase in membrane potential). Hyperpolarisation makes subsequent depolarisation more difficult.

Proteins that form ion channels exhibit ion selectivity and allow only specific ions to pass through the channels. Specific channels for Na^+, K^+, and Ca^{2+} have been identified. The permeability of a channel depends on the size, extent of hydration and charge on the ion.

Acetylcholine (ACh) receptor

Receptors that bind ACh are known as cholinergic receptors, of which there are two classes - nicotinic and muscarinic. The nicotinic ACh receptor is a ligand-activated ion-channel stimulated by the plant alkaloid *nicotine*. As shown in Figure 11.2, the nicotinic receptor at the neuromuscular junction, like most other ligand-activated ion-channel receptors, is a glycoprotein containing five subunits ($\alpha_2\beta\gamma\delta$), each of which has four transmembrane segments.

Muscarinic ACh receptors are stimulated by the plant alkaloid *muscarine*. They are linked to G-protein, and are found at post-ganglionic parasympathetic cells. Binding of ACh to muscarinic receptors can result in excitatory or inhibitory responses depending on cell type. For example, activation of muscarinic receptors on smooth muscle of the gut results in contraction and peristalsis, while activation of receptors on the heart decreases heart rate.

RECEPTORS LINKED TO G-PROTEINS

G-proteins form a large family of GTP-binding proteins of the *ras* superfamily. G-protein-coupled receptors mediate the cellular responses to a large number of structurally and functionally different types of hormones, neurotransmitters and local mediators, as well as to light. Over 300 different G-protein-linked receptors have been identified so far. The same ligand can in several instances activate many different types of G-proteins. For example, *adrenaline* can activate at least nine distinct G-proteins while *serotonin* can activate about 15.

G-protein receptors share common structural features and appear to be evolutionarily related. All are single polypeptide chains, each having an extracellularly located amino terminus, connected by several (usually seven) hydrophobic, transmembrane helixes to the C-terminus located on the cytoplasmic side of the membrane; a large loop facing the cytosol (between helixes 5 and 6), composed mainly of hydrophilic amino acids; and a hydrophilic segment at the C-terminus (Figure 11.3). The receptor protein is thought to interact with the G-protein via these hydrophilic regions. Although there appears to be a common overall structure of the G-protein linked receptors, there is much variation in the amino acid sequences of these receptors. For example, only 50% of the amino acid sequences are identical in the closely related β_1 and β_2 adrenergic receptors. The difference in the amino acid sequence determines the ligand specificity of the receptors and also shows how they interact with different types of G-proteins.

G-proteins are involved in the transduction of extracellular signals and are trimeric, containing an α, a β, and a γ-subunit. These proteins can alternate between an activated state and an inactive state, according to cellular needs; they are activated by the binding of GTP, and inactivated by an exchange of the GTP for GDP.

According to similarities in the amino acid sequence of the α-subunit, G-proteins can be grouped into several families:

- G_s family – G-proteins that increase the intracellular concentration of cAMP by activating the membrane bound enzyme, adenyl cyclase

- G_i family – G-proteins that inhibit adenyl cyclase activity

- G_q family – G-proteins that activate the membrane bound phospholipase C

MECHANISMS BY WHICH G-PROTEINS FUNCTION IN SIGNAL TRANSDUCTION

The binding of a ligand to a G-protein-linked receptor induces a conformational change in the receptor protein that in turn activates the coupled G-protein by promoting the binding of a GTP to the G-protein. The activated G-protein then triggers a cellular response by either altering the concentration of one or more small intracellular signalling molecules (often referred to as *second messengers*) that initiate a cascade of events that result in an alteration in the behaviour of cellular proteins, or the activity of an ion channel (Figure 11.1).

Alteration in the concentration of second messengers *cAMP* and *cGMP* involves a G-protein mediated activation or inhibition of the membrane bound *adenyl*

A

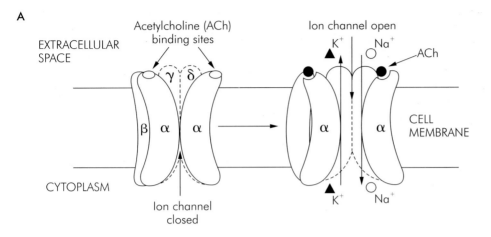

B

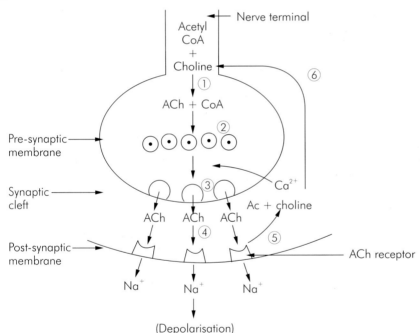

Figure 11.2 – A. An outline of the nicotonic acetylcholine receptor at the neuromuscular junction. Each α-subunit of the receptor binds one molecule of acetylcholine (ACh), before channel opening.
B. Major steps involved in the transmission of a nerve impulse by ACh across the neuromuscular junction:
① – Synthesis of ACh from choline and acetyl CoA, catalysed by *choline-acetyl transferase*
② – Storage of ACh in synaptic vesicles.
③ – Ca²⁺ enters from the synaptic space into the nerve terminus during transmission of a nerve impulse, and promotes release of ACh from synaptic vesicles by exocytosis.
④ – ACh binds to receptors on post-synaptic membrane, and permits entry of Na⁺ across the membrane, depolarising muscle membrane.
⑤ – On termination of nerve impulse, ion channels close and ACh is hydrolysed to acetate and choline by *acetylcholinesterase* (present in basal lamina of synaptic space)
⑥ – Reutilisation of choline for synthesis of more ACh.

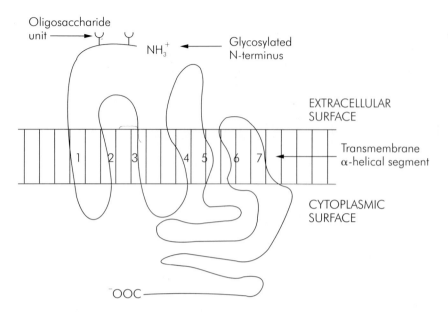

Figure 11.3 – Schematic representation of the β-adrenergic receptor. The three extracellular loops of the receptor are connected by seven trans-membrane helical segments to three cytoplasmic loops. Phosphorylation of specific C-terminal serine and threonine residues permits the interaction of the receptor with G-proteins.

cyclase and *guanyl cyclase* respectively. G-protein-mediated changes in the activity of *phospholipase C* will result in alterations in the concentrations of *1,2-diacylglycerol (DAG), inositol 1,4,5-triphosphate (IP₃)* and *Ca²⁺* that can function as second messengers.

cAMP-DEPENDENT SIGNAL TRANSDUCTION

In cells, cAMP is synthesised from ATP by the action of the plasma membrane-bound enzyme *adenyl cyclase*, and it is destroyed by the actions of one or more *cAMP phosphodiesterases* (Figure 11.4).

Signalling associated with an increase in cAMP production

On hormonal stimulation, the cellular cAMP concentration needs to be altered rapidly for it to function as an effective second messenger; it must also be equally rapidly destroyed. The activation of adenyl cyclase by the binding of a single hormone molecule to its receptor results in the generation of many molecules of cAMP, which in turn can phosphorylate many enzymes or other proteins. The extreme sensitivity of metabolic responses to small changes in hormone concentration is partly due to this amplification cascade.

cAMP mediates its physiological actions by activating a single protein kinase – *protein kinase* A (PKA). Each

PKA contains two regulatory (R) chains and two catalytic (C) chains. In the absence of cAMP, the R_2C_2 complex is catalytically inactive. Binding of cAMP results in an activation of PKA due to a release of the catalytic chains which are enzymatically active on their own. The active PKA promotes the phosphorylation of serine or threonine residues on many target proteins and alters their activities. A decrease in cAMP concentration results in a reassociation of the catalytic and regulatory chains. Activated PKA can also stimulate the expression of specific genes by phosphorylating a transcriptional activator called the cAMP-responsive element binding protein (CREB).

One of the best characterised examples of a G-protein receptor coupled to the activation of adenyl cyclase is the β-adrenergic receptor that mediates some of the actions of adrenaline. This receptor, which triggers the adenyl cyclase cascade, is a 7-helix G-protein receptor that spans the plasma membrane of target cells. Adrenaline binds to a pocket formed by the transmembrane helixes. The C-terminus of the receptor that lies on the cytosolic side of the membrane contains reversibly phosphorylatable serine and threonine residues. Phosphorylation of these residues prevents the interaction between the receptor and the G-protein.

The binding of adrenaline to the receptor triggers an exchange of GTP for the bound GDP in the

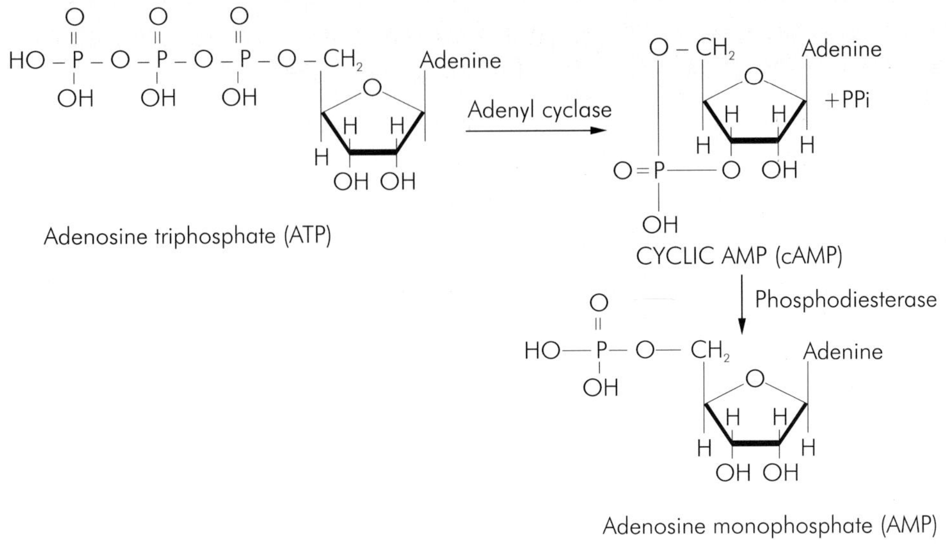

Figure 11.4 – Synthesis and degradation of cyclic AMP.

G-protein. This results in a dissociation of the α_s subunit bearing GTP from the $\beta\gamma$ dimer of the G-protein. The GTP-α_s subunit can activate the membrane-bound adenyl cyclase to generate cAMP that participates in signal transduction within the target cell. Each molecule of bound hormone results in the generation of many activated α_s subunits, thus producing an amplified response. On removal of the extracellular signal, the G-protein action can be terminated by hydrolysis of the GTP by the intrinsic GTPase activity in the protein. In addition, phosphorylation of the C-terminal serine and threonine residues of the receptor protein by the *β-adrenergic receptor kinase* results in a deactivation of the hormone-receptor complex. The ability of the receptor to interact with the G-protein is further diminished by the capping of the phosphorylated receptor by *β-arrestin*. Prolonged exposure to adrenaline results in a desensitization of the β-adrenergic receptor by phosphorylation and β-arrestin binding.

cAMP serves as an intracellular messenger for many different types of signalling molecules. Table 11.1 shows some examples of the variety of hormones that mediate their actions via a G-protein mediated increase in the cellular concentration of cAMP.

Signalling associated with an inhibition of cAMP production

Binding of certain ligands (e.g. *prostaglandin PGE$_1$* and

adenosine) to their receptors results in an activation of G-protein (G$_i$) that inhibits the activity of adenyl cyclase and decreases the cellular concentration of cAMP. As exemplified by adrenaline, the same signalling molecule can either increase or decrease the intracellular concentration of cAMP, depending on the type of receptor to which it binds. The ability of adrenaline to increase cAMP production when bound to a β-adrenergic receptor, and decrease cAMP production when bound to an α-adrenergic receptor, is due to the differences in the type of α-subunit in the G-protein that couples the receptor to the adenyl cyclase (α_s in the G-protein of the α-adrenergic receptor and α_i in the G-protein coupled to the α-adrenergic receptor). Dopamine is another catecholamine that can activate or inhibit adenyl cyclase according to the type of receptor it binds to.

When an activated α_2-adrenergic receptor interacts with G$_i$, the α_i subunit of the G-protein, binds GTP and dissociates from the $\beta\gamma$ dimer. Both the α_i and $\beta\gamma$ dimer are thought to be involved in the inhibition of adenyl cyclase. α_i can directly influence enzyme activity, while $\beta\gamma$ can inhibit the cyclase in one of two ways: by direct binding to the enzyme or by mediating a change in the enzyme activity indirectly by binding to any free stimulatory α_s subunits within the cell. Inhibitory G-protein activity has also been shown to result in the opening of K$^+$channels in the plasma membrane; this function is considered to play a more important role in G$_i$ protein action than adenyl cyclase inhibition.

METABOLIC RESPONSES MEDIATED IN DIFFERENT TISSUES BY HORMONES VIA G-PROTEIN DEPENDENT INCREASES IN INTRACELLULAR CYCLIC AMP (cAMP) CONCENTRATIONS.		
Tissue	Hormone	Metabolic response
Adipose	Adrenaline, Glucagon,	Increased lipolysis
Adrenal cortex	Adrenocorticotrophic hormone	Increased synthesis of cortisol
Bone and kidney	Parathyroid hormone	Increased resorption of Ca^{2+} from bone; increased Ca^{2+} and decreased phosphate reabsorption in kidney
Cardiac muscle	Adrenaline	Increase in rate of contraction
Kidney	Antidiuretic hormone	Reabsorption of water
Liver	Adrenaline, Noradrenaline, Glucagon	Increased glycogenolysis, inhibition of glycogenesis, increased uptake of amino acids and increased gluconeogenesis
Ovarian follicles	Follicle stimulating hormone Luteinizing hormone	Increase in synthesis of oestrogen and progesterone
Pituitary	Thyrotropin-releasing hormone	Increased secretion of thyroid stimulating hormone
Platelets	Prostacyclin (Prostaglandin I)	Inhibition of aggregation and secretion
Skeletal muscle	Adrenaline	Increased glycogenolysis
Thyroid	Thyroid stimulating hormone	Release of thyroid hormones

Table 11.1

SIGNAL TRANSDUCTION MEDIATED VIA AN INCREASE IN CELLULAR cGMP CONCENTRATION

Nitric oxide (NO) is a signal molecule known for many years as the *endothelium-derived relaxation factor (EDRF)* and produced in a variety of cells including endothelium, smooth muscle, cardiac muscle, macrophages and cells of the central nervous system. NO has a number of different roles in the body. It acts as a local tissue regulator and promotes the relaxation of smooth muscles of blood vessels, it helps the cytotoxic activity of macrophages and it acts as a neurotransmitter in the central (CNS) and peripheral nervous (PNS) systems. In the PNS, NO is released by some neurons that innervate the gastrointestinal tract, penis, respiratory

passages and cerebral blood vessels, and promotes smooth muscle relaxation and engorgement of these organs with blood. The relaxing effect of NO on blood vessels is associated with an increase in the amount of cGMP produced by the stimulation of the soluble form of *guanyl cyclase* (this enzyme can also exist in a particulate form), resulting from a binding of NO to a haem group on the enzyme (Figure 11.5). The cGMP in turn activates *protein kinase G* allosterically and mediates the phosphorylation of proteins that relax smooth muscle cells and cause vasodilation. In the brain, the neurotransmitter actions of NO are believed to be implicated in the processes of learning and memory.

Although low concentrations of NO can be beneficial, high concentrations of NO can inhibit several enzymes in the body (Table 11.2) and also be neuro-toxic. The neurotoxicity of high concentrations of NO is thought to be due to an interaction with the superox-ide anion to produce *peroxynitrite* that can nitrosylate many proteins as well as initiate lipid peroxidation.

NO is produced from arginine by the action of *nitric oxide synthase*. At least three forms of NO synthase have been identified — neuronal, constitutive (present in endothelium), and inducible. The neuronal and con-stitutive forms are activated by Ca^{2+} (e.g. during action of ACh on muscarinic receptors on vascular endothe-lial cells). The inducible form of NO synthase is active in the absence of Ca^{2+}. Some bacterial endotoxins and cytokines increase the production of the inducible form of NO synthase in vascular smooth muscle cells, vascular endothelium, myocardium and other cells. The development of shock in septicaemia and during

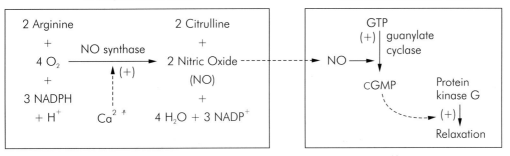

Figure 11.5 – Schematic representation of the synthesis of nitric oxide (NO) in an endothelial cell, and the subsequent relaxation of a smooth muscle cell. NO mediates an activation of *guanylate cyclase* in the muscle cell, to produce cyclic GMP (cGMP) that can cause relaxation of the muscle cell via stimulation of *protein kinase G*.
★ = Ca^{2+} generated by the phosphoinositide pathway (e.g. by binding of an agonist such as Ach, to its receptor) activates NO synthase.
(+) = Enzyme activation.

EXAMPLES OF ENZYMES THAT CAN BE ACTIVATED OR INHIBITED BY NITRIC OXIDE	
Enzyme	Function
Activation	
Cyclooxygenase*	Eicosanoid synthesis
Soluble guanylate cyclase	cGMP formation
Inhibition	
Aconitase	Citric acid cycle
Cyclooxygenase*	Eicosanoid synthesis
Glyceraldehyde 3-phosphate dehydrogenase	Carbohydrate metabolism
NADH-ubiquinone reductase	Electron transfer
NADPH oxidase	Oxygen radical generator
Ribonucleotide reductase	DNA synthesis
Succinate-ubiquinone reductase	Electron transfer
*Low concentrations of NO stimulate the inducible form of cyclooxygenase, while high concentrations of NO can inhibit this enzyme.	

Table 11.2

antitumour therapy with some cytokines is associated with vasodilation resulting from an increased production of NO by the inducible NO synthase.

Because of its muscle relaxing properties, NO has been used clinically to treat pulmonary hypertension as well as respiratory distress syndrome (NO-releasing drugs such as sodium nitroprusside and nitroglycerine have been used for years to promote vasodilation). On the other hand hypotension in certain conditions (e.g. septic shock) is apparently mediated by NO and has been successfully treated with drugs that inhibit NO synthase.

INOSITOL TRIPHOSPHATE AND CALCIUM ION-MEDIATED SIGNAL TRANSDUCTION

Binding of certain signal molecules (e.g. *antidiuretic hormone*) to cell surface receptors results in the activation of membrane bound *phosphoinositide specific phospholipase C* (PLC-β). PLC-β hydrolyses phosphoinositol bisphosphate (PIP$_2$) to generate two intracellu-

lar messengers (Figure 11.6), *inositol 1,4,5-triphosphate (IP$_3$)* and *diacylglycerol (DAG)*, that operate through different mechanisms (but synergistically), to mediate a common metabolic response.

Inositol triphosphate (IP$_3$). In a resting cell, most of the intracellular Ca^{2+} is bound in mitochondria, endoplasmic reticulum (ER), or to the plasma membrane. The cytosolic Ca^{2+} concentration is usually maintained at $< 0.1\mu$mol/L by the action of ATP-dependent Ca^{2+} pumps (which extrude Ca^{2+} in exchange for H$^+$) in the plasma membrane, and by 'pump-leak' systems in the ER and inner mitochondrial membrane.

The cytosolic Ca^{2+} concentration has to be maintained low, to prevent the formation of insoluble calcium phosphate esters. IP$_3$ generated by hormone stimulation of PCL-β passes into the cell cytoplasm and binds to Ca^{2+} receptors on the ER and causes the opening of ion channels, resulting in a rapid release of Ca^{2+} into the cytoplasm that triggers processes such as smooth

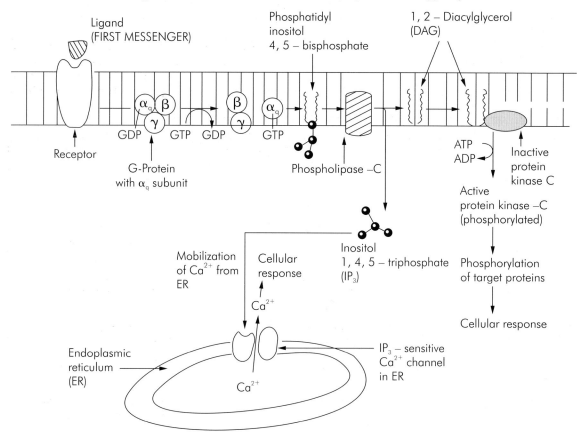

Figure 11.6 – G-protein mediated signal transduction via cyclic AMP as a second messenger. Hydrolysis of GTP to GDP is catalyzed by the intrinsic GTPase activity in the α$_s$-subunit of the G-protein. This step is inhibited by cholera toxin; PKA – Protein kinase A.

muscle contraction, glycogenolysis, and vesicle release by exocytosis (Table 11.3).

The action of IP_3 is very short-lived and within a few seconds IP_3 is inactivated by degradation directly to inositol by the sequential action of phosphatases, or indirectly via inositol 1,3,4,5-tetrakisphosphate.

Diacylglycerol (DAG). This compound remains in the plasma membrane and activates a *protein kinase C* (PKC, Figure 11.6). In unstimulated cells, PKC is located in the cytoplasm, but in stimulated cells the increased cytosolic Ca^{2+} concentration enables the enzyme to bind to the plasma membrane where it is activated by DAG. Activated PKC, like PKA, phosphorylates serine and threonine residues in specific target proteins, and thereby alters the activities of these proteins.

DAG action is short-lived because it is rapidly phosphorylated to phosphatidate or hydrolysed to glycerol and its constituent fatty acids.

ROLE OF CALMODULIN IN CA²⁺-MEDIATED ACTIONS

Many cellular effects of Ca^{2+} are mediated by complexing with the small cytosolic protein *calmodulin*. It contains four calcium-binding. Binding of Ca^{2+} to calmodulin alters the conformation of the protein in such a manner as to enable the Ca^{2+}-calmodulin complex to bind to specific target protein kinases that can modify the actions of other cellular enzymes by the addition of phosphate groups. Two important target proteins activated by the Ca^{2+}-calmodulin complex are (i) the multifunctional, *calmodulin-dependent protein kinase II (CAM kinase II)* that controls the activity of many enzymes involved in fuel metabolism (e.g. cAMP phosphodiesterase that decreases cAMP concentration, and terminates its effects) and (ii) the Ca^+-ATPase pump in the plasma membrane that pumps Ca^{2+} out of cells to restore its low basal cytosolic concentration.

The Ca^{2+}-binding proteins, *troponin C* in skeletal and cardiac muscle, and *myosin light chain* in smooth muscle function in a similar manner to calmodulin when acting as mediators for the action of Ca^{2+}.

SIGNAL TRANSDUCTION VIA G-PROTEIN-MEDIATED ALTERATIONS IN ION CHANNEL ACTIVITY

The binding of a signal molecule to some receptors results in the activation of a particular G-protein, which can cause either directly or indirectly the opening or closing of an ion-channel in the plasma

EXAMPLES OF CELLULAR PROCESSES CONTROLLED BY INOSITOL TRIPHOSPHATE AND CALCIUM ION MEDIATED SIGNAL TRANSDUCTION		
Extracellular signal	Target tissue	Cellular response
Acetylcholine	Pancreas (acinar cells)	Secretion of digestive enzymes (e.g. *amylase, trypsinogen*)
	Pancreas (islet cells) Parotid (salivary gland) Smooth muscle	Insulin release Secretion of amylase Contraction
Antigens	Lymphoblasts Mast cells	DNA synthesis Histamine secretion
Epidermal growth factor (EGF)	Fibroblasts	DNA synthesis, cell division
Thrombin	Blood platelets	Aggregation, shape change, secretion of hormones

Table 11.3

membrane. In *direct G-protein gating of ion channels,* the activated G-protein itself interacts with the ion channel and alters the net diffusion across the plasma membrane of the ion, or ions specific to that channel and thereby causes a change in membrane excitability (membrane potential). The binding of acetylcholine to muscarinic receptors in the heart and in certain neurons leads to the activation of a particular type of K^+ channel via the activation of a G-protein.

In *indirect G-protein gating of ion channels,* the activated G-protein controls the activity of the ion channel by either (i) regulating the phosphorylation of channel proteins by kinases, or (ii) by altering the concentrations of cyclic nucleotides (cAMP or cGMP) that directly activate or inactivate ion channels. Cyclic nucleotide gated ion channels play important roles in vision and olfaction.

Olfaction is mostly mediated by G-proteins of the G_{olf} subclass. The activation of G_{olf} results in a cAMP-mediated opening of ion channels that allow an influx of Na^+; this results in a depolarization of the cell, and initiates an impulse that travels along the axon to the brain.

Vision depends on a decrease in cellular cGMP concentration resulting from a G-protein-mediated activation of cGMP *phosphodiesterase* that degrades cGMP. The photoreceptor cells in the retina are *rods* (that function in dim light) and *cones* (that function in bright light). There are four different photopigments in the retina: *rhodopsin* is found in the rods while each of the other three are found in each of the three types of cones. Each photopigment is comprised of one type of a group of integral proteins, collectively known as *opsin,* bound to a chromophore molecule *11-cis retinal* (a derivative of vitamin A). These photopigments are arranged as stacks of membranous sacs in the outer segments of rod cells.

The plasma membrane of a rod cell contains cation-specific channels that are open in the dark. Entry of Na^+ and Ca^{2+} into the cell through these channels depolarises the plasma membrane, resulting in an increased release of neurotransmitter from these cells. Activation of retinal rod cells by light results in a change in shape due to the conversion of 11-*cis* retinal to *all-trans retinal.* This change facilitates the binding of opsin to a G-protein, *transducin* (G_t), causing the dissociation of the subunit (α_t) that activates cGMP phosphodiesterase, which hydrolyses cGMP. This results in a closure of plasma membrane ion channels controlled by cGMP. The decrease in Na^+ and Ca^{2+} influx that

occurs due to ion channel closure, results in a hyperpolarisation of the plasma membrane (more negative on the inside). This hyperpolarisation is conducted passively to the end of the photoreceptor cell where it decreases the rate of neurotransmitter release from the cell. The decreased neurotransmitter concentration signals to those neurons that synapse with the photoreceptor that light has been absorbed by the receptor. Thus, a light signal is converted to an electric signal via the action of transducin.

CLINICAL IMPORTANCE OF G-PROTEIN ACTIVITY

Inhibition of the activities of G-proteins, or mutations in G-protein coupled receptor genes, have been implicated in the pathogenesis of a variety of human disorders.

Diseases associated with inhibition of G-protein activity

Cholera – is an intestinal disorder caused by the action of a toxin produced by the gram-negative bacterium *Vibrio cholerae* that thrives in contaminated water. On entry of the toxin into cells, one of its subunits (A_1) catalyses the transfer of ADP-ribose from intracellular NAD^+ to a specific arginine residue of the α_s subunit of G-proteins, thus blocking the GTPase activity. Adenyl cyclase molecules activated by this α_s therefore remain in an active state indefinitely, leading to the production of abnormally high concentrations of cAMP in intestinal cells and phosphorylation of membrane proteins involved in active transport. There is inhibition of absorption of NaCl by a NaCl cotransport system and stimulation of Cl^- secretion resulting in massive secretion of Na^+ and water, producing severe diarrhoea.

Pertussis (Whooping cough) – *Bordetella pertussis,* a gram-negative bacterium, causes whooping cough due to the production of the *pertussis* toxin which catalyses the ADP ribosylation of a specific cysteine in the α_i subunit of the G-protein G_i and prevents the interaction of this G-protein with its receptors. Cells cannot therefore inhibit adenyl cyclase or open K^+ channels under physiological conditions and signal transduction is impaired.

Endocrine disorders assoiated with G-protein coupled receptor gene (GPCR) mutations

GPCR mutations underlie a number of endocrine disorders, for example, in X-linked nephrogenic diabetes insipidus, there is impaired cAMP generation due to failure of the vasopressin receptor to couple with G_s.

Cancer

The presence of altered forms of G-proteins and other proteins involved in signal transduction (e.g protein kinases, steroid receptors, growth factors and growth factor receptors) have been shown in a wide variety of tumour cells.

ENZYME-LINKED RECEPTORS

Enzyme-linked receptors either act directly as enzymes or are associated with enzymes (usually protein kinases that phosphorylate specific proteins in target cells). Five classes of enzyme-linked receptors have so far been identified (Table 11.4).

The majority of enzyme-linked receptors are either *tyrosine kinase* or *tyrosine kinase associated receptors*.

Receptors for insulin and other growth factors

Insulin and many other growth factors mediate their actions via *receptors that contain intrinsic tyrosine kinase activity*.

MAJOR CLASSES OF ENZYME-LINKED RECEPTORS AND THEIR BIOCHEMICAL FUNCTIONS		
Classes of enzyme-linked receptors	Function of activated receptor	Examples of receptor
Transmembrane receptor guanylcyclases	Direct generation of cGMP (from GTP) that binds and activates a cGMP-dependent protein-kinase (G-kinase) that phosphorylates serine or threonine residues in specific proteins	Atrial natriuretic peptide receptor on kidney cells and smooth muscle cells of blood vessels
Receptor tyrosine phosphatases	Removal of phosphate from phosphotyrosine side chains of specific proteins	CD-45 protein found on the surface of white blood cells; important in activation of both T and B lymphocytes by foreign antigens
Receptor serine/ threonine kinases	Addition of phosphate group to serine and threonine side chains on target proteins	Transforming growth factor-β receptors
Tyrosine-specific receptor protein kinases	Transfer of phosphate group from ATP to selected tyrosine residues	Insulin receptor; receptors for several growth factors (e.g. epidermal growth factor, nerve growth factor, hepatocyte growth factor)
Tyrosine kinase associated receptor (Kinase domain is encoded by separate gene and is non-covalently associated with receptor protein	Phosphorylation of various target proteins on binding of ligand to the receptor	Receptor for some local mediators (e.g. cytokines), growth hormone, prolactin and antigen-specific receptors on T and B lymphocytes

Table 11.4

The insulin receptor is found in most human cells and consists of two extracellular α-chains with ligand binding sites, connected by disulphide bonds to two β-subunits with tyrosine kinase activity, located on the cytosolic side of the plasma membrane (Figure 11.7). Binding of insulin to the α-subunits, switches on the tyrosine kinase activity of the β-subunits by inducing an allosteric interaction of the two receptor halves. Activation of the kinase results in the cross-phosphorylation (autophosphorylation) of multiple tyrosine residues of the two β-subunits in the cytoplasmic domains of the receptor.

Receptors for growth factors are monomers. Ligand binding induces a conformational change in the extracellular domain of the receptor that allows dimerisation followed by autophosphorylation.

Phosphorylated tyrosine residues in activated tyrosine kinase receptors become the binding sites for several intracellular signalling proteins. Special domains known as SH_2 domains on these proteins help them to recognise phosphorylated tyrosine residues. The SH_2-adaptor proteins serve to couple the activated phosphorylated tyrosine kinase receptor to other target cell proteins involved in cell growth and promote the phosphorylation of these proteins, thereby activating them. Autophosphorylation of receptor tyrosine residues therefore act as a switch that triggers the assembly of a multienzyme signalling complex that relays the signal into the cell interior to mediate the required physiological alteration. Tyrosine kinase activity is terminated by removal of the phosphate groups by *tyrosine phosphatase*.

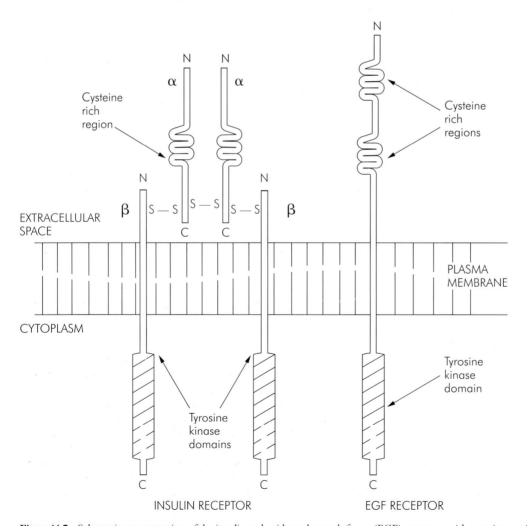

Figure 11.7 – Schematic representation of the insulin and epidermal growth factor (EGF) receptors with protein tyrosine kinase activity.

SIGNAL TRANSDUCTION VIA INTRACELLULAR RECEPTORS

Steroid hormones, vitamins D and A, and thyroid hormones are all small, non-polar molecules that pass easily through the plasma membranes of target cells. Each compound can bind to a specific receptor protein within the cells (cytoplasmic or nuclear receptor, depending on the ligand), and activate gene transcription.

Steroid hormones and related compounds

Steroid hormones, vitamin D and vitamin A (retinoic acid) interact with *cytoplasmic receptor proteins* in the target cells (Figure 11.8). This hormone-receptor complex is translocated into the nucleus, where it attaches by means of the receptor proteins to the chromatin at specific sites called acceptor sites, determined by non-histone (acidic) proteins in the chromatin. As illustrated in Figure 11.8, the glucocorticoid–receptor complex binds to the glucocorticoid response element or GRE located in an enhancer, close to a gene that responds to glucocorticoids. Steroidal regulation of the activity of most target genes appears to be mediated via enhancer activation. The attachment of the steroid hormone-receptor complex to the DNA results in the promotion of gene transcription and the synthesis of RNA that codes for the production of specific proteins that have major effects on growth, tissue development, and body homeostasis. All steroid activated receptors appear to bind to DNA at sequences rich in cysteine, arginine and lysine.

1,25-dihydroxycholecalciferol increases the concentration of mRNA that codes for the *calcium-binding protein* responsible for calcium absorption at the intestine, and protection of cells against increased cytosolic calcium that might otherwise occur. In *vitamin D-dependent rickets, type II*, in which serum concentration of 1,25-dihydroxycholecalciferol is high and is further increased with vitamin D, the receptor protein that binds 1,25-dihydroxycholecalciferol may be defective or absent.

Thyroid hormones

Thyroid hormones bind to triiodothyronine (T_3) receptor proteins already attached to chromatin in the nucleus. Thyroxine (T_4) that enters cells, is enzymatically converted to T_3. As with steroid hormones, the attachment of T_3 to the chromatin bound receptor protein, results in the production of new proteins by gene activation.

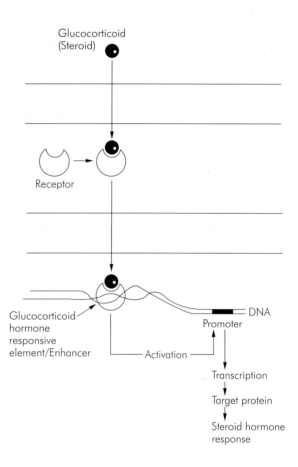

Figure 11.8 – Steroid mediated signal transduction via binding to intracellular receptors. Steroid hormones bind to cytoplasmic receptors which then pass into the nucleus and bind to DNA.

BIOCHEMISTRY AND PHYSIOLOGY OF SELECTED SIGNAL MOLECULES

HORMONES

According to the relationship of hormones generated by endocrine glands to the central nervous system, three levels of hormones can be recognised (Figure 11.9). Detailed accounts of the biochemistry and physiology of hormones produced by the hypothalmus, pituitary, thyroid, adrenal glands, gonads and parathyroids are presented later. This section will therefore focus only on insulin and related peptide hormones produced by pancreatic cells, and the eicosanoids, that can act both as hormones and local mediators.

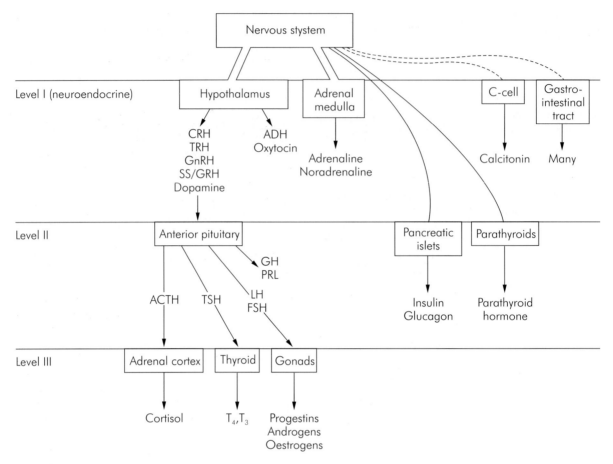

Figure 11.9 – Organization of the endocrine system.
Level I includes hormones generated by endocrine tissue derived embryologically from nervous tissue.
Level II include hormones generated by endocrine tissues directly or indirectly influenced by the nervous system.
Level III includes hormones generated by endocrine tissues that exhibit strong dependence on the anterior pituitary; they usually affect gene transcription in target cells.
(Adapted with kind permission from Bhagavan, N.V. *Medical Biochemistry*. Jones and Bartlett Publishers London, 1992, Fig 30–10, p 748).

PEPTIDE HORMONES SYNTHESISED BY PANCREATIC CELLS

The peptide hormones *glucagon, insulin, somatostatin* and *pancreatic polypeptide* are produced by the α (or A), β (or B), δ (or D), and E cells respectively, of the pancreatic islets of Langerhans. Each of the above hormones is synthesised as part of a larger molecule (*pre-prohormone*) that each have a leader sequence (signal peptide) of hydrophobic amino acids at its amino terminal end, that directs the polypeptide into the cisternae of the endoplasmic reticulum. After entry of the polypeptide into the endoplasmic reticulum lumen, the leader sequence is released, and the resultant *prohormone* undergoes further post-translational processing such as proteolytic cleavage (both

endoproteolytic and exoproteolytic) at specific sites before the mature hormone is released into the circulation.

Insulin

Proinsulin contains the B- and A-chains found in mature insulin, joined together by a connecting peptide known as the *C-peptide*. This molecule undergoes site specific cleavages catalysed by the Ca^{2+}-requiring enzymes, *prohormone convertase 2 (PC2)* and *prohormone convertase 3/1 (PC3/1)*, and *carboxypeptidase H*, to yield equimolar amounts of the mature insulin, and the C-peptide. The mature insulin molecule consists of an A-chain of 21 amino acid residues, and a B-chain of 30 residues, linked covalently by two disulphide bonds. The C-peptide has no known biological activity, and is not destroyed by anti-insulin antibodies. Assay of C-peptide may be used to distinguish insulin secreted endogenously from insulin administered exogenously.

Insulin is released from the pancreatic β-cells in response to high circulating concentrations of glucose. Its major sites of action for the regulation of blood glucose are liver and skeletal muscle. Insulin secretion is also markedly increased by chronic exposure to excessive concentrations of growth hormone, cortisol, placental lactogen, oestrogens and progestins (e.g. in late pregnancy). On the other hand, α-adrenergic agonists (mainly adrenaline), inhibit insulin release from the pancreas.

Its effects on intermediary metabolism (carbohydrate, protein and lipid metabolism) and the clinical consequences of insulin deficiency, have already been discussed in detail. Long-term effects of insulin require internalisation of the hormone-receptor complex by endocytosis, and phosphorylation of serine and threonine residues of specific enzymes (e.g. enzymes involved in glycogen metabolism and triacylglycerol synthesis), as well as alterations in the concentrations of specific proteins (e.g. phosphoenolpyruvate carboxykinase, glucokinase and pyruvate kinase), by influencing the rates of transcription of the corresponding mRNAs .

Insulin has a short plasma half-life (3–5 minutes under normal conditions) and is rapidly metabolised by liver, kidneys and placenta, by two enzyme systems – (i) an *insulin-specific protease,* and (ii) *glutathione-insulin transhydrogenase.*

Glucagon

Glucagon is a single-chain polypeptide hormone containing 29 amino acid residues. Secretion of glucagon from the pancreatic α-cells, is inhibited by glucose. It is not clear whether this inhibition is mediated via insulin or insulin-like growth factors, that are produced by the pancreatic islet cells.

The actions of glucagon are usually opposed to those of insulin. For example, glucagon stimulates glycogenolysis and gluconeogenesis in the liver by binding to specific plasma membrane receptors and stimulating adenyl cyclase activity in cells of these tissues, while insulin has opposite effects. Similarly, glucagon increases the rate of transcription of the key gluconeogenic enzyme phosphoenolpyruvate carboxykinase, while insulin inhibits its transcription.

Somatostatin and Pancreatic polypeptide

Somatostatin is a 15 amino acid polypeptide, and pancreatic polypeptide is a 36 amino acid peptide. The biochemical and molecular actions of these hormones are not well known. Somatostatin inhibits the release of other pancreatic hormones, and decreases the delivery of nutrients from the gastrointestinal tract into the circulation. The secretion of pancreatic polypeptide is increased by a protein meal, fasting, exercise, and acute hypoglycaemia.

EICOSANOIDS

The eicosanoinds are a family of signal molecules produced from the polyunsaturated, 20-carbon fatty acid, *arachidonic acid,* generated from plasma membrane phospholipids, by the enzyme-mediated reactions shown in Figure 11.10. The principal eicosanoids generated from arachidonic acid are the *prostaglandins (PGs), prostacyclins, thromboxanes,* and *leukotrienes.* The synthesis of PGs and thromboxanes depends on the actions of the microsomal protein *prostaglandin endoperoxide synthase* complex that contains a *cyclooxygenase* that requires two oxygen molecules for activity, and a *peroxidase,* that requires reduced glutathione for activity.

The conversion of the parent prostaglandin H_2 (PGH_2) (Figure 11.10) to *prostacyclin* is catalysed by *prostacyclin synthase* present in arterial walls. *Thromboxane* synthesis that occurs in blood platelets is catalysed by *thromboxane synthase.* The action of *5-lipoxygenase* on arachidonic acid in leucocytes, mast cells, platelets, and macrophages, in response to both immunologic and non-immunologic stimuli results in the production of *leukotrienes.* Unlike the actions of hormones produced by endocrine glands, the physiologic effects of most eicosanoids are exerted on cells and tissues near sites of synthesis (paracrine) rather than at distant sites.

Each of the major eicosanoid sub-divisions can be divided further, into several groups according to structural differences among its members. For example, prostaglandins (that are characterised by the presence of a cyclopentane ring in their structure) can be grouped into several series, depending on the substituents on the cyclopentane ring. Each series of PGs is designated a letter (e.g. PGE and PGF for prostaglandins of the E and F series respectively). Depending on the number of double bonds present in

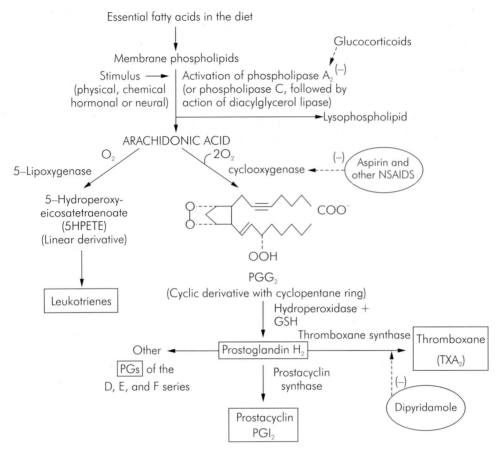

Figure 11.10 – An outline of the routes by which prostaglandins and other major eicosanoids are synthesised in the body. PG = Prostaglandin; NSAIDs = Non-steroidal anti-inflammatory drugs; (-) = Inhibition of enzyme activity.

its structure, each PG within a series is denoted by a subscript numeral (e.g. PGE_1, PGE_2 and PGE_3 that contain 1, 2, and 3 double bonds respectively).

PGs of the E and F series (physiologically, the most important series) are produced in most tissues. The actions of PGs in platelets, thyroid, corpus luteum, fetal bone, adenohypophysis and lung, are promoted by a receptor mediated increase in cAMP; in renal tubules and adipose tissue, their actions are mediated via a decrease in cAMP.

Inhibition of eicosanoid synthesis

Non-steroidal anti-inflammatory drugs (NSAIDs) such as *aspirin* and *indomethacin*, block the synthesis of endoperoxides, PGs and thromboxanes. Aspirin blocks

eicosanoid synthesis by acetylating a serine residue at the active site of *cyclooxygenase*, and inhibiting the enzyme irreversibly. Inhibition of cyclooxygenase by other NSAIDs is not covalent or irreversible as with aspirin. The ability of aspirin to inhibit cyclooxygenase (and therefore thromboxane production) is thought to be the basis for the use of low doses of aspirin to reduce the incidence of myocardial infarction and stroke in patients.

Steroidal hormones (e.g. *cortisol*) *produced by the adrenal glands*, that are used as anti-inflammatory drugs, also block the synthesis of all eicosanoids, by inhibiting *phospholipase A_2.*

Biomedical importance of eicosanoids

Eicosanoids possess diverse and potent biological

EXAMPLES OF THE BIOLOGICAL ACTIONS OF EICOSANOIDS		
Eicosanoid type	Major site of production	Biological action
Prostaglandins (PGs)		
PGE_2	Most tissues, especially kidney	Vasodilation, relaxation of smooth muscle
PGF_2	Most tissues	Vasoconstriction, contraction of smooth muscle, stimulation of uterine contraction
PGI_2	Endothelium	Vasodilatation, inhibition of platelet aggregation, increased formation of cAMP
Thromboxanes (TXs)		
TXA_2	Platelets	Promotion of platelet aggregation, decreased formation of cAMP, vaso-constriction, mobilisation of intracellular calcium, contraction of smooth muscle
Leukotrienes (LTs)		
LTA_4	Leucocytes, platelets, mast cells, heart and lung vascular tissue	*After conversion to LTE_4,* causes contraction of smooth muscle, bronchoconstriction, vasoconstriction, increase in vascular permeability, act as components of slow reacting substances of anaphylaxis *After conversion to LTB_4* Increases chemotaxis of polymorphonuclear leucocytes, release of lysosomal enzymes, and adhesion of white blood cells

Table 11.5

activities, affecting cell function in most organ systems. These actions are summarized in Table 11.5.

As shown in Table 11.5, thromboxanes and prostacyclins derived from arachidonic acid, have antagonistic actions; thromboxanes cause vasoconstriction and platelet aggregation while prostacyclins are potent inhibitors of platelet aggregation. The ability of *fish oil* to reduce the incidence of heart disease, diminish platelet aggregation and prolong clotting times in humans, is thought to be due to the presence of 20:5 ω3 (EPA or eicosapentanoic acid) fatty acids which give rise to the series 3 PGs (PG_3) and thromboxane TX_3. PG_3 and TX_3 inhibit the release of arachidonate from phospholipids, and therefore, the formation of PG_2 and TX_2. The inhibitory activity of PGI_3 on platelet aggregation is similar to that shown by PGI_2, but TX_3 is a weaker aggregator than TX_2; the balance of activity is therefore shifted towards non-aggregation.

Based on the various actions of PGs, they have many therapeutic applications. Potential therapeutic uses of PGs include:

- induction of labour at term and termination of pregnancy, because of the stimulatory actions of some PGs on uterine contraction (e.g. PGE_2 and PGF_2)

- prevention and treatment of peptic ulcers, because of the inhibitory activities on HCl secretion by gastric cells (e.g. PGE_1)

- inhibiting the effect of ADH in the kidney (e.g. PGE_1)

- treatment of bronchial asthma, due to bronchodilatory actions (e.g. PGEs)

- decreasing the risk of blood clotting during surgery (e.g. prostacyclins can inhibit platelet aggregation)

- control of inflammation and of blood pressure (e.g. PGEs and PGAs have vasodilatory and hypotensive effects)

NEUROTRANSMITTERS

The modes of action, and disorders associated with abnormal metabolism of selected neurotransmitters are summarised in Tables 11.6 and 11.7.

GROWTH FACTORS

Growth factors are generally defined as substances that control cell proliferation; they are produced by many different cells in the body. Most growth factors are peptides, although some non-protein classes of molecules (e.g. steroid hormones) also function as growth factors. Growth factors exert a *mitogenic response* in many different types of cells (e.g. cells from blood, nervous system, mesenchymal cells, and epithelial tissue) through a complex of intracellular signalling cascades, which ultimately regulate gene transcription and the functioning of the cell cycle control system.

Some examples of the better known peptide growth factors and their actions are summarized in Table 11.8. As stated in the section on enzyme-linked receptors, at target tissues, peptide growth factors bind to plasma membrane receptors that exhibit tyrosine kinase activity, and mediate their actions through the phosphorylation of tyrosine residues in specific proteins. Most growth factors are local mediators, and can act in an autocrine or paracrine manner, although some growth factors (e.g. epidermal growth factor or EGF) can function in an endocrine manner.

Growth factor activity can be blocked by *growth inhibitory factors* in the body (e.g. transforming growth factor-β or TGF-β, that inhibits growth of most cell types, except fibroblasts). The balance of cell growth can therefore be altered by chronic exposure to increased amounts of a growth factor or to decreased amounts of a growth inhibitory factor.

CYTOKINES

Interleukins and *transforming growth factors* (Table 9.8), are members of the *cytokine family* that include a heterogeneous group of water soluble polypeptides produced in response to inflammatory stimuli, and exercise specific receptor-mediated effects in an autocrine, or paracrine manner. The *tumour necrosis factors* (α and β), and the *interferons* (α, β, and γ) are two other types of well known and important cytokines that have been characterised. Until recently, cytokines were thought to be the products of phagocytic immune cells; however, it is now known that they can also be produced by T and B lymphocytes, fibroblasts, and various endothelial cells. Cytokines are not only produced as a part of the non-specific immune response to invasion of parasites and bacteria, but also in inflammatory diseases such as *Crohn's disease* and *rheumatoid arthritis,* which do not involve pathogens. They are also produced in conditions of physiological change, such as during the menstrual cycle, or after strenuous exercise. A great number of cytokines have been identified and characterised. A detailed knowledge of cytokines can be obtained by reference to any standard text book of immunology.

Cytokines have short half-lives, and are present in the plasma in very low concentrations, but they have very high biological specific activities (i.e. active at picomolar concentrations). Cytokines can themselves be influenced by other regulators (e.g. hormones and other cytokines) in either antagonistic or synergistic ways. Because cytokines are potent stimulators for the production of other cytokines, patients exposed to an inflammatory response may experience a cascade of cytokine production.

A single cytokine can act on many different target cell types by binding to specific receptors at the plasma membranes of these cells. The receptors for cytokines belong to several sub-families. For example, many cytokines mediate their actions via protein tyrosine kinase receptors; some cytokines such as *erythropoietin* (Table 11.8), mediate their effects by binding to receptors that are single, transmembrane proteins that lack protein-tyrosine kinase or other enzyme activity. Binding of erythropoietin to these receptors activates a membrane associated non-receptor protein tyrosine kinase called JAK 2 (Janus kinase 2); JAK 2 is also involved in the signal transduction of growth hormone and some interleukins (eg IL_2 and IL_5). Other interleukins (e.g. IL_8) mediate their actions via receptors with 7-transmembrane segments that interact with G-proteins, and activate phospholipase C. It is not clear which cytosolic enzymes these receptors influence.

Although cytokines are essential for recovery processes, they are lethal in high doses. Mechanisms must therefore exist in the body to down-regulate their pro-

SELECTED NEUROTRANSMITTERS AND NEUROHORMONES AND THEIR BIOLOGICAL FUNCTIONS		
Signal molecule	Function and remarks	Receptor type and mechanism of signal transduction
Acetylcholine	Excitatory neurotransmitter at neuromuscular junction and at pre- and post-ganglionic parasympathetic and preganglionic sympathetic nervous system junctions	*Nicotinic* (2 types) Formation of ion channels at neuro-muscular junction or autonomic ganglion in the central nervous system *Muscarinic* (5 types) Inhibition of adenyl cyclase coupled to activation of K^+ channels or activation of phospholipase C
Adrenaline	Excitatory neurotransmitter; participates in regulation of arterial pressure	α_1 activates phospholipase C α_2 inhibits adenyl cyclase β_1,β_2,β_3- activate adenyl cyclase
Dopamine	Excitatory neurotransmitter	Several receptors types; activation or inhibition of adenyl cyclase depending on type; adenyl cyclase inhibitors open K^+ channels
GABA (γ-aminobutyric acid)	Chief inhibitory neurotransmitter in brain	$GABA_A$- increase Cl^- conductance; contains allosteric sites for diazepam and barbiturates $GABA_B$ – inhibit adenyl cyclase and affect Ca^{2+} and K^+ channels via G-protein action
Glycine	Chief inhibitory neurotransmitter in spinal cord	Similar to $GABA_A$ receptor; Increases Cl^- flux and hyperpolarises post-synaptic neurons
Glutamate	Chief excitatory neurotransmitter in central nervous system; also plays a role in learning and memory	Several receptor types; some function as ligand activated cation channels, some activate phospholipase C; some activate cyclic nucleotide phosphodiesterase in retina
Histamine	Possible function in the sleep-wake cycle	H_1 receptor – linked to G-protein and Phospholipase action H_2-receptor – linked to G-protein and adenyl cyclase activation (blocked by Cimetidine and related H_2 antagonists)
Noradrenaline	Transmission of nerve impulses in the post ganglionic sympathetic nervous system	Ligand activated cation channel receptor
Serotonin	Excitatory neurotransmitter in brain; participates in sleep and arousal	Several receptor types; some inhibit adenyl cyclase(with or without opening of K^+ channels); others activate adenyl cyclase (and close K^+ channels) or activate phospholipase C (and close K^+ channels)
Opioids	Neuromodulators produced in the central and peripheral nervous systems, gut and adrenal medulla	Receptors linked to G_i-proteins; actions mediated via inhibition of adenyl cyclase

Table 11.6

EXAMPLES OF DISORDERS ASSOCIATED WITH ALTERATIONS IN THE ACTIVITY OF NEUROTRANSMITTERS		
Neurotransmitter	Functional defect and cause	Disorder and remarks
Acetylcholine	Decreased activity due to development of autoantibodies (IgG) against nicotinic receptors at neurotransmitter junctions	*Myasthenia gravis* Treatment may include administration of acetyl-choline esterase inhibitors (e.g. *pyridostigmine, neostigmine*) to prolong activity of acetylcholine at motor end plates *Alzheimer's disease* *Tacrine* used in treatment of Alzheimer's disease is a long-acting cholinesterase inhibitor
Dopamine	Decreased activity due to increased uptake into, and degradation of dopamine in neurons of the dopaminergic nigrostriatal pathway in the brain	*Parkinson's disease* Treatment may involve administration of (i) drugs such as *deprenyl* that inhibit the degradation of dopamine and other biogenic amines by *monoamine oxidase type B* (ii) *L-dopa* that can cross the blood-brain barrier and serve as a substrate for dopamine biosynthesis in striatal cells *Schizophrenia* Circumstantial evidence links defects in dopamine metabolism to schizophrenia. Most drugs used for treatment (e.g. *chlorpromazine*) are dopamine D_2 receptor antagonists
Serotonin	Decreased activity due to increased uptake and degradation in brain cells	*Depression* Treatment may include administration of *tricyclic anti-depressants* that inhibit uptake of both noradrenaline and adrenaline into brain cells, or other antidepressants such as *fluoxetine (Prozac)* that preferentially inhibit serotonin uptake Inhibitors of *monoamine oxidase A* that convert serotonin to an inactive aldehyde may also be used

Table 11.7

duction and actions. A number of studies have shown that glucocorticoids and prostaglandins are each able to inhibit cytokine production, although the biological significance of these effects remains to be determined. Recent investigations have also revealed the presence of a naturally occurring IL_1 receptor antagonist (IL - 1ra) that can block the inflammatory actions of IL_1.

Cytokines as therapeutic agents

Interferons are currently being evaluated as *antiviral and anticancer agents*. The antiviral effects of interferons are due to the stimulation of a protein kinase and an oligonucleotide synthetase which inhibit viral protein synthesis.

Interleukins are used for the *treatment of cancer*. In most cancer patients, the number of cytotoxic T-cells (CD8[+] cells) is insufficient to fight against the tumour cell population. One of the methods used to overcome this involves the removal of T-cells from the patient, and their culture *in vitro* with IL_2. Limited success has been reported with such lymphokine activated killer cell therapy (LAK therapy).

Attempts are also being made to use cytokines for *osteoinduction*. Bone for transplantation is in short supply, and attempts are being made to try and exploit the bone forming properties of some cytokines to try and increase the quantity of bone available.

GROWTH FACTORS AND THEIR BIOLOGICAL FUNCTIONS	
Growth factor	Function
Epidermal growth factor Transforming growth factor-α	Stimulate growth of many epidermal and epithelial cells and some neuroglial cells
Erythropoietin	Regulates development of early erythropoietic cells
Fibroblast growth factor	Stimulates proliferation of many cell types; inhibits differentiation of some stem cell types; acts as inductive signal in embryonic development
Haematopoietin A	Stimulates proliferation of hepatocytes
Insulin-like growth factor-1	Promotes cell survival; stimulates cell metabolism; stimulates cell proliferation in collaboration with other growth factors
Interleukin-1 Interleukin-2	Stimulates production of IL-2 by T-cells Stimulates growth of T-cells.
Interleukin-3 Haemopoietic colony stimulating factors	Stimulate proliferation and survival of various types of blood cell precursors
Nerve growth factor Brain derived neurotrophic fator; neutrophins	Trophic effects on sympathetic and certain sensory neurons
Transforming growth factor-β, Bone morphogenetic proteins Activins	Exert both stimulatory and inhibitory effects on responses of many cells to other growth factors; regulate differentiation of some cell types

Table 11.8

SELECTED READING

Alberts, B., Bray, D., Lewis, J., Raff, M., Roberts, K., and Watson, J.D. – *Molecular Biology of the Cell*, 3rd ed. Garland Publishing Inc., London, 1994.

Billiar, T.R. – Nitric oxide: novel biology with clinical relevance. *Annals of Surgery* 1995; **221**: 339–349.

Bredt, D.S. and Snyder, S.H. – Nitric oxide, a physiological messenger molecule. *Annual Review of Biochemistry* 1994; **63**: 175–195.

Galvani, D.W. – Cytokines: biological function and clinical use. *Journal of the Royal College of Physicians* 1988; **22**: 226–231.

Matfin, G. – The role of cytokines in normal and pathological bone states. *British Journal of Hospital Medicine* 1993; **49**: 407–415.

Mathews, C.K. and Van Holde, K.E. – *Biochemistry*, 2nd ed. The Benjamin/Cummings Publishing Co. Inc., N.Y., 1996.

Voet, D. and Voet, J.G. – *Biochemistry*, 2nd ed. John Wiley and Sons Inc., N.Y. 1995.

12

SODIUM, WATER AND POTASSIUM

BODY WATER

The minimum daily water requirement is about 1L. This is obtained from the diet and from oxidative metabolism. Water loss occurs from the kidney – a urine volume of about 0.5L being the minimum urine volume for waste product excretion. The gut, lungs and skin are also sources of water loss.

About 60% of body weight in men is due to water, slightly less in women due to their increased proportion of body fat. Intracellular fluid (ICF) comprises about two thirds of body water and the remainder is the extracellular fluid (ECF). Plasma contains less than 10% of body water.

The ECF and ICF differ in their electrolyte composi-

tion. The principle cation in the ECF is sodium and that of the ICF is potassium. The action of Na^+, K^+-ATPase at the cell membrane maintains this difference. The movement of body water between ECF and ICF is related to their relative osmotic pressures. The colloid osmotic, or oncotic, pressure is the osmotic pressure due to the difference in protein concentration between plasma and interstitial fluid – albumin being the major contributor. Capillary endothelium is not freely permeable to protein and, as the interstitial fluid protein concentration is less than that of plasma, colloid osmotic pressure is important in the distribution of ECF between intra- and extravascular compartments.

Almost all cell membranes are water permeable but the solute content of cells is essentially fixed. ICF volume is therefore determined by body water. Control of both water output and input exists. Control of renal water output is exerted via antidiuretic hormone (ADH) acting on the distal tubules. Control of water input is via both osmotic and non-osmotic control of thirst.

ECF volume is dependent on its sodium content which is controlled via conservation of sodium within the kidney and by sodium appetite. Sodium conservation within the kidney is the result of intrinsic renal control, the renin-angiotensin-aldosterone system and by natriuretic hormones. About four fifths of sodium filtered in the kidney are reabsorbed in the proximal tubules. The renin-angiotensin-aldosterone system is summarised in Figure 12.1.

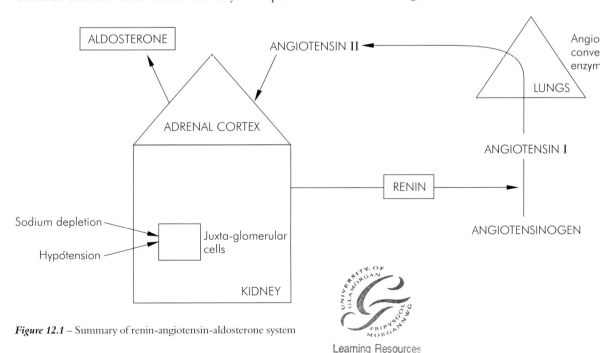

Figure 12.1 – Summary of renin-angiotensin-aldosterone system

Renin is secreted from the juxtaglomerular cells of the kidney in response to a decrease in blood pressure or to sodium depletion. Renin catalyses the formation of angiotensin I from the α_2-globulin angiotensinogen. During its passage through the lungs angiotensin I is metabolised to angiotensin II by angiotensin converting enzyme. Angiotensin II then acts to stimulate aldosterone release from the adrenal cortex and has other effects on sodium homeostasis. Aldosterone acts to stimulate reabsorption of sodium ions in the distal tubules of the kidneys in exchange for potassium and hydrogen ions. Atrial natriuretic peptide is secreted from the heart in situations of increased atrial pressure. Its exact physiological role is uncertain but it can decrease plasma renin activity and aldosterone concentration resulting in increased sodium excretion. In situations of severe sodium loss, a salt appetite can occur.

DISORDERS OF SALT AND WATER HOMEOSTASIS

In all situations of deficiency or excess of sodium there is a co-existing abnormality of water homeostasis, however certain circumstances exist in which features

are attributable more to abnormality of one than the other.

SODIUM AND WATER DEPLETION

The clinical effects of predominant sodium depletion are largely a result of decreased ECF volume. The response to this is an increased secretion of aldosterone which stimulates sodium reabsorption in the distal tubule. Glomerular filtration rate decreases and antidiuretic hormone secretion increases resulting in production of a small volume of highly concentrated urine. Haematocrit and plasma protein concentration are increased and clinical signs are of circulatory failure.

Predominant water depletion results in an increased ECF osmolality, in spite of compensatory water movement from the ICF. Stimulation of thirst mechanisms and antidiuretic hormone excretion occur. Hypernatraemia results but haematocrit and plasma protein concentration are not usually markedly abnormal. Cerebral dehydration can occur in severe water depletion.

Causes of sodium and water depletion are compared in Table 12.1.

CAUSES OF SODIUM AND WATER DEPLETION		
	Predominant sodium depletion	Predominant water depletion
Increased loss:		
From kidney	diuretics	renal tubular disorders
	diuretic phase of acute tubular necrosis	diabetes insipidus
	mineralocorticoid deficiency	increased osmotic load e.g. diabetes mellitus
From gut	vomiting	diarrhoea
	diarrhoea	
	fistulae	
	ileus	
	intestinal obstruction	
From skin	sweating + + +	sweating
	burns	
	dermatitis	
	cystic fibrosis	
From lungs		hyperventilation
Inadequate intake:		
Rare except when inadequate to balance excessive loss		unconsciousness
		infancy, old age
		dysphagia

Table 12.1

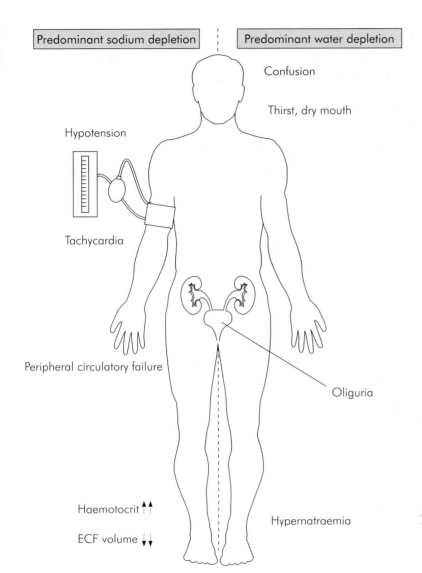

Predominant sodium depletion   Predominant water depletion

Confusion

Thirst, dry mouth

Hypotension

Tachycardia

Peripheral circulatory failure

Oliguria

Haemotocrit ↑↑

ECF volume ↓↓

Hypernatraemia

Figure 12.2 – Clinical effects of sodium and water depletion.

Sodium depletion occurs more frequently than pure water depletion. Clinical features of sodium and water depletion are compared in Figure 12.2.

SODIUM AND WATER EXCESS

As with deficiency, sodium and water excess involve both components but one may predominate. Sodium excess is most frequently due to secondary hyper-aldosteronism but is then often accompanied by hyponatraemia. Causes of sodium and water excess are shown in Table 12.2.

Water excess is usually related to impaired ability of water excretion although rarely can be caused by exces-

sive intake. Clinical features of sodium and water excess are shown in Figure 12.3.

HYPONATRAEMIA

Hyponatraemia has many causes and is relatively common. It is more often related to water excess than to sodium deficiency. However, due to the complex relationships between sodium and water balance hyponatraemia can occur in states of sodium excess. In hospital patients, hyponatraemia is often thought to be the result of the "sick cell syndrome" – a reduction in cellular osmotic pressure may underlie this syndrome but its aetiology is multifactorial. Causes of hyponatraemia are shown in Figure 12.4.

CAUSES OF SODIUM AND WATER EXCESS	
Predominant sodium excess	**Predominant water excess**
Increased intake:	
Excessive parenteral administration	excessive parenteral administration
	excessive enteral administration (rare)
	absorption from bladder irrigation
Decreased excretion:	
Acute renal failure	renal failure
Increased tubular reabsorption:	cortisol deficiency
1°mineralocorticoid excess-Conn's syndrome	ectopic or inappropriate secretion of ADH
Cushing's syndrome	
2°mineralocorticoid excess-congestive cardiac failure	
liver disease & ascites	
nephrotic syndrome	
renal artery stenosis	

Table 12.2

Spurious hyponatraemia occurs when venous sampling is performed close to the site of an intravenous infusion of fluid with a sodium concentration less than that of plasma. The infusion fluid usually contains dextrose, therefore spurious hyperglycaemia usually co-exists. Pseudohyponatraemia occurs, with some methods of laboratory analysis, when the plasma contains a high concentration of lipid or protein replacing some of the plasma water. Sodium content of the plasma water is unchanged but the plasma sample contains less water, the osmolality (mmol/kg) of the sample is normal. Hypoaldosteronism in adrenal failure can cause hyponatraemia due to renal sodium loss, and a dilutional effect secondary to lack of glucocorticoid action as cortisol has a permissive effect on water excretion. In secondary hyperaldosteronism there are clinical features such as oedema suggestive of increased ECF volume with redistribution of fluid between the extravascular and vascular compartments – such patients are often hyponatraemic. The syndrome of inappropriate ADH (SIADH) can result for example from pulmonary, neurological and therapeutic causes. Ectopic ADH secretion, most commonly from bronchiogenic carcinoma, can also be the cause. The syndrome occurs in the presence of normal renal and adrenal function and with no oedema on clinical examination. Laboratory investigation reveals hyponatraemia and a sodium-containing urine the osmolality of which is inappropriately high.

Correction of disorders of sodium and water home-ostasis should be slow as cerebral damage has been associated with rapid restoration of plasma sodium to the reference range.

LABORATORY INVESTIGATION OF DISORDERS OF SODIUM AND WATER HOMEOSTASIS

Measurement of plasma sodium concentration, whilst useful, is not a reliable guide to body sodium status as it can be low, normal or even high in sodium deficiency. Measurement of urinary sodium concentration can be a useful investigation, a low value (< 20 mmol/L) in the presence of hyponatraemia indicating sodium depletion. Osmotic pressure can be thought of in terms of osmolarity (mmol/L) or osmolality (mmol/kg). Plasma osmolality can be measured and osmolarity can be calculated from the formula $2([Na^+]+[K^+])+[Urea]+[Glucose]$. The measured and calculated values are usually comparable but a difference, the osmolar gap, can occur in the presence of extreme hyperlipidaemia or hyperproteinaemia or of abnormal substances such as mannitol or alcohol.

The laboratory investigation of hyponatraemia should exclude a spurious result by the measurement of a plasma osmolality initially but this does not need to be repeated. Measurement of urine sodium is useful, a low concentration being found in sodium deficiency,

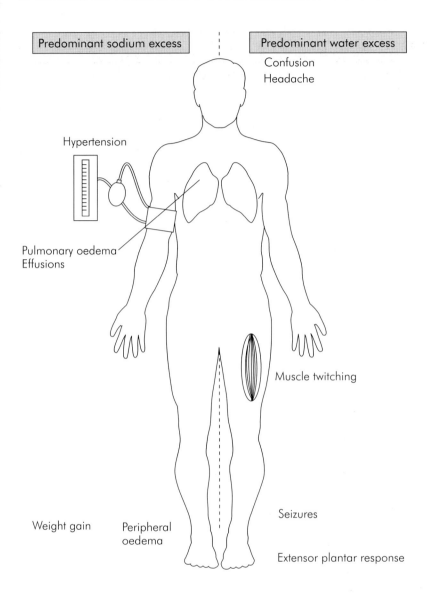

Predominant sodium excess

Predominant water excess

Confusion
Headache

Hypertension

Pulmonary oedema
Effusions

Muscle twitching

Weight gain   Peripheral
oedema

Seizures

Extensor plantar response

Figure 12.3 – Clinical features of sodium and water excess.

and natriuresis in adrenal failure and SIADH. An inappropriately high urine osmolality is also found in SIADH. Thyroid function tests should be performed as hypothyroidism can lead to ADH release and a Synacthen test may need to be carried out to investigate the state of the adrenal glands.

POTASSIUM

Potassium homeostasis is achieved mainly in the kidney with reabsorption of almost all filtered potassium in the proximal tubule. In the distal tubules potassium and hydrogen ions are secreted in response to the electrochemical gradient engendered by aldosterone-mediated sodium reabsorption. The amount of potassium actually secreted in the urine is therefore in part linked with that of sodium and hydrogen ions. It follows that alkalosis tends to be associated with hypokalaemia and acidosis with hyperkalaemia. The colon plays a small part in potassium homeostasis by alteration of its potassium secretion. Potassium is the main intracellular cation and as such measurement of plasma potassium is not an accurate reflection of total body potassium.

CAUSES OF HYPONATRAEMIA
Spurious sampling above dextrose infusion hyperproteinaemia hyperlipidaemia **With increased ECF volume** renal failure congestive cardiac failure hypoproteinaemic states "sick cell syndrome" **With normal ECF volume** acute water intoxication SIADH chronic renal failure glucocorticoid deficiency **With low ECF volume** gastrointestinal loss renal loss skin loss

Figure 12.4

HYPOKALAEMIA

Hypokalaemia is a common clinical problem. Causes of hypokalaemia are shown in Figure 12.5.

Diuretics are a frequent cause of hypokalaemia and concomitant treatment with potassium-sparing diuretics or supplements may be necessary. In renal tubular acidosis abnormality of bicarbonate absorption (type 1) or hydrogen ion excretion (type 2) results in acidosis with hypokalaemia.

Clinical features of hypokalaemia are shown in Figure 12.6.

Hypokalaemia can underlie a wide range of symptoms and signs but, even when severe, may be asymptomatic.

Treatment of hypokalaemia is by replacement, either oral or intravenous, and should usually be considered when plasma potassium concentration is < 3mmol/L.

HYPERKALAEMIA

Hyperkalaemia does not always imply surfeit of total body potassium and can occur in the face of total body potassium depletion, for example in diabetic ketoacidosis. Causes of hyperkalaemia are shown in Figure 12.7.

CAUSES OF HYPOKALAEMIA
Decreased intake parenteral oral (rare) **Increased loss** renal diuretics mineralocorticoid excess – Conn's syndrome   Cushing's syndrome renal tubular acidosis **Gastrointestinal** diarrhoea laxative abuse vomiting fistulae **Transcellular movement** alkalosis rapid cellular proliferation

Figure 12.5

Spurious causes of hyperkalaemia are common in clinical practice and should always be excluded before clinical significance is attached to a result.

Clinical effects of hyperkalaemia are shown in Figure 12.8

The most serious effects of hyperkalaemia are on the cardiovascular system and ECG changes can be exacerbated by co-existing hypocalcaemia, hyponatraemia and hypermagnesaemia.

Intravenous glucose infused with insulin promotes uptake of potassium into cells, as does salbutamol and both are used as treatments for hyperkalaemia. Intravenous calcium gluconate can be used as therapy to oppose the effect of hyperkalaemia on the myocardium but has no effect on plasma potassium concentration.

Reference ranges
Sodium 135–145 mmol/L *Potassium 3.5–5.0 mmol/L* *Osmolality 282–295 mmol/kg*

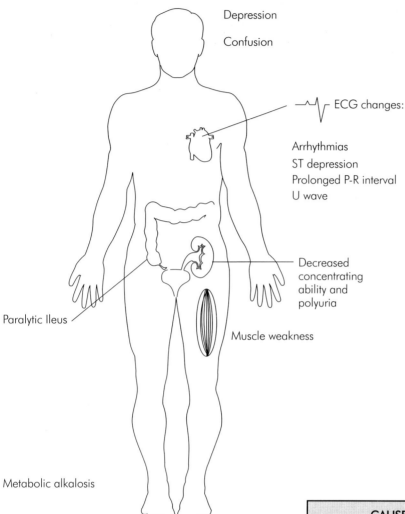

Depression

Confusion

ECG changes:

Arrhythmias
ST depression
Prolonged P-R interval
U wave

Decreased
concentrating
ability and
polyuria

Paralytic Ileus

Muscle weakness

Metabolic alkalosis

Figure 12.6 – Clinical features of hypokalaemia.

CAUSES OF HYPERKALAEMIA
Spurious haemolysis delay in separation of sample
Increased intake parenteral oral (rare) transfusion of old blood
Decreased loss renal failure mineralocorticoid deficiency e.g. Addison's disease
Transcellular movement acidosis rapid tissue breakdown

Figure 12.7

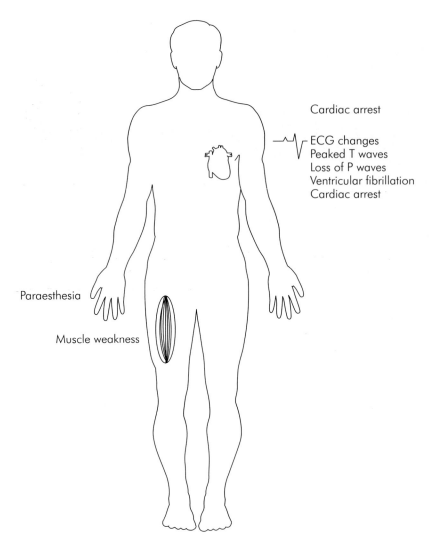

Figure 12.8 – Clinical effects of hyperkalaemia.

SELECTED READING

Marshall, W.J. and Bangert, S.K. (eds). *Clinical Biochemistry: Metabolic and Clinical Aspects*. Churchill Livingstone, Edinburgh. 1995.

13

HYDROGEN ION HOMEOSTASIS

Objectives

To understand:

- The physiology of hydrogen ion homeostasis

- The laboratory investigation of disorders of hydrogen ion homeostasis

- The pathogenesis of disorders of hydrogen ion homeostasis – acidosis and alkalosis

An acid is a substance that can dissociate to produce hydrogen ions. A base is a substance that can accept hydrogen ions.

pH is defined as $\log_{10}$ of the reciprocal of the hydrogen ion activity. A buffer system consists of a partially dissociated (weak) acid and its conjugate base. An example is the bicarbonate-carbonic acid system:

$$H^+ + HCO_3^- \rightleftharpoons H_2CO_3$$

If hydrogen ions are added to this system the amount of carbonic acid formed is increased. If the hydrogen ion concentration decreases hydrogen ions are generated by the dissociation of carbonic acid. Thus, the buffer system acts to reduce the potential effect of a change in hydrogen ion concentration. Other buffer systems of physiological importance include the monohydrogen phosphate (HPO_4^{2-}) and dihydrogen phosphate ($H_2PO_4^-$) system, haemoglobin and other proteins.

THE PHYSIOLOGY OF HYDROGEN ION HOMEOSTASIS

Daily metabolism results in the production of about 60 mmol of hydrogen ions which are excreted into the urine. There is also massive endogenous turnover of hydrogen ions. This turnover makes no permanent change to hydrogen ion formation – for example lactic acid arises as a result of glycolysis and may accumulate in exercise but it is then used for gluconeogenesis, a process which consumes hydrogen ions. More than 15,000 mmol of carbon dioxide are produced per 24 hours as a result of oxidative metabolism and are lost from the body in expired air. In the presence of water CO_2 can form carbonic acid:

$$H_2O + CO_2 \rightleftharpoons H_2CO_3$$

This explains why those types of respiratory diseases in which carbon dioxide retention occurs, frequently cause acidosis. Acid-base balance is carefully controlled to maintain body hydrogen ion concentration within narrow limits. In health, potential imbalances in acid-base status can be limited by buffering and compensated for by changes in respiratory rate and hydrogen ion excretion.

HYDROGEN ION EXCRETION AND BICARBONATE REABSORPTION

Hydrogen ions are excreted in the urine. However, for urine to be acidified, bicarbonate present in the filtrate must first be absorbed. In health, urine is virtually free of bicarbonate and has an acid pH. In the kidney, direct absorption of bicarbonate cannot take place as it cannot permeate the luminal surface of the renal tubular cells. Within the tubular cells the enzyme carbonate dehydratase catalyses the formation of carbonic acid which dissociates to bicarbonate and hydrogen ions. The bicarbonate ions pass into the interstitial fluid and hydrogen ions pass into the tubular lumen in exchange for sodium ions. Within the tubular lumen carbonic acid is formed from hydrogen and bicarbonate ions and dissociates into carbon dioxide and water. The carbon dioxide which is not excreted in urine diffuses back into the tubular cells.

There is no actual excretion of hydrogen ions during the reabsorption of bicarbonate. The presence of urinary buffer systems is essential for hydrogen ion excretion. Phosphate is the most important urinary buffer:

$$H^+ + HPO_4^{2-} \rightleftharpoons H_2PO_4^-$$

Ammonia is produced by deamination of glutamine in the cells of the renal tubule and diffuses readily across cell membranes. During buffering, ammonium ions are formed:

$$H^+ + NH_3 \rightleftharpoons NH_4^+$$

Ammonium ions are not freely diffusible and so passive reabsorption cannot occur.

CARBON DIOXIDE TRANSPORT

Carbon dioxide is produced as a result of aerobic metabolism. This carbon dioxide diffuses out from cells to dissolve in the extracellular fluid. Virtually no carbon dioxide is formed within erythrocytes as their metabolism is anaerobic. Carbon dioxide diffuses down its concentration gradient into erythrocytes and carbonic acid formation is catalysed by carbonate dehydratase. The carbonic acid dissociates to bicarbonate and hydrogen ions, the latter are then buffered by haemoglobin. The bicarbonate ions diffuse out of the erythrocytes and chloride ions move inwards to maintain electrochemical neutrality. Within the lungs carbon dioxide is formed from bicarbonate and diffuses outwards to be excreted in expired air. Whilst the majority of carbon dioxide in the blood is in the form of bicarbonate, carbon dioxide is also carried as carbonic acid, some is dissolved and some is in the form of carbamino compounds.

LABORATORY INVESTIGATION OF ACID BASE STATUS

Acid base status is normally evaluated using a sample of arterial blood from which are determined the hydrogen ion concentration, the pCO_2 and the pO_2. The sample should be analysed promptly having been sent to the laboratory on ice. The bicarbonate concentration is calculated from the formula:

$$[H^+] = K \frac{pCO_2}{[HCO_3^-]}$$

K is a constant, its value being approximately 180 when $[H^+]$ is expressed in nmol/L, $[HCO_3^-]$ in nmol/L and pCO_2 in kPa.

DISORDERS OF HYDROGEN ION HOMEOSTASIS

Acidosis occurs in situations where there is a tendency for the hydrogen ion concentration to increase and alkalosis occurs when there is a tendency for it to decrease. Disorders of hydrogen ion homeostasis involve the bicarbonate buffer pair. In respiratory acidosis or alkalosis the primary abnormality is a change in pCO_2.

RESPIRATORY ACIDOSIS

Respiratory acidosis is, by definition, an acidosis whose cause is an increase in pCO_2. The tendency to acidosis tends to be corrected by an increase in renal H^+ excretion with a consequent increase in plasma bicarbonate concentration. This renal compensation occurs slowly and in respiratory acidosis of acute onset plasma bicarbonate is usually normal. Causes of respiratory acidosis are shown in Table 13.1.

CAUSES OF RESPIRATORY ACIDOSIS
Respiratory depression
cerebral damage
sedative drugs
Neuromuscular abormalities
motor neurone disease
myasthenia gravis
Pulmonary disorders
thoracic cage trauma
severe pneumonia
severe asthma
chronic obstructive airways disease

Table 13.1

METABOLIC ACIDOSIS

This can arise due to increased production or decreased excretion of H^+ ions or to loss of bicarbonate. Buffering of the excess H^+ occurs resulting in carbonic acid formation with the CO_2 produced lost from the lungs. The increased H^+ concentration itself stimulates the respiratory centre resulting in hyperventilation and lowering of the pCO_2 / $[HCO_3]$ ratio, thus compensating in part for the acidosis. Complete compensation cannot occur in this way as it is the elevated H^+ concentration that stimulates the respiratory centre and the increased action of the respiratory muscles itself increases CO_2 production. Causes of metabolic acidosis are shown in Table 13.2.

Ketoacidosis occurs most often in diabetes mellitus due to increased lipolysis and ketogenesis. Ketosis can also occur in association with alcohol excess, its aetiology being multifactorial. Lactate is formed from pyruvate in muscle and is converted to glucose in the liver. In type A lactic acidosis hypoxia is the initiating event whereas type B can be the result of ingestion of drugs or ethanol or as the result of inherited metabolic disease. Other metabolic defects can result in accumulation of organic acids. In renal failure acidosis occurs as the glomerular filtration reduces the amount of sodium that is filtered and therefore available to be exchanged with H^+ in the distal convoluted tubule. In proximal renal tubular acidosis (Type II) there is incomplete reabsorption of bicarbonate and in distal renal tubular acidosis (Type I) the underlying abnormality is a defect in H^+ excretion.

In metabolic acidosis the bicarbonate concentration falls and electrochemical balance is achieved by other

CAUSES OF METABOLIC ACIDOSIS
Increased hydrogen ion formation
ketoacidosis
lactic acidosis
toxins – salicylate, ethylene glycol
Decreased hydrogen ion excretion
renal failure
renal tubular acidosis
Bicarbonate loss
diarrhoea
loss of alkaline secretions -biliary, pancreatic, intestinal

Table 13.2

CAUSES OF RESPIRATORY ALKALOSIS
Stimulation of the respiratory centre
cerebral damage
drugs e.g. aspirin
voluntary hyperventilation
hepatic failure
Gram negative septicaemia
Hypoxia
severe anaemia
decreased pCO_2 of inspired air
Pulmonary disease
pulmonary embolism

Table 13.3

anions. These anions may be produced in parallel with the increase in H^+ ions, otherwise chloride ions correct the defect.

The anion gap (not to be confused with the osmolar gap!) is defined as the difference between the concentrations of sodium and potassium ions and chloride and bicarbonate ions and is usually of the order of 14–8 mmol/l due to the net negative charge of circulating proteins.

$$\text{Anion gap} = ([Na^+]+[K^+]) - ([Cl^-]+[HCO_3^-])$$

Calculation of the anion gap may be an aid to diagnosis in some cases of acidosis. If the acidosis is due to loss of bicarbonate the anion gap is unchanged but if it is due to generation of acid, for example in ketoacidosis, the associated anions replace bicarbonate which is consumed by buffering, resulting in an increased anion gap.

RESPIRATORY ALKALOSIS

This results from a decrease in pCO_2. Compensation occurs due to decreased excretion of H^+ by the kidney resulting in a decreased serum bicarbonate concentration. This compensation takes several days to become established. Causes of respiratory alkalosis are shown in Table 13.3.

METABOLIC ALKALOSIS

This is associated with an increased ECF bicarbonate and therefore a decreased H^+ concentration. Causes of metabolic alkalosis are shown in Table 13.4.

Excess mineralocorticoid action results in alkalosis secondary to increased H^+ secretion in the distal tubule in exchange for increased sodium reabsorption. Similarly in potassium deficiency there is a decreased amount of K^+ for exchange with Na^+ in the distal tubule and H^+ excretion is increased resulting in alkalosis. Vomiting usually results in loss of both gastric acid and small intestinal contents containing bicarbonate. However, with gastric aspiration or vomiting in association with pyloric stenosis, only acidic secretions are lost resulting in alkalosis.

The expected mechanism of compensation for a metabolic alkalosis would be hypoventilation leading to an increase in pCO_2. However carbon dioxide is a respiratory stimulant thus limiting the effectiveness of this mechanism. In chronic metabolic alkalosis there may be a decrease in sensitivity of the respiratory centre such that a degree of compensation can occur via this mechanism.

OXYGEN DELIVERY TO THE TISSUES

The delivery of oxygen from the atmosphere to the tissues depends on the amount of oxygen within arterial blood and on the blood supply to the tissues. Oxygen is essential for cell metabolism and disturbance of this oxygen delivery mechanism leads to hypoxaemia.

The processes involved begin with alveolar ventilation but for adequate tissue oxygenation the actual oxygen content of the blood is important. This is determined by both the haemoglobin concentration and by the oxygen affinity of the blood. The tissue blood supply is a function of the cardiac output and the vascular resistance within the tissue concerned. The causes of hypoxaemia are shown in Table 13.5.

CAUSES OF METABOLIC ALKALOSIS

Increased intake of alkali
    excessive administration
    injudicious correction of acidosis

Increased loss of hydrogen ions
    renal loss
        Conn's syndrome
        diuretics
        hypokalaemia
    gastrointestinal loss
        gastric aspiration
        vomiting in presence of pyloric stenosis

Table 13.4

CAUSES OF HYPOXAEMIA
Decreased inspired oxygen   high altitude
Decreased alveolar ventilation   respiratory depression
Decreased diffusion   pulmonary fibrosis
Abnormalities of ventilation/perfusion   pulmonary embolus
Venous to arterial shunting   cyanotic congenital heart disease

Table 13.5

SELECTED READING

Cohen, R.D. The metabolic background to acid-base homeostasis and some of its disorders. In: Cohen, R.D., Lewis, B., Alberti, K.G.M.M. and Denman, A.M. (eds). *The Metabolic Basis of Aquired Disease*. Ballière Tindall, 1995.

Reference ranges	
$[H^+]$	35–46 nmol/L (arterial blood)
Oxygen (pO_2)	11–15 kPa
Carbon dioxide (pCO_2)	4.5–6 kPa
Bicarbonate (total CO_2)	22–30 mmol/L

14

THE CARDIOVASCULAR SYSTEM

The heart is a muscular organ whose function is the pumping of blood around the body. It consists of four chambers separated by valves. Disorders of the heart may affect the heart muscle (myocardium), the valves or the coronary arteries which supply blood to the heart muscle itself.

MYOCARDIAL INFARCTION

Ischaemic heart disease is a major health problem. It may present as angina – chest pain caused by a decreased blood flow in the coronary arteries – which typically occurs on exercise. It may also present acutely as infarction of the heart muscle, and as sudden death. The diagnosis of myocardial infarction (MI) is usually made from the clinical history, supplemented by electrocardiographic changes and biochemical tests. Mortality and morbidity due to MI are reduced by the administration of thrombolytic therapy which breaks down blood clots in the coronary arteries, thus re-establishing blood flow. Ideally this therapy should be given within four hours of the onset of chest pain, thus making a rapid diagnosis of MI essential. Various substances are released from the ischaemic myocardium and can be measured in the blood. The most commonly measured markers of MI are the so-called 'cardiac enzymes' – creatine kinase (CK), aspartate transaminase (AST) and lactate dehydrogenase (LDH). Other markers include troponins T and I and myoglobin.

THE LABORATORY DIAGNOSIS OF MI

After myocardial infarction the time from the onset of chest pain to release of marker enzymes varies, as does the duration of rise. Due to the nature of the changes, the combination of measurement of different enzymes can be used to diagnose MI from about four hours to several days after the onset of chest pain. Details of these changes are shown in Figure 14.1.

Creatine kinase is found in heart muscle, skeletal muscle and in the brain. CK exists as a dimer made from the monomers M and B. These monomers can combine to form three isoenzymes — MB, MM and BB. MB is found principally in the heart, MM in skeletal muscle and BB in the brain. The plasma activity of CK begins to rise before that of the other cardiac enzymes, so it is the most widely used marker of MI. As CK is present in skeletal muscle even minor damage to skeletal muscle can cause diagnostic difficulty. To increase the specificity of CK as a marker for heart muscle damage carefully timed CK measurements can be made and the increment calculated or the activity of the MB isoenzyme may be estimated. CK MM, the skeletal muscle isoenzyme, usually comprises 95% of that detectable in the plasma, thus CK MB levels > 5% are indicative of myocardial damage.

Aspartate transaminase in the plasma rises to a concentration of four to five times the upper limit of the reference range after myocardial infarction. As AST is found in tissues other than heart, other factors such as liver disease or haemolysis may decrease the usefulness of the test.

Lactate dehydrogenase activity may be elevated three to four times above the upper limit of the reference range after MI. LDH has a widespread tissue distribution and as well as the heart it is found in erythrocytes, liver and skeletal muscle. However, there are tissue specific isoenzymes, the measurement of which increases the specificity of LDH as a marker. The enzyme is composed of four subunits of two types, either H or M. Thus there are five possible combinations — the

Enzyme	Activity		
	Start of rise (hours)	Peak (hours)	Duration (days)
CK	4-6	12-24	3-5
AST	6-8	20-30	3-6
LDH	12-24	48-72	7-12

Figure 14.1 – Plasma enzyme changes after myocardial infarction.

cardiac form being M_4 or LDH_1. LDH_1 is able to catalyse conversion of α-hydroxybutyrate, this being known as HBD activity and is a more specific marker of myocardial damage.

Although measurement of cardiac enzymes is useful, no single measurement, or combination of measurements, can give a diagnosis within 4 hours of the infarct occurring – the optimal time for thrombolysis.

Troponins are proteins associated with the contractile apparatus of muscle cells. Troponin T may have a particular role in unstable angina as a predictor of patients likely to progress to myocardial infarction. Troponin I is thought to be more specific for cardiac muscle damage than creatine kinase or troponin T.

Myoglobin may have a specific role in the assessment of infarct size.

HYPERTENSION

Hypertension may be defined as a blood pressure of greater than 140/90 mmHg on at least three occasions. The mortality of those with hypertension is more than double that of those with a normal blood pressure. The high pressure on the arteries increases the risk of coronary artery disease, stroke, renal damage and retinal damage. In about 95% of patients there is no obvious cause for the raised blood pressure; this is termed essential hypertension. Rarely a cause can be found, in which case it is termed secondary hypertension. The diagnosis of essential hypertension is one of exclusion. To this end potassium, creatinine and calcium should be measured on all patients while they are not on treatment. Particular effort to find a cause should be directed to young patients with no family history of hypertension and in those patients whose hypertension is resistant to treatment. Causes of secondary hypertension are listed in Table 14.1.

In addition to a search for a secondary cause of hypertension, associated vascular risk factors such as an abnormal lipid profile and diabetes mellitus should be screened for.

In some cases of secondary hypertension there may be a surgically remediable cause; however in the majority of patients with hypertension requiring treatment antihypertensive drugs are used. Lifestyle advice such as decreasing salt and alcohol intake may be beneficial in hypertension, together with attention to other cardiac risk factors such as smoking and obesity.

CAUSES OF SECONDARY HYPERTENSION	
Renal	renal artery stenosis
	renal parenchymal disease
Endocrine	Cushing's syndrome
	Conn's syndrome
	phaeochromocytoma
Hypercalcaemia	
Alcohol excess	

Table 14.1

The modes of action of some anti-hypertensive drugs are shown in Table 14.2.

CARDIAC FAILURE

Cardiac failure is the inability of the heart to maintain an output of blood sufficient for the needs of the body. It may be due primarily to failure of the left ventricle or to failure of the right ventricle. Causes of ventricular failure are shown in Table 14.3.

Left ventricular failure may be chronic or acute. When it is of gradual onset there is shortness of breath on exertion followed later by shortness of breath on lying flat. Tiredness and weakness occur secondary to the low cardiac output associated with poor peripheral perfusion. There is retention of salt and water due to imbalance between the glomerular filtration and tubular reabsorption of sodium. The salt and water retention causes an increase in blood volume and excess fluid accumulates in tissue spaces. The distribution of this fluid is affected by gravity and so it accumulates as oedema in the ankles and legs of those who are ambulant and over the sacrum in patients confined to bed. In right ventricular failure the liver becomes enlarged and tender and this may eventually lead to jaundice.

PLASMA PROTEINS

Plasma contains a number of proteins, functions of which are shown in Table 14.4.

The plasma proteins are synthesised mainly in the liver, although the complement proteins are also synthesised by macrophages and immunoglobulins are derived from B cells.

THE MODE OF ACTION OF COMMON ANTIHYPERTENSIVE DRUGS	
Drug type	Mode of action
β-blockers (e.g. propranolol)	Blockade of β-adrenergic receptors thus decreasing cardiac output and dilating arteries and arterioles
α-blockers (e.g. prazocin)	Post-synaptic blockade of α- adrenergic receptors and vasodilatation
Thiazide diuretics (e.g. bendrofluazide)	Reduction of smooth muscle tone and blood volume
Calcium channel blockers (e.g. nifedipine)	Reduction in cardiac and smooth muscle excitability due to prevention of influx of calcium into cells
Angiotensin converting enzyme inhibitors (e.g. captopril)	Inhibition of the renin-angiotension system

Table 14.2

CAUSES OF VENTRICULAR FAILURE	
Causes of left ventricular failure	Causes of right ventricular failure
Hypertension	Secondary to left ventricular failure
Myocardial infarction	Some forms of congenital heart disease
Disease of the aortic or mitral valves	Disease of the tricuspid or mitral valves
Cardiac muscle disorders	Secondary to pulmonary disease

Table 14.3

The concentration of a plasma protein depends on the relative rates of synthesis and catabolism. A raised concentration of total protein may occur when there is loss of protein-free fluid and is also seen in conditions such as myeloma where the immunoglobulin fraction is increased massively. Low total protein concentration may occur if there is severe immunoglobulin deficiency or in hypoalbuminaemia.

Albumin is the plasma protein present in highest concentration. It has a molecular weight of 66,000 and a half life of about 30 days. Albumin is the most important protein contributing to the plasma oncotic pressure. To maintain blood pressure fluid must be retained in the intravascular compartment. Hydrostatic pressure acts to force fluid into the extravascular space and this is opposed by the opposing oncotic pressure. Hypoalbuminaemia is a very common finding, causes of which are shown in Table 14.5.

α_1-antitrypsin is a protease inhibitor (P_i) limiting the action of enzymes released from phagocytes. There are a number of genetic variants of α_1-antitrypsin inherited as codominant alleles some of them resulting in proteins with altered function. ZZ homozygotes may present with prolonged neonatal jaundice or cirrhosis in later life. They and SS homozygotes are also prone to lung damage resulting in basal emphysema exacerbated by tobacco smoking due to the unopposed action of proteases.

FUNCTIONS OF PLASMA PROTEINS	
Function	Example
Transport	Albumin and specific binding proteins e.g. cortisol binding globulin, Caeruloplasmin, apolipoproteins
Control of infection	Immunoglobulins
Control of extracellular fluid volume via oncotic pressure effect	All proteins, especially albumin
Buffering	All proteins
Enzymes	Renin, Complement proteins
Haemostasis	Clotting factors

Table 14.4

CAUSES OF HYPOALBUMINAEMIA
Decreased synthesis
malnutrition
malabsorption
liver disease
Increased volume of distribution
overhydration
increased capillary permeability
Increased loss
nephrotic syndrome
burns
extensive skin disease
protein losing enteropathy
Increased catabolism
trauma
sepsis
malignant disease

Table 14.5

LABORATORY INVESTIGATION OF PLASMA PROTEINS

The plasma proteins may be quantified by measurements of total protein or, more usefully, by assessment of individual proteins. Changes in individual proteins may be quantified by electrophoresis followed by densitometry, an assay of concentration may be carried out or estimation of the activity of a protein may be assessed – for example, prothrombin time may be measured to assess clotting factors. Electrophoresis is a technique that can be used to separate proteins according to differences in size and electrical charge. By electrophoresis plasma proteins can be separated into five groups – albumin and α_1-, α_2-, β- and γ-globulins. Each fraction may contain more than one protein as shown in Table 14.6.

In the past, characteristic patterns found on electrophoresis have been used in the diagnosis of specific diseases, however the main use of protein electrophoresis is for the detection of paraproteins.

ELECTROPHORETIC SEPARATION OF PLASMA PROTEINS	
Fraction	Proteins
Albumin	Albumin
α_1-globulin	α_1-antitrypsin
	α_1-acid glycoprotein
α_2-globulin	α_2-macroglobulin
	Haptoglobin
	Caeruloplasmin
β-globulins	Transferrin
	Low density lipoprotein
	C3 fraction of complement
γ-globulins	Immunoglobulins

Table 14.6

THE ACUTE PHASE RESPONSE

Injury to tissues, whatever its cause, results in a complex sequence of reactions which constitute the acute phase response. This comprises fever and a raised white cell count, together with an increase in vascular permeability. The acute phase reaction includes changes in the concentrations of plasma proteins which serve to limit inflammatory damage by enhancing phagocytosis and counteracting the effect of proteolytic enzymes. There is a rise in the α_1 and α_2 fractions due to increased amounts of α_1-antitrypsin, haptoglobin and C-reactive protein. The increase in plasma proteins begins about six hours after the inflammatory stimulus reflecting the time required for the proteins to be synthesised and released. The time course of the increase in concentration of different proteins varies. C-reactive protein (CRP) is an opsonin which binds to foreign particles helping to initiate activation of the complement system. The concentration of CRP increases very early on in the acute phase response, reaching a maximum concentration by 48 hours after the onset of the inflammatory process. The measurement of CRP is particularly useful as an early indicator of inflammation. The cytokines are an important component of the acute inflammatory response. They are polypeptides which help to regulate the immune response.

IMMUNOGLOBULINS

Immunoglobulins are proteins involved in various ways in the immune response. They are made up of two heavy and two light chains linked by disulphide bonds to form a Y-shaped molecule. Immunoglobulins have antibody activity, each immunoglobulin having two antigen binding sites. Each chain has variable and hypervariable regions, associated with the antigen-binding sites, and constant regions with conserved amino acid sequences which mediate the activation of complement. There are five different classes of heavy chain – γ, α, μ, δ and ε – and two types of light chain – κ and λ. There are five classes of immunoglogulins, which in order of their concentration in the plasma, are IgG, IgA, IgM, IgD and IgE, the class being determined by the type of heavy chain. IgG is present in the highest concentration and is the major antibody involved in secondary immune responses. IgA exists as two subunits, joined by a J chain, together with a secretory piece produced by epithelial cells. IgA is present in the secretions of the intestinal and respiratory systems and in tears and colostrum. IgM is made up of five subunits stabilised by a glycoprotein J chain. IgM is confined to the intravascular compartment due to its large size and is therefore an important component of the primary immune response. IgD is found on B lymphocytes and is important in antigen recognition. IgE binds to mast cells and basophils, When antigen combines with IgE on the surface of these cells various chemical mediators are released, thus explaining the role of IgE in immediate hypersensitivity reactions.

PARAPROTEINAEMIA

On antigenic stimulation B cells produce a polyclonal response. However, if one B cell proliferates, a clone of similar cells is formed. A paraprotein is an immunoglobulin produced by such a clone and can be visualised as an abnormal dense band on electrophoresis, most commonly in the γ-region. The presence of a paraprotein is often, but not always, associated with malignancy. Common causes of a paraprotein are shown in Table 14.7.

Bence-Jones protein consists of free monoclonal light chains which, due to their low molecular weight, are filtered by glomeruli. The presence of Bence-Jones protein in the urine is highly suggestive of malignant proliferation of B cells. Examination of the urine is essential where myeloma is suspected as in almost one quarter of cases only light chains are produced. Light chains may not be detected in serum due to their rapid clearance from the blood.

Myeloma results from a malignant proliferation of plasma cells and may present with symptoms of hypercalcaemia, bone pain or renal failure. It is typified by the appearance of a paraprotein, bone destruction and

CAUSES OF PARAPROTEINAEMIA
Malignant
multiple myeloma
lymphoma
chronic lymphocytic leukaemia
Waldenstrom's macroglobulinaemia
Non-malignant
benign
transient
immune complex disease

Table 14.7

abnormal bone marrow containing neoplastic cells. The levels of immunoglobulins other than the paraprotein are depressed (immune paresis) thus increasing susceptibility to infection.

Waldenstrom's macroglobulinaemia is characterised by the presence of an IgM paraprotein. The concentration of IgM leads to a hyperviscosity syndrome with such clinical manifestations as visual disturbance and neurological problems.

Benign paraproteinaemia is a diagnosis of exclusion and requires regular reassessment of the patient even after ruling out other more serious causes. Transient paraproteinaemia occurs most often in the immunocompromised and usually disappears within a month. Immune complex disorders such as rheumatoid arthritis may also lead to paraproteinaemia.

PROTEINS IN THE CEREBROSPINAL FLUID

About 500 mL of cerebrospinal fluid (CSF) are formed each day but as its mean turnover is about six hours, the CSF occupies a volume of only about 150 mL. Solutes enter the CSF in a number of ways but 80% of the CSF protein content is from plasma proteins which have diffused across the blood-brain barrier. A small amount of protein is synthesised within the central nervous system itself. A sample of CSF can be obtained by lumbar puncture. In suspected bacterial meningitis a CSF protein concentration > 0.4 g/L would support the diagnosis. The mechanism for the increased protein being that inflammation decreases the integrity of the blood CSF barrier. The examination of CSF is also important in the diagnosis of multiple sclerosis (MS). This is a progressive neurological condition where episodes of demyelination occur separated in time and site. MS is associated with a B cell response and the immunoglobulins produced may be detected by electrophoresis of the CSF. In 90% of those with MS CSF electrophoresis shows a few discrete (oligoclonal) bands not present in serum.

Reference ranges	
Creatine kinase	<150 IU/L
Total protein	60–80 g/L
Albumin	35–50 g/L

SELECTED READING

Roitt, I.M. *Essential Immunology*, 9th Edition. Blackwell Science Inc. 1997.

15

HAEMOGLOBIN, PORPHYRIN AND IRON

Objectives

To understand:

- The synthesis of haemoglobin

- The nature of abnormal haemoglobin derivatives

- Congenital abnormalities of haemoglobin – haemoglobinopathies, thalassaemia

- Factors in erythrocyte development

- Iron deficiency and iron overload

- Porphyrias

Haem is an important molecule which can be synthesised by all mammalian cells. Haem is incorporated into haemoglobin, myoglobin, the cytochromes, catalases and peroxidases and is therefore essential to oxygen transport, protein synthesis and cellular respiration.

HAEMOGLOBIN

Haemoglobin is the oxygen carrying pigment of blood and is an iron-containing protein made up of four polypeptide chains, two of α-globin and two β-globin each polypeptide binding one haem molecule.

HAEMOGLOBIN SYNTHESIS AND CATABOLISM

Haem is made up of a tetrapyrrole ring, protoporphyrin IXa, to which one iron (II) (Fe^{2+}) is bound. Haem synthesis takes place at the erythroblast and reticulocyte stages of red cell development and is outlined in Figure 15.1.

Glycine and succinyl CoA are converted to ALA by ALA synthase which is the rate-limiting step in the pathway and is regulated by negative feedback from haem itself. Two molecules of ALA combine to form PBG, four molecules of which combine to form uro-

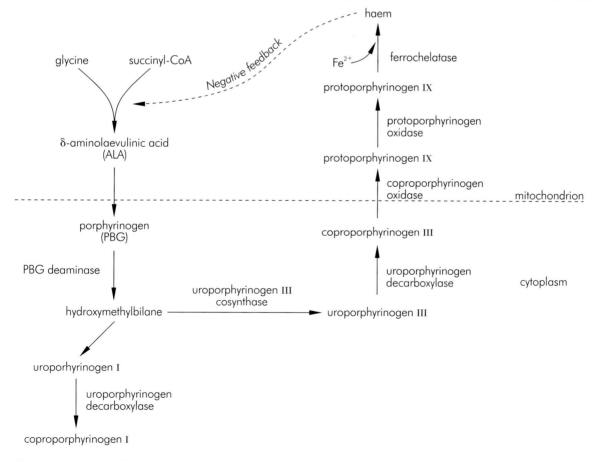

Figure 15.1 – Synthesis of haem.

porphyrinogen. Porphyrinogens are colourless, unstable compounds and are oxidised to red-coloured porphyrins when excreted in faeces or urine. Two isomers of uroporphyrinogen are formed, I and III. The major pathway is that involving the III isomer and it is only this pathway that leads to haem formation. Excess intermediates along the pathway are excreted – ALA, PBG and uroporphyrin in the urine and protoporphyrin in the bile and thus in the faeces.

When the erythrocyte reaches the end of its lifespan haem is removed from globin and spontaneously oxidized to the iron (III) (Fe^{3+}) state. The enzyme haem oxidase then acts to open the porphyrin ring producing biliverdin and carbon monoxide.

Haemoglobinaemia and haemoglobinuria

Haemolysis may be classified as intravascular, in which red blood cell destruction occurs within the circulation and extravascular where the destruction is within the reticuloendothelial system and where iron accumulates. In intravascular haemolysis, haemoglobin is released into the plasma (haemoglobinaemia) and when the renal threshold for haemoglobin is exceeded, haemoglobin is excreted in the urine (haemoglobinuria).

Fetal haemoglobin

The fetus and neonate possess their own forms of haemoglobin which have different structures and oxygen affinities from the adult form. In the first three months *in utero* the main form of haemoglobin consists of two ζ and two ε chains. Later ζ subunits are replaced by α and ε subunits by γ. This results in fetal haemoglobin with an $\alpha_2\gamma_2$ structure which is itself replaced by adult type haemoglobin between one month before and three months after birth. In some haemoglobinopathies, such as sickle cell disease, genetically determined high levels of fetal haemoglobin may ameliorate the effect of the disease.

CONGENITAL ABNORMALITIES OF HAEMOGLOBIN

Structural haemoglobin variants (haemoglobinopathies)

There are more than 500 haemoglobin variants in which the haemoglobin molecule has an altered structure and sometimes an altered function. One of the most common abnormal haemoglobins is HbS which has a reduced solubility resulting in sickling of erythrocytes causing them to become fragile and less deformable than usual. The clinical features of the resulting sickle cell disease may be either acute or chronic. The most common acute manifestation is a painful 'crisis' secondary to vaso-occlusion, most commonly in bone, resulting in avascular necrosis of the bone marrow. Chronic problems may involve progressive bony destruction, infection and lung disease due to repeated infarction.

Thalassaemias

The thalassaemias together are the most common autosomal recessive condition worldwide. They result from a defect in either the α-globin gene (α thal) or that of the β-globin (β thal). As there are two α-globin genes, five possible types of α thal exist. Deletion of all four α globin genes is not compatible with life, affected infants dying *in utero*. Deletion of three α genes results in a chronic haemolytic anaemia named HbH disease and those individuals with deletion of one or two α genes are asymptomatic.

β thalassaemia

In the homozygous state (β thalassaemia major) there is virtual absence of β chain production and ineffective erythropoiesis. Treatment of β thalassaemia consists of frequent blood transfusion coupled with administration of the chelating agent desferroxamine to decrease the risk of damaging iron accumulation.

HAPTOGLOBIN

Haptoglobin is a plasma protein which binds free haemoglobin. The haemoglobin-haptoglobin complex is then removed by the reticuloendothelial system. Haptoglobin levels are decreased in haemolytic disease and may also be lowered in the presence of hepatocellular disease. Raised levels may occur in malignancy and chronic inflammatory conditions.

ABNORMAL HAEMOGLOBIN DERIVATIVES

Carboxyhaemoglobin (COHb)

COHb is formed in the presence of carbon monoxide whose oxygen affinity for haemoglobin is about 200 times greater than that of oxygen. The presence of COHb therefore decreases the capacity of the blood to carry oxygen. A small amount of COHb is a common occurrence in the blood of town dwellers, with higher amounts being present in the blood of smokers.

Methaemoglobin

Methaemoglobin is unable to carry oxygen, being oxidized haemoglobin containing iron (III). A small quantity is found in normal red blood cells and is reduced enzymatically to haemoglobin. Increased methaemoglobin can occur with ingestion of drugs, for example sulphonamides and in some congenital haemoglobinopathies. In congenital methaemoglobinaemia there is cyanosis. In toxic methaemoglobinaemia methaemalbumin is formed due to the haemolysis of erythrocytes containing methaemoglobin; methaemalbumin gives a brown colour to plasma.

Haematin

Haematin, oxidised iron (III) haem, can be formed from free haemoglobin in situations of severe intravascular haemolysis or it can be released from methaemoglobin after haemolysis of methaemoglobin-containing red cells.

Glycated haemoglobin

Haemoglobin undergoes an irreversible non-enzymatic glycation. The amount of this glycated haemoglobin can be used in diabetes mellitus as an index of glycaemic control.

FACTORS IN ERYTHROCYTE DEVELOPMENT

Erythropoietin

Erythropoietin is a glycoprotein hormone, secreted by the kidney in response to the oxygen level in the blood, that stimulates maturation of red cell precursors.

Vitamin B_{12}

Vitamin B_{12} is a group of related cobalamins found in products of animal origin and necessary for coenzyme activity in the synthesis of nucleic acids. Vitamin B_{12} is absorbed in the terminal ileum, a process which requires intrinsic factor from gastric parietal cells. Deficiency can occur in vegans and in those with deficiency of intrinsic factor due to gastric abnormalities or pernicious anaemia where auto-antibodies to parietal cells are formed. As intestinal bacteria require vitamin B_{12} deficiency may occur in situations of bacterial overgrowth such as blind loop syndrome. Deficiency of vitamin B_{12} may cause megaloblastic anaemia and a specific neurological lesion – subacute degeneration of the spinal cord, together with a peripheral neuropathy.

Folate

Folate is also essential to erythropoiesis, deficiency causing megaloblastic anaemia. Folate is found in meat and green vegetables and dietary deficiency may occur. Absorption takes place in the small intestine and deficiency may occur in malabsorption.

Iron

Iron is essential for haem synthesis. Iron deficiency results in anaemia — other iron containing molecules such as myoglobin, cytochromes and some enzymes are not usually affected.

Iron absorption is responsible for the control of body iron. Iron absorption takes place by active transport in the upper part of the small intestine. The protein apoferritin complexes with iron in intestinal cells to form ferritin. About 10% of dietary iron is absorbed each day, about 1 mg, but this is influenced by the extent of the body's iron stores, oxygen tension within the cells of the intestine and by the degree of erythropoiesis within the bone marrow. Women have greater iron requirements than men due to losses resulting from menstruation and pregnancy and they absorb slightly more iron than men. Increased absorption of dietary iron occurs in children and adolescents who have increased requirements due to the demands of growth.

Excretion of iron from the body occurs due to desquamation of ferritin containing cells in the gut and the skin and amounts to about 1mg each day.

Transferrin is an iron binding protein transporting iron within the plasma as iron (III). Transferrin is normally about one third saturated and carries iron to the bone marrow and to iron stores where it is incorporated into ferritin and haemosiderin.

About three quarters of body iron is found in the circulating red blood cells as haemoglobin. Most of the rest of the iron is stored as ferritin and haemosiderin in the reticuloendothelial system of the liver, spleen and bone marrow.

IRON DEFICIENCY AND IRON OVERLOAD

Iron deficiency causes a microcytic, hypochromic anaemia. This causes pallor and symptoms of tissue hypoxia such as fatigue and breathlessness. Iron deficiency occurs whenever absorption does not meet requirements, for example in pregnancy, menorrhagia, chronic blood loss and after acute haemorrhage. Iron overload may be due to increased intestinal absorption of iron or to parenteral administration as shown in Table 15.1.

```
┌──────────────────────────────────────┐
│        CAUSES OF IRON OVERLOAD         │
├──────────────────────────────────────┤
│ Parenteral administration             │
│   excessive blood transfusion         │
│                                        │
│ Increased intestinal absorption       │
│   dietary excess                      │
│   idiopathic haemochromatosis         │
│   anaemia associated with ineffective erythropoesis │
│   liver disease                       │
│   inappropriate oral administration   │
└──────────────────────────────────────┘
```

Table 15.1

The accumulated iron may be distributed in two distinct patterns. Reticuloendothelial overload may result from excessive parenteral administration. There is accumulation of iron in the liver, spleen and bone marrow which is occasionally severe enough to cause actual parenchymal damage. Haemochromatosis is an autosomal recessive condition in which there is increased intestinal absorption of iron gradually leading to increased iron stores deposited in a parenchymal pattern. It presents more frequently and at an earlier age in men, due to the greater iron losses in women. Tissue damage by iron may lead to cirrhosis, diabetes mellitus, hypogonadism and pigmentation of the skin. The condition can be treated by venesection.

The treatment of anaemia, for example in thalassaemia, by multiple blood transfusions is associated with iron overload.

Plasma ferritin and iron are usually low in iron deficiency and raised in iron overload. Illness, even if minor, usually results in a decrease in the plasma iron concentration. In chronic inflammation and infection, iron stores and plasma ferritin are usually normal but associated with a normochromic, normocytic anaemia, not responsive to iron therapy. Plasma iron concentrations alone are not useful in the diagnosis of iron deficiency or iron overload. Plasma ferritin is usually decreased in iron deficiency and raised in iron overload but can also be raised in chronic inflammation, malignancy and in liver disease. The total iron binding capacity (TIBC) reflects transferrin concentration and both are increased in iron overload and decreased in conditions of low plasma iron and remain unchanged in acute illness.

PORPHYRIAS

The porphyrias are a group of disorders of haem biosynthesis which may be either congenital or acquired. They may be classified into acute and non-acute.

Acute porphyrias

Acute porphyrias are inherited in an autosomal dominant manner. Some people with the disorder will never experience an acute attack and remain in a latent phase. Others are liable to acute attacks precipitated by factors including infection, decreased caloric intake, alcohol and drugs. A number of drugs are implicated and it is hard to predict from its chemical structure the potential of a drug to precipitate an acute attack. The clinical features of an acute attack are variable with abdominal pain, tachycardia and hypertension being the most common. Nervous system involvement may cause psychiatric disturbance, seizures and peripheral neuropathy. In VP and HCP the skin may be involved with development of photosensitivity. Management of the acute attack is essentially symptomatic. A high carbohydrate intake is encouraged and any known precipitating factors removed. However it is possible to supply haem (as haem arginate) – the end-product of the haem pathway – and thus decrease the activity of ALA synthase, the rate limiting step in the pathway.

Non-acute porphyrias

Patients with PCT experience increased skin sensitivity, particularly on the hands and face which are exposed to light. Blistering on the backs of the hands may occur and, more rarely, facial hair or increased pigmentation may develop. The disorder may be inherited in an autosomal manner or may be sporadic in association with environmental factors such as a high alcohol intake. CEP and EPP are both characterised by the accumulation of porphyrins in red blood cells. In CEP mild photosensitivity and hepatocellular damage occur. CEP is a severe disorder, inherited autosomally. There is severe photosensitivity, haemolytic anaemia and the deposition of porphyrins in bones and teeth.

The porphyrin concentrations in red cells, urine and faeces may be measured to diagnose and classify the porpyrias. These features are shown in Table 15.2.

```
┌──────────────────────────────────────┐
│ Reference ranges                       │
│                                        │
│ Haemoglobin        Females 12–15 g/dL  │
│                    Males 13–17 g/dL    │
└──────────────────────────────────────┘
```

Type	Deficient enzyme	Inheritance	Symptoms	Porphyrins present		
				Urine	Faeces	Red cells
Acute						
Acute intermittent porphyria (AIP)	PBG deaminase	AD	N	ALA, PBG	–	–
Variegate porphyria (VP)	Protoporphyrinogen oxidase	AD	N, P	ALA, PBG copro	copro, proto	–
Hereditary coproporphyria (HCP)	Coproporphyrinogen oxidase	AD	N, P	ALA, PBG copro	copro	–
Chronic						
Porphyria cutanea tarda (PCT)	Uroporphyrinogen decarboxylase	AD	P	uro	isocopro	–
Congenital erythropoietic porphyria (CEP)	Uroporphyrinogen cosynthase	AR	P	uro, copro	uro, copro	yes
erythropoietic protoporphyria (EPP)	Ferrochelatase	AD	P	–	proto	yes

N=neurological, P=photosensitising

Table 15.2 Diagnostic features of porphyria.

SELECTED READING

Hoffbrand, A.V. and Peltif, J.E. *Essential Haematology*, 3rd Edition. Blackwell Science Inc. 1991

16

THE LIVER

Objectives
To understand:

- The functions of the liver
- The classification of jaundice
- The laboratory assessment of liver disease
- Biochemical features of liver disease

The liver is a wedge shaped organ situated in the right upper quadrant of the abdomen, protected by the rib cage. Functionally the liver consists of groups of cells each fed by a terminal portal venule and hepatic arteriole. Biliary canaliculi are formed from hepatocyte membranes and coalesce to form a system of bile ducts which drains, via the common bile duct, into the small intestine.

FUNCTIONS OF THE LIVER

The liver is a vital organ involved in numerous metabolic processes. Functions of the liver are summarised in Table 16.1.

BILIRUBIN METABOLISM

The liver excretes bile whose contents include lipid, bile acids and bile pigments. Bile is essential for the absorption of lipid constituents from the gut. Bile pigments are derived from bilirubin the principal source of which is haem from the breakdown of haemoglobin from red blood cells. Bilirubin is also derived from the breakdown of myoglobin and cytochromes. Essential features of bilirubin metabolism are shown in Figure 16.1.

Unconjugated bilirubin is insoluble in water and is therefore solubilised by binding to albumin within the circulation. In the liver, bilirubin is taken up by an active carrier-mediated mechanism and then undergoes conjugation with glucuronic acid within the smooth endoplasmic reticulum forming diglucuronides. Once conjugated the bilirubin is water soluble and reaches the small intestine via the biliary system. Gut bacteria then convert the bilirubin to urobilinogen which is colourless. Most urobilinogen becomes oxidised to the brown pigment urobilin within the gut and is excreted in the faeces. A small amount of urobilinogen is absorbed from the gut into portal blood. However, hepatic uptake of this is not complete with the result that a small amount of

FUNCTIONS OF THE LIVER	
Carbohydrate metabolism	glycogen synthesis and breakdown gluconeogenesis
Protein metabolism	deamination of amino acids urea synthesis synthesis of plasma proteins (not immunoglobulins)
Fat metabolism	synthesis of cholesterol, bile acids, lipoproteins and fatty acids
Bilirubin conjugation and excretion	
Metabolism of hormones	polypeptide hormones 25-hydroxylation of vitamin D
Storage	glycogen vitamins iron
Kuppfer cells	contribute to activities of the reticuloendothelial system
Metabolism and excretion of drugs and toxins	
Hydrogen ion homeostasis	decrease in ureagenesis and increased glutamine synthesis in acidosis

Table 16.1

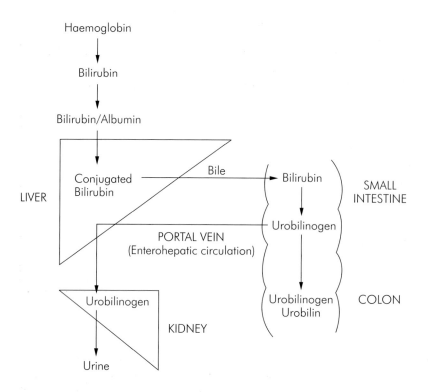

Figure 16.1 – Bilirubin metabolism.

urobilinogen reaches the urine. In health, plasma bilirubin is almost entirely unconjugated and, because of its protein binding, filtration in the glomerulus does not occur hence bilirubin is not found in urine. Urobilinogen is found in the urine and its absence is an indicator of biliary obstruction. Bilirubinuria is always abnormal and is due to an increase in the amount of conjugated bilirubin in the plasma.

The clinical classification of jaundice

Jaundice is a yellowish discolouration of tissues due to deposition of bilirubin. This can be detected clinically when plasma bilirubin is greater than about 50 μmol/L. Jaundice may be classified as pre-hepatic, hepatic and post-hepatic as shown in Table 16.2.

Patients with haematological conditions causing haemolysis or ineffective erythropoiesis, for example sickle cell disease and thalassaemia, are often slightly jaundiced. Gilbert's disease is a common condition characterised by mild, fluctuating jaundice due to increased unconjugated bilirubin in plasma. It is usually asymptomatic and is often revealed by a blood test taken for an intercurrent illness. In Dubin-Johnson syndrome there is defective excretion of conjugated bilirubin and the liver appears dark brown due to pigment deposition. Rotor syndrome is similar to Dubin-Johnson syndrome but there is no hepatic pigmentation.

As many as half of all normal babies develop 'physiological jaundice' after 48 hours of age which is essentially due to immaturity of the hepatic conjugating system. The excess bilirubin is unconjugated and if its concentration rises very high it can cross the blood-brain barrier and be deposited in the brain causing a specific form of brain damage (kernicterus). If neonatal jaundice persists for more than ten days further investigations should be done, particularly determination of whether the hyperbilirubinaemia is conjugated or unconjugated. Causes of neonatal jaundice are shown in Table 16.2.

CLASSIFICATION OF JAUNDICE

Pre-hepatic
  when the liver is presented with bilirubin in an amount that exceeds the conjugating mechanism
  haemolysis
  ineffective erythropoiesis
  Gilbert's syndrome

Hepatic
  when the causal abnormality is in the liver
  diffuse hepatocellular damage – hepatitis, toxins
  intra-hepatic cholestasis – drugs
  Dubin-Johnson syndrome, Rotor syndrome

Post-hepatic
  when there is obstruction to the biliary system
  gallstones
  carcinoma of the head of the pancreas

Table 16.2

LABORATORY ASSESSMENT OF LIVER DISEASE

The standard tests used in the assessment of liver disease are measurement of plasma bilirubin concentration, total protein and albumin and the activity of certain enzymes – notably aspartate transaminase (AST), alanine transaminase (ALT), alkaline phosphatase (ALP) and γ-glutamyl transferase (GGT). This group of tests will correctly divide patients into liver disease/non-liver disease groups in 75% of cases.

An increase in plasma bilirubin concentration does not always occur in liver disease and it may be present in extrahepatic disorders. AST and ALT indicate damage to hepatic cytoplasmic or mitochondrial membranes. However they are not specific to the liver, occurring in other tissues also. The liver synthesises ALP and secretes it into the bile. In both hepatic and post-hepatic jaundice the ALP is raised, the increase tending to be higher with post-hepatic causes. ALP is also produced by bone and in some circumstances it may be necessary to perform electrophoresis to separate the tissue specific isoforms and therefore clarify the tissue of origin. GGT activity may be increased due to enzyme induction by alcohol or drugs, for example some anticonvulsants. GGT may also be found to be elevated in hepatitis and in non-hepatic conditions such as pancreatic carcinoma.

As the synthesis of albumin occurs in the liver its plasma concentration is an indicator of hepatic function. However, it is not only the rate of synthesis of albumin which affects its plasma concentration. In chronic liver disease plasma albumin may be decreased, but due to its long half life of about 30 days the concentration is usually not decreased in acute liver disease. Measurement of prothrombin time (PT) provides an assessment of the activity of the liver derived vitamin-K dependent clotting factors. One of these, Factor VII, has a half life of about five hours. An increase in PT is therefore a sensitive indicator of liver function. However, an increased PT may also occur secondary to vitamin K deficiency due to decreased fat absorption because of decreased bile salt availability. If this is the cause the PT will correct after the administration of parenteral vitamin K.

There are more specialized tests for use in special circumstances. For example, the bromosulphthalein excretion test and the ^{14}C-caffeine breath test assess microsomal activity. The measurement of glutathione-S-transferase is a more specific and sensitive indicator of hepatic damage than measurement of transaminases. Specific biochemical tests may also help determine the cause of liver dysfunction for example α_1-antitrypsin phenotyping if deficiency is suspected; caeruloplasmin and copper measurement in Wilson's disease and increased transferrin saturation in haemochromatosis.

BIOCHEMICAL FEATURES OF LIVER DISEASES

Hepatitis, cirrhosis and tumours are the most common disorders affecting the liver.

HEPATITIS

This is the result of damage to liver cells. It is most often caused by viruses — predominantly hepatitis A or B but also Epstein-Barr, cytomegalovirus and a number of other agents. Drugs, for example paracetamol and toxins such as alcohol can also induce hepatitis, as can autoimmune processes. The associated biochemical abnormalities are a large rise in transaminase activity, a less pronounced rise in ALP and hyperbilirubinaemia and bilirubinuria. Characteristically the increase in transaminases occurs before the peak rise in bilirubin concentration. In the majority of cases hepatitis resolves completely. In <1% of cases there is progression to acute liver failure. Progression to chronic hepatitis can also occur in which the clinical or biochemical features of liver disease are present for more than 6 months. On histological criteria chronic hepatitis can be divided into chronic persistent hepatitis and chronic active hepatitis, the latter commonly progressing to cirrhosis.

CIRRHOSIS

This is a histological diagnosis based on the presence of increased fibrous tissue formation and nodular regeneration leading to disruption of the normal architecture of the liver. Causes include alcohol excess, chronic active hepatitis, autoimmune disease and some forms of metabolic liver disease. Conventional liver function tests may remain completely normal in the early stages of the disease as the liver has a high functional reserve and the cirrhosis is then said to be compensated. Decompensation can be precipitated by drugs, infection or gastrointestinal bleeding. Decreased albumin production and increased portal and hepatic venous pressure contribute to the development of ascites.

TUMOURS

Tumours occurring in the liver are most commonly metastases. Primary liver tumours often occur in association with cirrhosis or persistent hepatitis B infection. Alpha-fetoprotein is elevated in most cases of primary hepatocellular carcinoma and measurement of its plasma concentration may be a useful screening test for tumour development in high risk patients. As metastatic lesions are fairly well localised there may be sufficient functional tissue for biochemical tests to remain normal. Elevation of ALP is often the first detectable abnormality.

METABOLIC LIVER DISEASE

This occurs in a number of inherited disorders and may progress to cirrhosis. α_1-antitrypsin deficiency may result in neonatal hepatitis progressing to cirrhosis. Less severely affected individuals may develop perturbation of liver function tests in adult life. Wilson's disease is a disorder of copper metabolism in which accumulation of copper in the liver can cause hepatic damage. Haemochromatosis is an abnormality of iron metabolism resulting in iron deposition in the liver.

LIVER FAILURE

Any of these conditions may predispose to liver failure. Liver failure is defined as acute when it occurs within six months and fulminant when it occurs within eight weeks of the development of liver disease. The most common cause of fulminant hepatic failure (FHF) in the UK is paracetamol overdose. Clinically FHF is characterised by the development of hepatic encephalopathy which may be severe enough to cause coma. The plasma ammonia concentration is raised in encephalopathy but does not necessarily correlate with severity. Other biochemical abnormalities include hypoglycaemia and hyponatraemia. Renal failure (hepato-renal syndrome) may develop and there may be a disparity between the urea and creatine concentrations, urea being disproportionately low due to decreased hepatic synthesis. FHF predisposes to disturbances of acid-base balance of various types. Accumulated toxins can cause respiratory stimulation with resulting alkalosis. Lactic acidosis may occur secondary to decreased hepatic gluconeogenesis and urinary loss of hydrogen ions due to secondary hyperaldosteronism may lead to a metabolic alkalosis.

GALL STONES

These are common and may be clinically silent or present with biliary colic, acute cholesystitis or bile duct obstruction. They usually consist of cholesterol, bilirubin and calcium; however, radiological investigation is usually unhelpful as only about 1% of gall stones contain enough calcium to be radio-opaque. Pigment stones are small and multiple and consist of bile pigments. They are usually found in chronic haemolytic states.

Reference ranges	
Bilirubin (total)	2 -20 μmol/L
AST	10 – 60 IU/L
ALP (adult)	30 – 100 IU/L
GGT	5-55 IU/L

SELECTED READING

Bircher, J. *Oxford Textbook of Clinical Heptology*, 2nd Edition. Oxford University Press, 1999.

17

THE GASTROINTESTINAL SYSTEM

Objectives

To understand:

- The processes leading to absorption of food

- Disorders of the gastrointestinal tract – malabsorption, abnormalities of increased and decreased secretions, short bowl syndrome

- Laboratory investigation of gastrointestinal function

The major functions of the gastrointestinal system are the digestion and absorption of food. However, it also has other functions, gut lymphoid tissue being involved with protection against micro-organisms and parasites and intestinal bacteria contributing to the vitamin K available from the gut. The colon is involved with water reabsorption and via the action of aldosterone, in sodium and potassium homeostasis.

DIGESTION AND ABSORPTION OF FOOD

During digestion, dietary components are broken down to smaller molecules and absorption of these digested constituents from the gut then occurs. Efficient gut motility is essential to bring about mixing and forward propulsion of gut contents and a complex combination of processes leading to absorption is integrated by hormonal and neuronal mechanisms.

CARBOHYDRATE DIGESTION

Carbohydrate digestion commences in the mouth with the action of salivary amylase and is continued by pancreatic amylase resulting in the formation of oligosaccharides and some larger branched saccharides. Absorption of these oligosaccharides is brought about by three disaccharidases within the brush border of the cells of the small intestine – lactase, maltase and sucrase-isomaltase. The resulting monosaccharides – glucose, galactose and fructose are then absorbed.

PROTEIN DIGESTION

Protein digestion begins with the action of pepsin in the stomach and is continued by proteases secreted from the pancreas. These proteases are trypsin, chymotrypsin, elastase and carboxypeptidase which are all secreted as inactive proenzymes. An enterokinase from the brush border acts on the proenzyme trypsinogen to produce trypsin which then activates the other proenzymes. Peptidases within the brush border continue protein digestion and a combination of amino acids, dipeptides and tripeptides are absorbed.

FAT DIGESTION

Fat digestion begins with emulsification resulting from chewing and stomach motility. Phospholipid from the diet and from bile, together with bile salts, help to stabilise this emulsion. Pancreatic lipase hydrolyses triglycerides to release free fatty acids. Pancreatic phospholipase and esterase digest phospholipids and cholesteryl esters respectively. These products, together with bile salts, then form mixed micelles. Within these micelles insoluble cholesterol, monoglycerides and free fatty acids are held as an emulsion. Within enterocytes these components are reformed into chylomicrons and absorbed, although some medium chain fatty acids can be absorbed intact.

DISORDERS OF THE GASTROINTESTINAL TRACT

Disorders of the gastrointestinal tract may be generalised or be related to specific functions or anatomical regions.

GASTROENTERITIS

Gastroenteritis is a very common disorder and may present with nausea, vomiting, abdominal pain and diarrhoea. Gastroenteritis may be the result of infection or from the effects of bacterial toxins ingested with food.

MALIGNANCY

Carcinoma of the oesophagus, stomach, colon and rectum are common but small bowel malignancies are rare.

COELIAC DISEASE

Coeliac disease is an enteropathy resulting from gluten sensitivity. It may present with diarrhoea and failure to thrive in infancy but less severe forms may go undetected until later life, presenting with growth failure, anaemia and abdominal pain.

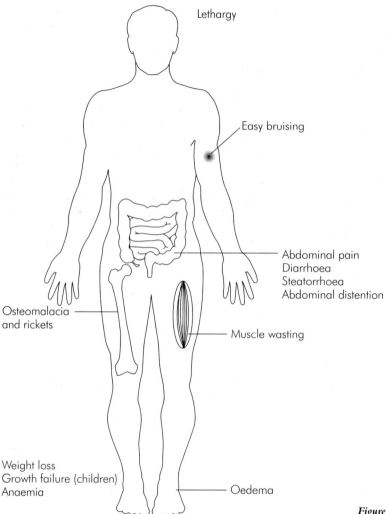

Lethargy

Easy bruising

Abdominal pain
Diarrhoea
Steatorrhoea
Abdominal distention

Osteomalacia
and rickets

Muscle wasting

Weight loss
Growth failure (children)
Anaemia

Oedema

Figure 17.1 – Clinical features of malabsorption.

MALABSORPTION

A large number of disorders of the gastrointestinal tract present as malabsorption. Malabsorption may be of a single dietary component, for example vitamin B_{12} resulting in pernicious anaemia, or a type of dietary component such as fat, or generalised. Clinical features of malabsorption are shown in Figure 17.1.

Malabsorption of carbohydrate may result in abdominal distension and diarrhoea whilst steatorrhoea – the passage of bulky, pale stools – occurs in fat malabsorption. Other presentations include anaemia, growth failure and weight loss. These clinical features are the result of a limited number of pathological processes – abnormal gastrointestinal secretions, defective enzyme production or abnormalities of the gastrointestinal mucosa.

Disorders of gastric secretion

The stomach produces acid, the resulting pH aiding the action of pepsin. The stomach secretes intrinsic factor which is essential for the absorption of vitamin B_{12}.

Decreased pancreatic secretions

Decreased pancreatic secretions may be the result of destructive processes such as chronic pancreatitis. Chronic pancreatitis is often related to excess alcohol consumption and can be associated with disorder of the endocrine pancreas. In the inherited disorder cystic fibrosis pancreatic involvement is usual and affected children may present with diarrhoea and failure to thrive. Pancreatic bicarbonate secretion is necessary to neutralise gastric acid and without an alkaline pH optimum activity of pancreatic lipase is not achieved. Exocrine pancreatic secretions are essential for the digestion of carbohydrate, protein and fat and so malabsorption resulting from defective pancreatic secretions tends to be severe. Treatment with enzyme supplements in an encapsulated form can be used to aid digestion.

Decreased biliary secretion

Decreased biliary secretion can be the result of primary hepatobiliary pathology or by extrinsic obstruction to bile flow, for example from carcinoma of the head of the pancreas. The result is malabsorption of fat and of fat soluble vitamins.

Decreased oligosaccharidase activity

Reduced activity of the enterocyte oligosaccharides maltase and sucrase-isomaltase is rare usually presenting in infancy with diarrhoea and failure to thrive. Congenital lactase deficiency is uncommon, deficiency of the enzyme occuring much more frequently secondary to disorders of the intestinal mucosa, for example, gastroenteritis and inflammatory bowel disease. It usually improves with resolution of the primary pathology but a period of milk free diet is often necessary.

Disorders of absorption of specific amino acids

An example of a disorder of the absorption of specific amino acids is Hartnup disease in which disordered renal tubular reabsorption coexists. Hartnup disease may manifest as pellagra due to a decrease in tryptophan absorption.

A generalised decrease in absorptive capacity in its most extreme form is exemplified by the short bowel syndrome. In adults the most frequent cause is surgical resection of bowel secondary to mesenteric vascular occlusion and in children secondary to necrotising enterocolitis. The effect of small intestinal resection is related to both the extent and nature of the remaining bowel. Resection of the jejunum is of less functional importance than loss of the proximal small bowel and preservation of the ileocaecal valve reduces the likelihood of contamination of the small bowel by colonic bacteria. The terminal ileum is essential for the absorption of bile salts which, if not absorbed, are irritative to the colon contributing to decreased transit time. The gut has a reserve capacity and in time adaptation to a shortened bowel can occur. Parenteral nutrition may be necessary during this adaptation process and in

some patients is a permanent requirement. In the future bowel transplantation may become a viable treatment option.

Disorders of increased gut secretions

Oversecretion from the gut can also cause dysfunction. Oversecretion of acid is implicated in the aetiology of duodenal, but not gastric, ulceration. Disturbances of gut function secondary to abnormal endocrine secretions can occur, examples being the Zollinger-Ellison syndrome secondary to excess gastrin, usually from a pancreatic tumour and the Verner-Morrison syndrome which is the result of excessive vasoactive-intestinal polypeptide. Increased secretion may be the result of bacterial infection, for example with *Vibrio cholerae*, or by ingestion of toxins which stimulate secretion.

Bacterial overgrowth

Causes of bacterial overgrowth in the small bowel include diverticulae, strictures and blind loops. Fat malabsorption occurs as a result of deconjugation of bile acids by the bacteria.

LABORATORY INVESTIGATION OF DISORDERS OF GASTROINTESTINAL FUNCTION

Investigation of disorders of the gastrointestinal tract can be achieved by biochemical tests, radiography or direct visualisation by endoscopy. Histological examination of bowel biopsies remains an important diagnostic tool. Microbiological tests to detect the presence of bacteria, viruses or parasites may also be helpful.

The investigation of disorders of gastrointestinal function, like its physiology, can be considered in terms of its separate dietary components.

CARBOHYDRATE MALABSORPTION

Carbohydrate malabsorption has, in the past, been detected by sugar tolerance tests. However, glucose tolerance tests are unhelpful, absorption depending on related processes such as insulin secretion. Xylose and lactose tolerance tests have also been used but may not be informative. Absorption tests involving combinations of sugars are gaining acceptance. Unabsorbed carbohydrate within the gut is broken down by gut bacteria to methane and hydrogen. A hydrogen breath test assesses the hydrogen content of the breath after a test dose of carbohydrate. To establish a diagnosis of disaccharidase deficiency assessment of activity of the relevant enzyme in biopsy tissue may be helpful.

FAT MALABSORPTION

Fat malabsorption can be assessed in a quantitative fashion by measurement of faecal fat excretion. However, this is an unpleasant procedure for all involved and is not always diagnostic. It is being replaced by other investigations such as the ^{14}C-triolein breath test. This involves administration of fat containing ^{14}C-triolein, expired ^{14}CO$_2$ then being used as an indicator of fat absorption, decreased excretion indicating decreased absorption.

PROTEIN MALABSORPTION

Protein malabsorption is not usually specifically investigated. However protein-losing enteropathy can be investigated using faecal excretion of α_1-antitrypsin or by radio-isotope techniques.

PANCREATIC FUNCTION

The pancreolauryl and PABA tests can be used to assess pancreatic function. In the pancreolauryl test fluorescein dilaurate is ingested and the fluorescein released by the action of pancreatic enzymes is absorbed and excreted into the urine where it can be measured. To compensate for abnormalities of hepatic and renal function the test is then repeated with free fluorescein and the ratio expressed. The PABA test is similar in principle. Traditional tests involving the assessment of enzyme activity in duodenal aspirate after a standard test meal are now obsolete.

GASTROINTESTINAL BLOOD LOSS

The detection of gastrointestinal blood loss has previously been based on faecal occult blood testing. This is an extremely sensitive test and false positives are common but due to the episodic nature of blood loss false negative results are also common.

VITAMIN B$_{12}$ MALABSORPTION

The Schilling test can be used to investigate vitamin B$_{12}$ malabsorption. As malabsorption may be caused by decreased intrinsic factor production or by decreased absorption due to disease of the terminal ileum, the test assesses absorption of radio-labelled vitamin B$_{12}$ with and without oral administration of intrinsic factor.

DETECTION OF SPECIFIC DISEASES

Certain tests may be useful in the diagnosis of specific disorders – for example the detection of anti-gliadin and antiendomesial antibodies as a screening test for coeliac disease, the latter being more specific, and serological tests for *Helicobacter pylori* in the investigation of gastric ulceration.

Laboratory investigations of gastrointestinal function are summarised in Table 17.1.

LABORATORY INVESTIGATION OF GASTROINTESTINAL DISEASE	
Suspected diagnosis	**Laboratory investigation**
Carbohydrate malabsorption	Hydrogen breath test
Fat malabsorption	^{14}C-triolein breath test
Decreased pancreatic function	Pancreolauryl test ^{14}C-PABA test
Bacterial overgrowth	^{14}C-glycocholic acid breath test

Table 17.1

SELECTED READING

Spiller, R.C. Digestion and malabsorption of nutrients. In: Bouchier, I.A.D., Allan, R.N., Hodgson, H.J.K. and Keighley, M.R.B. (eds). *Gastroenterology: Clinical Science and Practice*. W.B. Saunders, London. 1993.

Stendall, C. *Practical Guide to Gastrointestinal Function Testing*. Blackwell Science Inc. 1997.

18

THE KIDNEYS

Objectives

To understand:

- The physiology of the kidney – the function of the glomeruli, tubules and collecting ducts

- Biochemical tests of renal function

- Disorders of the kidney – renal failure, tubular disorders, proteinuria, renal calculi

The kidneys are situated on the posterior wall of the abdomen, each contains about one million functional units called nephrons. The kidneys function to allow the excretion of waste products and the maintenance of extracellular fluid volume and ionic composition. They are also involved in hormone synthesis by the production of renin and erythropoietin, and the 1α-hydroxylation of 25-hydroxycholecalciferol.

THE PHYSIOLOGY OF THE KIDNEY

The kidneys receive about 25% of the cardiac output. The majority of this blood flows initially to capillary tufts in the glomeruli. Here the blood undergoes filtration. This is a passive process, the total filtration rate being determined by the difference between the blood pressure within the glomerular capillaries and the hydrostatic pressure within the lumen of the nephron, by the number of glomeruli and by the nature of the glomerular basement membrane. The ability of a molecule to pass through the glomerular filter depends upon both its size and electrical charge. Positively charged molecules are more easily filtered than those which are negatively charged. The glomerular filtrate has a similar composition to plasma except that it is almost protein free. Proteins with a molecular weight less than that of albumin are filterable. The normal urinary protein excretion is less than 150 mg/24 hours, as the majority of the protein in the glomerular filtrate is subsequently reabsorbed. The glomerular filtration rate (GFR) in health is about 170 L/day – 120 mL/minute. Only about 1–2 L of urine are produced each day as the majority of the glomerular filtrate is reabsorbed during its passage through the nephron.

The glomerular filtrate passes from the glomerulus into the proximal convoluted tubule where about 70% of its volume is reabsorbed. There are also energy-dependent processes which result in reabsorption of 75% of the sodium and virtually all the potassium,

bicarbonate, glucose and amino acids. The proximal tubule cannot dissociate the absorption of water and that of solute but the proportion of water absorption must be varied according to need in order to correct changes in extracellular osmolality.

This adjustment takes place in the loop of Henlé, distal convoluted tubule and collecting duct by the countercurrent mechanism. Countercurrent multiplication is an active process which occurs in the loop of Henlé. Chloride ions are actively pumped out of the ascending limb of the loop accompanied by sodium ions and diffuse from the surrounding interstitial fluid into the descending limb of the loop. The ascending limb of the loop is impermeable to water thus this movement of sodium and chloride ions, together with the flow of fluid around the loop, results in the production of a gradient of increasing osmolality on passing from the cortico-medullary junction to the deeper layers of the medulla. Urea also contributes to the hypertonicity of the medulla due to its diffusion from the collecting duct into the interstitium and thus into the loop of Henlé. The result of countercurrent multiplication is that the tubular fluid, which is isotonic at the end of the proximal tubule, is hypotonic on entering the distal tubule.

Further sodium reabsorption occurs in the distal tubule and collecting duct under the influence of aldosterone. The extra-cellular gradient resulting from the absorption of sodium is balanced by the secretion of potassium and hydrogen ions. ADH increases the permeability of the cells within the distal tubules and collecting duct allowing water to move passively along the osmolality gradient that has been established within the medulla. The collecting duct has a close relationship to the ascending vasa recta of the kidney, thus the absorbed water enters the blood-stream and is carried through the cortex to enter the general circulation. The normal plasma osmolality and thus the osmolality of the glomerular filtrate is 280–295 mmol/kg, however at the extremes of water intake the urine osmolality can vary between 40 and 1400 mmol/kg.

Events within the nephron are summarised in Figure 18.1.

LABORATORY TESTS OF RENAL FUNCTION

Tests of renal function include those which assess glomerular filtration rate, glomerular integrity and tubular function.

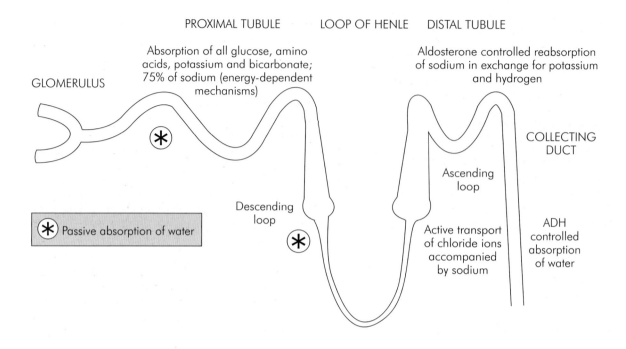

Figure 18.1 – Summary of events within the nephron.

GLOMERULAR FUNCTION

Three tests are commonly used in the assessment of GFR – estimation of clearance and measurement of plasma urea and creatinine.

Clearance

Clearance is an estimate of the GFR and can be made by measuring the removal from the blood of a substance which is completely filtered from the blood by the glomerulus and is not then secreted, metabolised or reabsorbed by the renal tubules. The clearance of such a substance is equal to the GFR and is defined as the volume of blood from which the substance is completely removed in one minute. The method of choice for the estimation of clearance is the injection of ^{51}Cr-EDTA, followed by measurement of the rate of fall of radioactivity as the isotope is cleared. The measurement of inulin clearance has been found to be useful for experimental purposes but for regular use creatinine clearance is usually estimated. Creatinine is an endogenous substance derived mainly from creatine phosphate within muscle, with a small contribution from dietary intake of meat.

Creatinine clearance may be calculated from the following equation:

$$\text{Creatinine clearance} = \frac{U \times V}{P \times T}$$

where

U = urinary creatinine concentration (μmol/L)
V = urine volume (mL)
P = plasma creatinine concentration (μmol/L)
T = collection period (minutes)

The usual period of collection is 24 hours but a shorter period is valid if accurately timed. Some creatinine is secreted by the renal tubules thus the creatinine clearance tends to slightly overestimate the GFR. This overestimate is not significant until the GFR is very low.

Plasma urea

Plasma urea arises principally as a by-product of amino acid deamination and is the main route of nitrogen excretion. Some tubular reabsorption occurs which becomes particularly significant at low urine flow rates. Thus, in dehydration the plasma urea concentration may rise when glomerular function is normal. The plasma urea concentration may also be increased by a high dietary protein intake, in states of hyper-catabolism and after gastrointestinal haemorrhage. The plasma urea concentration may be lowered in patients with liver disease or those on a low protein diet.

Plasma creatinine

Plasma creatinine concentration is a more reliable measure of glomerular filtration than plasma urea. The plasma creatinine is proportional to muscle bulk, hence the reference range is lower in infants and children than in adults. Changes in the plasma creatinine concentration may occur without change in renal function because of changes of muscle mass, for example in muscle wasting disorders, or in starvation. Theoretically, the plasma creatinine should be measured on a fasting blood sample to avoid a contribution from dietary meat intake.

GLOMERULAR INTEGRITY

If the integrity of the glomerulus is altered molecules normally retained are filtered. This can be assessed by the measurement of urinary protein, although protein-uria may occur in other situations, some of which are of no clinical significance.

The presence of blood in the urine can result from abnormalities throughout the urinary tract. However, when red cells are surrounded by protein they are termed red cell casts and their presence is usually due to glomerular dysfunction.

TUBULAR FUNCTION

The most commonly performed tests of tubular function are the water deprivation test which assesses the ability of the kidney to produce a concentrated urine and tests of urinary acidification in the diagnosis of distal (type I) renal tubular acidosis. Glycosuria, in the presence of a normal blood glucose concentration may occur in association with a proximal tubular abnormality. Chromatography can be used to assess amino-aciduria due to tubular defects.

DISORDERS OF THE KIDNEY

Renal disorders may affect glomerular function, glomerular integrity or tubular function, alone or in combination.

ACUTE RENAL FAILURE

Acute renal failure is characterised by a sudden decrease in renal function. It is usually, but not always, characterised by a renal flow rate <15 mL/hour.

Pre-renal renal failure

This occurs as a result of a reduction in renal blood flow and the homeostatic responses that follow. The decrease in renal blood flow may be due to severe haemorrhage or loss of fluid, or to a decrease in blood pressure secondary to cardiogenic shock or vasodilatation. In response to the decrease in renal blood flow there is an increase in ADH secretion and stimulation of the renin-angiotensin-aldosterone system which leads to the production of a reduced volume of urine that is highly concentrated and has a low sodium content. The decreased GFR leads to retention of substances such as urea and creatinine which are usually filtered. The function of the renal tubules is essentially unchanged however decreased delivery of sodium to the distal tubules impairs its exchange with hydrogen and potassium ions leading to acidosis and hyper-kalaemia. It is important to recognise pre-renal failure so that its progression to acute tubular necrosis can be prevented. In pre-renal failure urinary sodium is <20 mmol/L as sodium conservation is maximal in an attempt to increase the extracellular fluid volume.

Intrinsic renal failure

This is secondary to intrinsic kidney disease and may be precipitated by a number of causes including nephrotoxins e.g. aminoglycosides and renal diseases such as glomerulonephritis. Uncorrected renal under-perfusion and other renal insults, may result in acute tubular necrosis in which there is an initial oliguric phase, then a diuretic phase as the GFR increases but abnormalities of tubular function persist, followed by a recovery phase. Once tubular necrosis occurs the ability of the kidney to concentrate urine is lost. Urine passed is similar to plasma in its ionic composition, contains protein and may contain haem pigments, giving it a dark colour. Retention of urea, creatinine and hydrogen and potassium ions occurs and hypona-traemia is a frequent finding. There is retention and intracellular leakage of phosphate, the resulting hyper-phosphataemia inhibiting the production of calcitriol which leads to hypocalcaemia. In the diuretic phase there is an improvement in the GFR initially without change in tubular function, resulting in the passage of large volumes of dilute urine. As tubular function recovers, normal kidney function returns although minor abnormalities may persist. In very severe cases there may be no recovery of renal function.

Post-renal renal failure

This may result from prostatic enlargement, renal calculi, neoplasms of the renal tract and retroperitoneal fibrosis. Its presence may be suggested by complete anuria, although this is not an invariable finding. If the obstruction is relieved promptly, complete return of renal function may follow.

Acute renal failure results in considerable morbidity and mortality. The management of acute renal failure is initially directed towards correction of abnormalities of fluid and electrolytes and of acid-base balance. To preserve life it may be necessary to institute renal replacement therapy by haemodialysis or haemofiltration.

CHRONIC RENAL FAILURE

Renal failure may occur in a gradual fashion resulting in a progressive decrease in GFR – chronic renal failure (CRF). Eventually renal dialysis or transplantation become life-saving. Causes of chronic renal failure are shown in Table 18.1.

Clinical features of chronic renal failure are shown in Figure 18.2.

The clinical features of CRF (the 'uraemic syndrome') are varied and none is specific. These features are thought to be due to the retention of certain substances usually excreted, which are retained in excess — for example urea, creatinine, hippuric acid and peptides. Deficiencies of substances usually produced by the kidneys such as calcitriol and erythropoietin may also contribute.

A number of biochemical disturbances are found in CRF. High plasma concentrations of urea and creatinine are found, together with a decreased GFR. In

early CRF sodium balance may be maintained but sodium depletion may occur secondary to decreased tubular reabsorption. When the GFR falls very low sodium retention is characteristic. Hyperkalaemia is a life-threatening complication of CRF but may not occur until the GFR is considerably lowered. Acidosis occurs due to decreased renal H^+ excretion. As the kidneys fail calcitriol synthesis falls leading to decreased calcium absorption from the gut. Hypocalcaemia results, which is resistant to the action of PTH and is accompanied by a raised phosphate concentration. Many patients then go on to develop renal osteodystrophy. Factors contributing to the aetiology of this bone disease include decreased renal production of calcitriol, bone demineralisation due to buffering of hydrogen ions by bone and osteomalacia due to aluminium accumulation. Aluminium may be absorbed from the gut when given orally to bind phosphate and reduce its absorption and may also be absorbed from some types of dialysis fluid. Dyslipidaemia is another common biochemical complication of CRF. Endocrine effects occur — gonadal failure being common in both males and females and growth failure, thought to be multifactorial in origin, occurs frequently in children with CRF.

RENAL TUBULAR DISORDERS

Disorders of the renal tubules may affect single or multiple aspects of tubular function. The cause may be congenital or acquired with clinical effects due to loss of substances which are usually absorbed by the tubules.

Glycosuria

This can occur where there is proximal tubular dysfunction and be due to 'overflow' when the plasma glucose concentration is elevated. However, glycosuria is sometimes a finding of little significance due to a decreased renal threshold for glucose absorption. This tendency is sometimes hereditary.

Aminoaciduria

This may be secondary to elevated plasma amino acid concentrations which cause saturation of tubular reabsorption, as for example in phenylketonuria. Specific defects of tubular reabsorption also lead to aminoaciduria, as in cystinuria. This is a defect of the absorption of the aminoacids cystine, ornithine, arginine and lysine. Cystine is relatively insoluble, thus its

CAUSES OF CHRONIC RENAL FAILURE
glomerulonephritis
diabetes mellitus
pyelonephritis
hypertension
drugs and toxins

Table 18.1

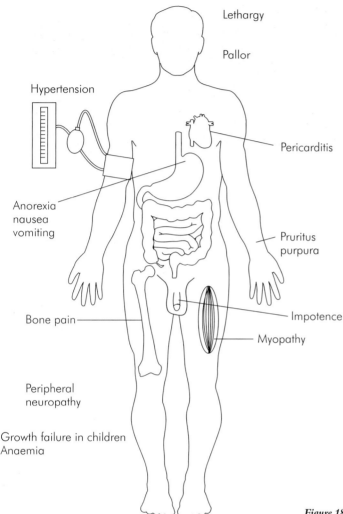

Lethargy

Pallor

Hypertension

Pericarditis

Anorexia
nausea
vomiting

Pruritus
purpura

Bone pain

Impotence

Myopathy

Peripheral
neuropathy

Growth failure in children
Anaemia

Figure 18.2 – Clinical features of chronic renal failure.

presence in high concentration in the renal tubules predisposes to the formation of renal calculi.

Renal tubular acidosis

This acidosis is classified into proximal (type II) and distal (type I). In proximal renal tubular acidosis there is impaired bicarbonate reabsorption due to a defect in the carbonate dehydratase mechanism. The loss of bicarbonate may lead to a systemic acidosis but the ability to form an acid urine is preserved. Treatment is by the administration of bicarbonate. Distal renal tubular acidosis is more common and comprises a defect in the excretion of hydrogen ions such that the urine cannot be acidified. In most acidotic states hyperkalaemia is found but in distal renal tubular acidosis the inability of the distal tubules to secrete hydrogen

ions results in increased potassium ion excretion in exchange for sodium reabsorption and thus acidosis and hypokalaemia co-exist. Diagnosis of distal renal tubular acidosis can be made on the finding of an inappropriately high urinary pH (usually ≥ 6.5) after an ammonium chloride load. Treatment consists of the administration of bicarbonate and potassium.

The Fanconi syndrome

This is a generalised disorder of proximal tubular function therefore resulting in glycosuria, aminoaciduria, phosphaturia and acidosis. The syndrome may be idiopathic or occur as part of an inherited metabolic disorder – for example tyrosinaemia or glycogen storage disorders. It may also be secondary to paraproteinaemia, amyloidosis or nephrotoxins.

Impaired urinary concentration occurs in diabetes insipidus CRF, and may occur in association with hypokalaemia and hypercalcaemia. Some drugs, for example lithium, may also impair urinary concentration.

PROTEINURIA

The normal urinary protein excretion is < 150 mg/24hr. In clinical situations the presence of proteinuria is usually screened for by the use of a reagent-impregnated 'dip-stick' which detects albumin at concentrations > 200 mg/L. If proteinuria is detected in this way a 24 hour urinary protein estimation should be carried out and simple tests of renal function performed. The presence of proteinuria is not always indicative of renal disease. Proteinuria may occur in those with normal renal function as a result of fever or excessive exercise. Orthostatic proteinuria is a benign condition, occurring principally in young people, in which proteinuria occurs only in the upright position due to increased hydrostatic pressure in the renal veins. A diagnosis of orthostatic proteinuria can be made if an early morning sample of urine does not contain protein.

Diabetic nephropathy

One of the most common disorders associated with proteinuria is diabetic nephropathy. Microalbuminuria is defined as a urinary albumin excretion of 20–200 μg/min (30–300 mg/24hr) and its detection is useful as an early indicator of diabetic nephropathy. Measurement of urinary albumin: creatinine ratio is a simple quantitative test by which to assess microalbuminuria.

Nephrotic syndrome

This syndrome is characterised by the presence of hypoproteinaemia, proteinuria and oedema. Other clinical features include an increased susceptibility to infection, as plasma concentrations of immunoglobulins and complement are reduced, hyperlipidaemia due to increased synthesis of apolipoproteins and a tendency to thrombosis because of lowered antithrombin III and increased fibrinogen concentrations. Nephrotic syndrome occurring in children is frequently the result of a 'minimal change' glomerulonephritis and often responds to steroids.

RENAL CALCULI

Renal calculi are usually composed of normal products of metabolism present at concentrations near to their maximum solubility. Minor alterations in urinary composition may then result in precipitation of these products within the renal substance itself or within the renal tract. Such alterations include changes in urine pH, usually due to bacterial infection and urinary stagnation due to outflow obstruction. A high urinary concentration of stone forming products may occur due to a low urinary volume or to a high excretion rate. At least three quarters of all renal calculi contain calcium, either as calcium oxalate or calcium phosphate, sometimes in combination with magnesium ammonium phosphate. The formation of calcium stones may be associated with hypercalcaemia, however, many patients with calcium containing calculi have a normal plasma calcium concentration. Uric acid, cystine and xanthine stones also occur. Uric acid stones may be associated with hyperuricaemia and with gout. Often no predisposing cause is found but precipitation is favoured in acid urine. Cystine and xanthine stones occur in patients who have the inherited metabolic diseases cystinuria and xanthinuria respectively. Hyperoxaluria predisposes to urinary calculi formation and usually results from increased intestinal absorption of dietary oxalate. Two inherited types of hyperoxaluria predisposing to stone formation have also been described.

The biochemical investigation of patients with renal calculi should include measurement of plasma calcium, urate and phosphate concentrations. Urine pH should be assessed, a qualitative test for cysteine performed and the 24 hour excretion of calcium, oxalate and uric acid assessed. If available the calculus itself should be analysed.

Reference ranges	
Urea	3.5–7.0 mmol/L
Creatinine	60–120 μmol/L
Urinary protein	<150 mg/24hours

SELECTED READING

Davison, A.M., Cameron, J.S. and Grunfeld J.–P. (eds). *Oxford Textbook of Clinical Nephrology*. Oxford University Press, 1998.

19

CALCIUM, PHOSPHATE, MAGNESIUM AND BONE

Calcium is the most abundant mineral in the body. About 99% of body calcium is found in bone, complexed with phosphate as hydroxyapatite. Most of the remaining 1% is of great importance due to its involvement in the processes of muscle contraction and neurotransmitter release.

PHYSIOLOGY OF CALCIUM, PHOSPHATE AND MAGNESIUM HOMEOSTASIS

The calcium requirement in adults is at least 10 mmol/24 hours but the usual intake is two to three times higher. Requirements are increased during rapid growth, pregnancy and lactation. Dietary calcium originates largely from milk and milk products.

CALCIUM ABSORPTION AND EXCRETION

Calcium absorption occurs mainly in the upper part of the small intestine and requires a metabolite of vitamin D which stimulates production of a calcium binding protein within the enterocyte. Calcium absorption may be decreased if complexes are formed, in the gut, with excess phosphate or fatty acids. This is made use of therapeutically as oral phosphate can be given in hypercalcaemia to decrease phosphate absorption. In steatorrhoea excess fatty acids in the intestinal lumen complex with calcium reducing absorption.

Calcium is lost from the body in faeces and urine. A large amount of calcium enters the gut in intestinal secretions. That which is not absorbed from the secretions is excreted in the faeces. The urinary excretion of calcium is dependent upon the quantity of calcium reaching the glomeruli, renal function and the levels of parathyroid hormone and 1,25 (OH_2) Vitamin D (calcitriol) and on the excretion of urinary phosphate.

CONTROL OF CALCIUM HOMEOSTASIS

Calcium is present in the plasma in three forms. Approximately 47% is bound to proteins, principally albumin, 46% exists as free ions and the remainder is complexed with phosphate or citrate. The free ions are the only form that is physiologically active. The plasma concentration of calcium is controlled by parathyroid hormone (PTH), a polypeptide hormone synthesised in the parathyroid glands, and calcitriol.

PTH

This is synthesised as pre-pro-PTH (115 amino acids) and is cleaved to pro-PTH (90 aminoacids) with cleavage before secretion to PTH (84 amino acids). PTH secretion is stimulated in response to a decrease in the concentration of plasma ionised calcium and acts to raise the plasma concentration of calcium and to decrease that of phosphate. PTH acts on bone to cause rapid release of calcium and increased osteoclastic resorption, thus increasing plasma calcium. PTH also causes increased calcium reabsorption in the kidney and decreased phosphate reabsorption. Changes in plasma phosphate have no effect on PTH secretion.

Calcitriol

This is derived from vitamin D3 (cholecalciferol). More cholecalciferol is derived from synthesis in the skin than is derived from dietary 7-dehydrocholecalciferol. Vitamin D undergoes 25-hydroxylation in the liver and then 1α-hydroxylation in the kidney. The 1α-hydroxylase enzyme is closely regulated and activity of the enzyme is stimulated by a low plasma phosphate and by an increase in plasma PTH concentration. Oestrogen, prolactin and growth hormone also stimulate 1α-hydroxylase thus increasing calcium absorption during pregnancy, lactation and growth. A high plasma phosphate concentration inhibits the enzyme. Calcitriol stimulates the absorption of dietary calcium and phosphate from the gut and promotes mineralisation of bone.

Calcitonin

This is produced from the C-cells of the thyroid. It decreases osteoclastic activity but its role in calcium homeostasis is uncertain. In medullary carcinoma of the thyroid gland calcitonin levels can be very high without disturbance of calcium homeostasis.

FUNCTIONS OF CALCIUM

Calcium has many functions as shown in Table 19.1.

As well as structural functions calcium has an important role as an intracellular signal for many processes such as metabolic changes, secretory activity and changes in cell motility and division.

LABORATORY ASSESSMENT OF CALCIUM CONCENTRATION

Most commonly total calcium is measured in the laboratory, although the free ionised fraction can be measured using an ion-specific electrode. The total calcium concentration is dependent on the plasma albumin concentration and formulae have been derived to calculate the calcium concentration when the plasma albumin level lies outside the reference range. One such formula is:

[albumin] < 40 g/L: corrected calcium (mmol/L) = $[Ca^{2+}] + 0.02 \times (40 - [albumin])$

[albumin] > 40 g/L: corrected calcium (mmol/L) = $[Ca^{2+}] + 0.02 \times ([albumin] - 40)$

Stasis during venepuncture may cause apparent hypercalcaemia and samples for calcium estimation should be taken without a tourniquet. Hypocalcaemia may result if blood is collected into a tube containing the anticoagulant EDTA.

PHOSPHATE

Dietary deficiency of phosphate rarely occurs on a normal diet. The majority of phosphate within the body is intracellular and is important as a component of phospholipids, phosphoproteins, nucleic acids and nucleotides. Phosphorylation/dephosphorylation reactions are important in the regulation of enzyme activity. Chemical energy is stored in the high energy phosphate bonds of substances such as adenosine triphosphate (ATP) and as diphosphoglycerate, an important regulator of oxygen transport in erythrocytes.

MAGNESIUM

The majority of magnesium is found in bone. Magnesium is the second most abundant intracellular cation – only about 0.5% of total body magnesium is found in the plasma, thus the measurement of plasma concentration does not accurately reflect total body magnesium status. Magnesium is an important cofactor for more than 300 enzymatic reactions, particularly those which require ATP. Magnesium is also essential to the structure of ribosomes, nucleic acids and some proteins and is required for replication of DNA and for the processes of transcription and translation. Owing to its association with calcium, magnesium is important in bone formation and in effects on excitable membranes.

DISORDERS OF CALCIUM, PHOSPHATE AND MAGNESIUM HOMEOSTASIS

HYPERCALCAEMIA

This is a common finding and is often spurious. Causes of true hypercalcaemia are shown in Table 19.2.

Malignancy and primary hyperparathyroidism are the most common causes of hypercalcaemia, once spurious hypercalcaemia has been excluded.

Malignancy is often associated with hypercalcaemia in patients both with and without bone metastases. Non-metastatic hypercalcaemia may result from the action of PTH-related peptides secreted by tumour cells. In myeloma there is production of cytokines which have osteoclast stimulating actions.

Hyperparathyroidism may be classified into primary, secondary and tertiary types. In the primary and tertiary forms plasma calcium is elevated, whereas in the

FUNCTIONS OF CALCIUM	
Role in bone formation	structural organ protection
Tooth formation	
Neuromuscular	muscle contraction neurotransmitter function
Hormonal	enzyme actions blood coagulation
Regulation of transmembrane ion transport	

Table 19.1

CAUSES OF HYPERCALCAEMIA

Spurious
Malignancy
Hyperparathydoidism
Endocrine causes
    thyrotoxicosis
    acromegaly
    adrenal failure
Granulomatous disease
    sarcoidosis
    tuberculosis
Immobilisation
    especially in Paget's disease
Iatrogenic
    thiazide diuretics
    lithium
Familial hypocalciuric hypercalcaemia
Vitamin D excess
Milk alkali syndrome

Table 19.2

secondary form plasma calcium is low. Primary hyperparathyroidism can result from hyperplasia of the glands or from benign or, rarely, malignant tumours of the parathyroid glands. A single adenoma is the most common cause. Parathyroid adenomas may be familial and may also occur as part of multiple endocrine neoplasia (MEN). There is increased PTH secretion leading to a raised plasma calcium with a decreased plasma phosphate.

In conditions such as chronic renal failure there is a decrease in calcitriol production. This leads to hypocalcaemia and PTH increases in an attempt to restore the plasma calcium level towards normal (secondary hyperparathyroidism). In prolonged secondary hyperparathyroidism the parathyroid glands may hypertrophy leading to hypercalcaemia (tertiary hypercalcaemia). This has been described in malabsorption, but is more common after successful renal transplantation.

In granulomatous diseases such as sarcoidosis and tuberculosis, hypercalcaemia can occur due to 1α-hydroxylase activity of macrophages in the granulomatous tissue.

Endocrine causes of hypercalcaemia include thyrotoxicosis due to increased osteoclastic activity. Excess growth hormone has a direct stimulatory effect on the renal 1α-hydroxylase enzyme and causes hypercalcaemia together with hyperphosphataemia.

Thiazide diuretics interfere with the secretion of calcium by the kidney. Familial hypocalciuric hypercalcaemia is an autosomal dominant disorder in which there is mild hypercalcaemia and usually hypophosphataemia. Urinary calcium excretion is reduced. Vitamin D excess may result in hypercalcaemia as may overenthusiastic treatment with vitamin D metabolites such as calcitriol.

Milk alkali syndrome is rarely seen now, but, before the onset of effective therapies for duodenal ulceration, it occurred due to excess consumption of alkaline preparations taken to neutralise gastric acid.

Clinical effects of hypercalcaemia are shown in Figure 19.1.

When the plasma free ionised calcium concentration is elevated, the solubility product of calcium phosphate may be exceeded resulting in its precipitation. Deposition in the kidney impairs urine concentrating mechanisms, thus resulting in polyuria. Calcium salts can also be deposited in the urine causing renal calculi. The raised calcium concentration depresses neuromuscular excitability in skeletal and smooth muscle resulting in hypotonia and muscle weakness as well as constipation and abdominal pain. Anorexia, nausea and depression may occur, probably as direct effects of the increased ionised calcium on the central nervous system. Gastrin secretion is stimulated by calcium, thus increasing gastric acid secretion which can lead to peptic ulceration. Pancreatitis may be a manifestation of hypercalcaemia. Hypercalcaemia also has effects on the cardiovascular system. Hypertension may occur but this may remit if normocalcaemia is achieved. Very high calcium levels cause ECG changes and may even result in cardiac arrest.

HYPERPHOSPHATAEMIA

The most common cause of hyperphosphataemia is renal failure but it is also observed in catabolic states, vitamin D intoxication and hypoparathyroidism. In excess, phosphate can inhibit calcitriol production and can combine with calcium with resulting metastatic deposition in the tissues. Both these effects tend to cause hypocalcaemia.

HYPERMAGNESAEMIA

This is rare except in renal failure and tends to cause cardiac and respiratory complications.

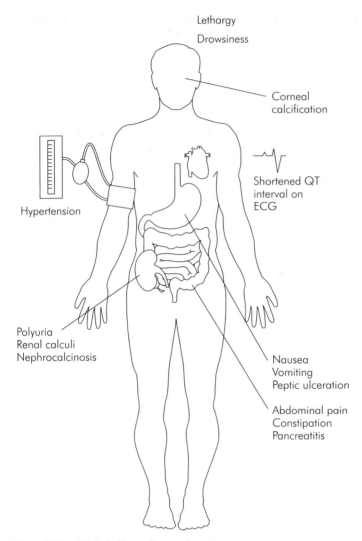

Lethargy
Drowsiness

Corneal
calcification

Shortened QT
interval on
ECG

Hypertension

Polyuria
Renal calculi
Nephrocalcinosis

Nausea
Vomiting
Peptic ulceration

Abdominal pain
Constipation
Pancreatitis

Figure 19.1 – Clinical effects of hypercalcaemia.

HYPOCALCAEMIA

The effects of hypocalcaemia are due to a decrease in free calcium concentration. Causes of hypocalcaemia are shown in Table 19.3.

Vitamin D deficiency may result from dietary inadequacy, malabsorption or inadequate exposure to sunlight. Vitamin D metabolism may be abnormal in renal failure, due to decreased 1α-hydroxylase activity and also in patients treated with anticonvulsants such as phenytoin or phenobarbitone which induce hepatic enzymes. In both vitamin D deficiency and in situations of altered metabolism there is decreased calcitriol synthesis resulting in decreased absorption of calcium

CAUSES OF HYPOCALCAEMIA
Vitamin D deficiency or abnormalities of vitamin D metabolism
Renal failure
Hypoparathyroidism
Magnesium deficiency
Acute pancreatitis

Table 19.3

from the gut. Hypocalcaemia commonly occurs in renal failure due to a decreased amount of functioning renal tissue and to inhibition of the 1α-hydroxylase enzyme due to the high plasma phosphate. Hypoparathyroidism may be congenital or acquired. The congenital form may occur in association with abnormalities of the aortic arch, thymic aplasia and immune deficiency (Di George syndrome). Acquired hypoparathyroidism may be idiopathic or autoimmune. The autoimmune type may occur alone or in association with other autoimmune disorders. Hypoparathyroidism may occur after thyroid surgery or due to infiltrative conditions such as haemochromatosis. Magnesium deficiency may result in hypocal-

caemia as magnesium is essential for PTH secretion. Acute pancreatitis may be accompanied by hypocalcaemia due to the formation of calcium salts by fatty acids released by the action of pancreatic lipase.

Clinical effects of hypocalcaemia are shown in Figure 19.2.

Hypocalcaemia leads to an increase in the excitability of muscles and nervous tissue. This may result in tetany with manifestations such as carpopedal spasm and perioral paraesthesiae. ECG changes occur with prolongation of the QT and ST intervals. If longstanding, hypocalcaemia may result in cataracts and calcification of the basal ganglia.

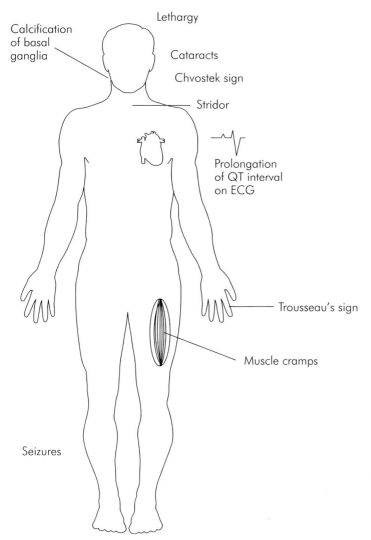

Figure 19.2 – Clinical effects of hypocalcaemia.

HYPOPHOSPHATAEMIA

This is common but replacement is usually only indicated when the serum concentration is < 0.3 mmol/L. Hypophosphataemia is detrimental to the function of many tissues due to their requirement for phosphate-containing compounds such as ATP and 2,3 DPG. Hypophosphataemia may occur on recovery from diabetic ketoacidosis, on re-feeding malnourished patients, alcohol withdrawal, in respiratory alkalosis, and hyperparathyroidism.

HYPOMAGNESAEMIA

Magnesium deficiency is common occurring in association with diuretic therapy, malnutrition, diarrhoea and alcoholism. Consequences include muscle weakness, seizures and cardiac arrythmias. As magnesium is necessary for PTH secretion, hypocalcaemia may result. Refractory hypokalaemia and hypophosphataemia may also occur prior to replacement.

BONE

The majority of body calcium is present in bone. The bony skeleton protects the internal organs and is an important part of the locomotor and respiratory systems. It also functions as a reservoir of calcium, phosphate and magnesium. Bone consists of about 60% mineral, 35% matrix and 5% cells. The matrix is made up of largely type I collagen and non-collagen proteins such as osteocalcin. The secretion of these proteins in the urine can serve a useful markers of bone disease. There are two cell types in bone – osteoclasts and osteoblasts. Osteoclasts are responsible for resorption of bone. PTH and calcitriol both stimulate this resorption. Osteoblasts carry out synthesis of the bone matrix and produce alkaline phosphatase which is essential to bone mineralisation.

OSTEOPOROSIS

Osteoporosis is characterised by a decrease in the amount of bone that is adequately mineralised. This results in an increased incidence of fractures, especially of the neck of the femur, wrist and vertebrae. Causes of osteoporosis are shown in Table 19.4.

Peak bone mass is reached in the third and fourth decades of life after which time it slowly decreases. This decrease is especially marked in postmenopausal women. There is evidence that heredity is linked to the

CAUSES OF OSTEOPOROSIS
Advanced age
Heredity
Endocrine
Cushing's syndrome
hypogonadism
hyperthyroidism
Drugs
glucocorticoids
heparin
Immobilisation
Idiopathic

Table 19.4

incidence of osteoporosis and may be due to variations in the vitamin D receptor gene. Glucocorticoids produce bone loss by inhibiting the activity of osteoblasts.

OSTEOMALACIA AND RICKETS

Osteomalacia and rickets are due to defective mineralisation of bone. Clinical features of osteomalacia include bone pain and myopathy. Defective mineralisation in children is termed rickets which may be associated with growth retardation, bowing of the tibia and enlargement of the costochondral junctions (rickety rosary). The underlying abnormality in these conditions may be a defect in homeostasis of calcium or phosphate or a defect in osteoblast function as shown in Table 19.5.

A low dietary calcium intake may lead to osteomalacia as may binding of calcium to phytates within the gut. Anticonvulsants which cause hepatic enzyme induction may cause osteomalacia due to increased clearance of 25-OH vitamin D. Phenytoin can also impair calcium uptake within the gastrointestinal tract. Deficiency of the 1α-hydroxylase enzyme is common in chronic renal failure and in the autosomal recessive disorder vitamin D dependent rickets type I. Type II is similar but results from target organ resistance to the hormone. Renal tubular disorders resulting in phosphate loss can cause osteomalacia. These may be inherited, for example cystinosis or acquired such as in lead nephropathy. Hypophosphataemic rickets is an X-linked dominant disorder in which an isolated defect of tubular phosphate reabsorption occurs. Acquired defects of osteoblastic function may be due to aluminium retention, which may occur in patients undergoing long-term renal dialysis. Hypophosphatasia has

CAUSES OF OSTEOMALACIA AND RICKETS
Calciopenic
Decreased calcium absorption
low intake
binding by phytates
malabsorption
Decreased production or action of 1,25-OH vitamin D
low exposure to sunlight
anticonvulsants
chronic liver disease
chronic renal failure
vitamin D dependent rickets
Phosphopenic
Renal tubular disorders
Fanconi's syndrome
X-linked hypophosphataemic rickets
Defective osteoblastic function
aluminium retention
fluorosis
hypophosphatasia

Table 19.5

Reference ranges	
Calcium (total)	*2.2 – 2.6 mmol/L*
Phosphate	*0.8 – 1.4 mmol/L*
Magnesium	*0.7 – 1.0 mmol/L*

an autosomal dominant mode of inheritance and is secondary to decreased alkaline phosphatase activity.

PAGET'S DISEASE

Paget's disease may affect one or many bones and is characterised by increased bone turnover, the resulting new bone being abnormal at these sites. Bone pain and deformity commonly arise. Characteristically in Paget's disease the alkaline phosphatase concentration is raised, the extent reflecting disease activity. Plasma calcium concentration is usually within the reference range but hypercalcaemia may occur during immobilisation.

SELECTED READING

Mundy, G.R. *Calcium Homeostasis: Hypercalcaemia and Hypocalcaemia*. Oxford University Press, 1991.

Avioli, L.V. and Krane, S.M. (eds). Metabolic Bone Disease and Clinically Related Disorders. Academic Press, N.Y. 1998.

20

THE HYPOTHALAMUS AND PITUITARY GLAND

The hypothalamus is located at the base of the brain and is connected to the pituitary gland by the pituitary stalk. The pituitary gland is divided into anterior and posterior parts. The anterior pituitary, or adenohypophysis, and the posterior pituitary, or neurohypophysis, have different embryological origins. The anterior pituitary secretes six hormones – growth hormone (GH), prolactin (PL), thyroid stimulating hormone (TSH), adrenocorticotrophic hormone (ACTH), follicle stimulating hormone (FSH) and luteinizing hormone (LH). TSH, ACTH, FSH and LH are trophic hormones, that is they exert their actions on a target endocrine gland. The posterior pituitary produces two hormones – oxytocin and antidiuretic hormone (ADH), also known as vasopressin.

PHYSIOLOGY OF THE HYPOTHALAMIC-PITUITARY AXIS

The hypothalamus produces hormones with both stimulatory and inhibitory effects on the pituitary. GH releasing hormone (GHRH) stimulates GH production and somatostatin inhibits it. The tripeptide thyroid releasing hormone (TRH) acts to stimulate secretion of TSH. TRH can also cause PL release but this is not thought to be of physiological significance. Corticotrophin releasing hormone (CRH) stimulates ACTH secretion and gonadotrophin releasing hormone (GnRH) increases secretion of both FSH and LH. Control of PL secretion is exerted by dopamine from the hypothalamus which inhibits PL secretion. There is no physiological PL releasing hormone.

ANTERIOR PITUITARY

The secretion of anterior pituitary hormones is influenced by hormones released from the hypothalamus. Other influences such as circadian variation, stress and drugs can exert influences which also affect pituitary secretion. The whole system, with the exception of PL which regulates its own secretion, is controlled by negative feedback at the level of the hypothalamus and pituitary. This is shown in Figure 20.1.

Connection between the hypothalamus and the anterior pituitary is achieved by a portal system of blood vessels.

POSTERIOR PITUITARY

The posterior pituitary hormones are synthesised in the hypothalamus, reaching the posterior pituitary via the neurons of the pituitary stalk, to be stored and released when required.

Plasma concentrations of hypothalamic and pituitary hormones can be assessed by immunoassay. As the release of these hormones is pulsatile, single measurements are not reliable for diagnosis. When measuring trophic hormones the pituitary hormone and the hormone produced by the target gland may be measured concurrently. For example, in the assessment of

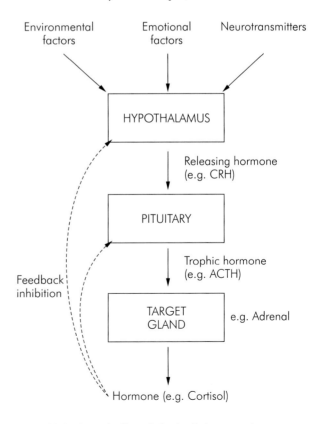

Figure 20.1 – Control of hypothalamic-pituitary secretions.

thyroid function TSH and thyroxine are frequently measured together. Dynamic tests are also used for the assessment of pituitary function, stimulation tests to assess suspected hypofunction and suppression tests to assess suspected hyperfunction.

PITUITARY HORMONES AND DISORDERS OF THEIR SECRETION

GROWTH HORMONE

Growth hormone is a polypeptide with both growth promoting and metabolic actions. It is released in a pulsatile fashion with maximum release occurring during sleep. The growth promoting action is mediated by insulin-like growth factor-I (IGF-I) which is produced in large quantities in the liver and also synthesised locally in growing tissues. IGF-I exerts negative feedback on GH secretion. GH is not the only hormone affecting growth – thyroxine is also essential and androgens play an important role in the pubertal growth spurt. Metabolic actions of GH are summarised in Table 20.1.

GH excess is usually the result of a GH secreting adenoma of the pituitary gland. In childhood excess GH leads to gigantism, after fusion of the epiphyses the condition is called acromegaly and results in increased bone and soft tissue growth evident by coarsening of facial features and increasing size of the hands and feet. There may be impaired glucose tolerance due to the anti-insulin effect of GH. The diagnosis of acromegaly may be made by failure of GH to suppress during a glucose tolerance test.

GH deficiency is a rare cause of short stature and if congenital usually manifests itself towards the end of the first year of life. Affected children have relatively fat bodies and faces and have a tendency towards hypoglycaemia. The treatment of GH deficiency in adults is often of benefit.

METABOLIC EFFECTS OF GH
Opposition of the effects of insulin
Increase in lipolysis
Increase in protein synthesis

Table 20.1

Random measurements of GH are generally unhelpful because of its pulsatile secretion, but IGF-I is proving a useful indicator of GH status.

PROLACTIN

The function of PL is to initiate and maintain lactation. The action of suckling stimulates its secretion. Inhibitory control of PL secretion is exerted by dopamine. Prolactin secretion is pulsatile, increasing during sleep and in stress. In pregnancy levels rise but have returned to normal by one week after birth if the woman chooses not to breast feed.

Hyperprolactinaemia may occur due to a PL secreting pituitary tumour. Because the major influence controlling PL secretion is inhibitory due to dopamine from the hypothalamus damage to the pituitary stalk or drugs with an anti-dopaminergic action such as phenothiazines and haloperidol may also cause hyperprolactinaemia. In severe primary hypothyroidism the plasma level of PL may be raised due to stimulation of its secretion by the increased concentration of TRH. Patients with hyperprolactinaemia may present with galactorrhoea. In women there may be amenorrhoea and both sexes may develop infertility due to the inhibitory effects of PL on the pulsatile release of GnRH together with a direct effect on the synthesis of gonadal steroids.

Diagnosis of hyperprolactinaemia may be made by the plasma level on a single occasion but this may be misleading as prolactin status is affected by stress and by oestrogen levels. The prolactin response to TRH may be used in the diagnosis of PL secreting tumours, being lessened in most cases of tumour. PL deficiency results in failure to initiate and sustain lactation.

THYROID STIMULATING HORMONE

TSH is a glycoprotein with α and β subunits. The β subunit is specific to TSH whilst the α subunit is identical to that of FSH, LH and human chorionic gonadotrophin. TSH secretion is stimulated by the tripeptide TRH which is released from the hypothalamus. Dopamine can inhibit TSH secretion but whether it has a physiological role is unclear.

The function of TSH is to act on the thyroid gland to stimulate the secretion of the thyroid hormones thyroxine and tri-iodothyronine. Excess TSH may result in hyperthyroidism but this is rare. Similarly hypothyroidism is occasionally secondary to a deficiency of TSH. Disorders of thyroid hormones are considered further in Chapter 21.

ADRENOCORTICOTROPHIC HORMONE

ACTH is a polypeptide hormone released from the pituitary in response to CRH. The function of ACTH is to stimulate the production of glucocorticoids from the adrenal gland. ACTH excess results in Cushing's syndrome whilst a deficiency of ACTH causes secondary adrenal hypofunction. This is dealt with further in Chapter 22.

FOLLICLE STIMULATING HORMONE AND LUTEINIZING HORMONE

FSH and LH control the development of germ cells and secretion of hormones from the gonads. FSH is the hormone primarily involved in the development of germ cells and LH is more involved with gonadal hormone production. FSH and LH secretion is controlled by GnRH. However FSH and LH concentrations do not always change in parallel as their secretion can be differentially modified. FSH and LH are discussed further in Chapter 23.

ANTIDIURETIC HORMONE

This is stored in the posterior pituitary and released in situations of relative decrease in body water. Its functions are considered more fully in Chapters 12 and 18.

OXYTOCIN

Oxytocin functions to control ejection of milk from the lactating breast. It may also play a part in the initiation of uterine contractions at the start of labour and is used therapeutically to induce labour.

HYPOPITUITARISM

Whilst isolated deficiencies of individual pituitary hormones may occur, in other situations there may be more widespread disturbance of pituitary function. In pituitary hypofunction GH is usually the first hormone whose secretion is interrupted, then the gonadotrophins, ACTH and lastly TSH. Causes of hypopituitarism are shown in Table 20.2.

Congenital hypopituitarism may be due to develop-

CAUSES OF HYPOPITUITARISM
Congenital
Tumours
Iatrogenic
Vascular
Infiltrative conditions
Infection
Trauma
Secondary to hypothalamic disorders

Table 20.2

ment abnormalities of the pituitary alone or to more widespread damage involving other midline structures. Functionless pituitary tumours may enlarge leading to hypofunction of the gland. Iatrogenic hypopituitarism may occur in patients who have had surgery or irradiation to the head. Such patients must be carefully followed-up as the hypopituitarism may not become manifest for some time after the initial insult. Sheehan's syndrome, now rare, is hypopituitarism secondary to post-partum haemorrhage. Infiltrative conditions, such as sarcoidosis and infections, particularly tuberculous meningitis, may affect the pituitary as can trauma to the head. Clinical features of hypopituitarism are shown in Figure 20.2.

The diagnosis of hypopituitarism may be made on the result of a combined pituitary stimulation test using the stress of insulin induced hypoglycaemia to stimulates GH and ACTH secretion, TRH to evaluate TSH release and GnRH to stimulate FSH and LH secretion. Because of the difficulty of measuring ACTH, due to its lability, estimation of cortisol concentration is used instead. Basal concentrations are measured and samples at intervals after the stimulus. Safer alternatives to insulin include glucagon for the evaluation of GH and ACTH and arginine or clonidine for the evaluation of GH alone.

SELECTED READING

Grossman, A. *Clinical Endocrinology*, 2nd Edition. Blackwell Scientific, Oxford. 1997.

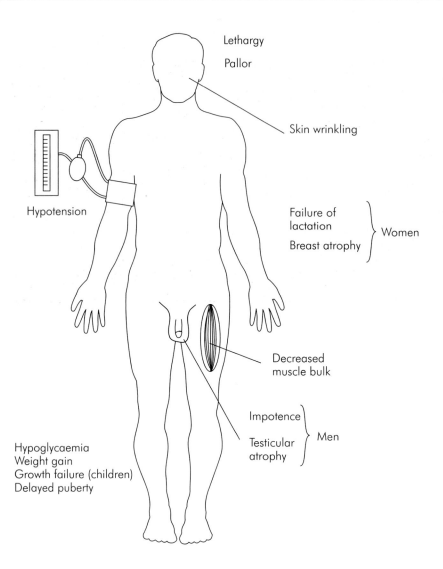

Lethargy

Pallor

Skin wrinkling

Hypotension

Failure of
lactation

Breast atrophy

⎫
⎬   Women
⎭

Decreased
muscle bulk

Impotence ⎫
⎬   Men
Testicular
atrophy   ⎭

Hypoglycaemia
Weight gain
Growth failure (children)
Delayed puberty

Figure 20.2 – Clinical features of hypopituitarism.

Reference ranges		
To exclude hypopituitarism		
		Serum
(stimulation test)	*Cortisol*	*>500 nmol/L*
	GH	*> 20 mU/L*
	FSH	*> 1.5 × basal**
	LH	*> 5 × basal**
	TSH	*>5 m U/L**
* increment		

21

THE THYROID GLAND

Objectives

To understand:

- The physiology of the thyroid gland
- The laboratory assessment of thyroid disease
- Disorders of thyroid function — hypothyroidism, hyperthyroidism

The thyroid gland is a bilobed structure situated in the neck just below the larynx. The thyroid consists of numerous follicles each comprising an outer layer of follicular cells and an inner portion containing colloid which consists mainly of thyroglobulin. In between the follicles lie the parafollicular, or C cells, which secrete calcitonin which may have a role in calcium homeostasis. The principal hormones produced by the thyroid gland are thyroxine (T_4) and triiodothyronine (T_3) whose structures are shown in Figure 21.1

THE PHYSIOLOGY OF THYROID HORMONES

Thyroid hormones influence many of the body's metabolic processes.The thyroid hormones increase basal metabolic rate and the sensitivity of the cardio-

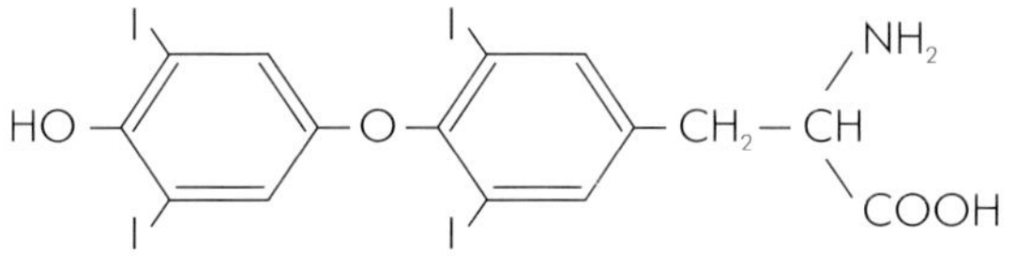

Thyroxine (T_4)

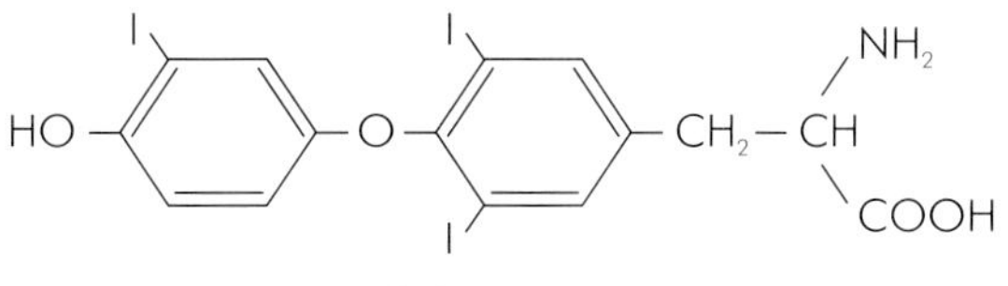

Triiodothyroxine (T_3)

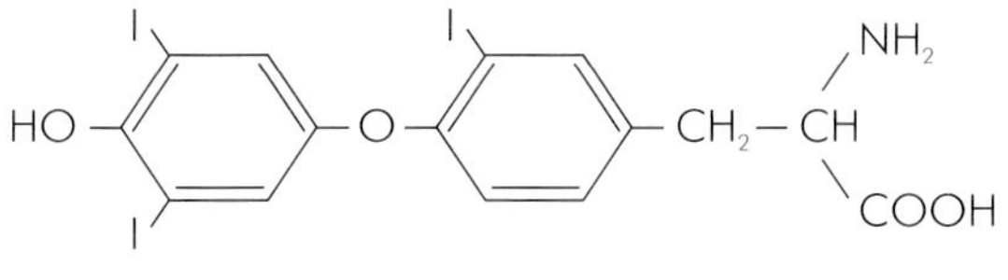

Reverse triiodotyronine (rT_3)

Figure 21.1 – Structures of thyroid hormones.

vascular and central nervous systems to catecholamines, thus affecting cardiac output and heart rate. They are also essential for normal growth and intellectual development.

SYNTHESIS

T_4 and T_3 are synthesised in the thyroid follicles. This process begins with the absorption of dietary iodine and the active uptake of iodide from the blood. The iodide is then oxidised to iodine within the thyroid gland. Thyroglobulin is a glycoprotein containing numerous tyrosyl residues which are iodinated to form mono-iodotyrosine (MIT) and di-iodotyrosine (DIT). Iodotyrosyl residues are then coupled to form T_4 (DIT+DIT) and T_3 (DIT+MIT). The thyroid hormones, still incorporated in thyroglobulin, are stored in colloid follicles. Colloid droplets fuse with lysosomes and then proteolytic degradation brings about the release of T_4 and T_3. More T_4 than T_3 is produced from the thyroid gland, the majority of T_3 being formed by peripheral deiodination of T_4. Peripheral deiodination may also result in production of reverse T_3 (rT_3) which is inactive – an increase in the relative proportion of rT3 occurring in a number of illnesses and in starvation. Control of synthesis of thyroid hormones is due to thyroid stimulating hormone (TSH) secretion from the pituitary gland, influenced by the hormone hypothalamic tripeptide thyroid releasing hormone (TRH). The thyroid hormones themselves exert negative feedback at the level of the pituitary and possibly the hypothalamus.

TRANSPORT OF THYROID HORMONES IN THE BLOOD

Once in the blood, thyroid hormones become almost completely bound to the plasma proteins thyroxine-binding globulin (TBG), thyroid binding pre-albumin and albumin. T_4 is bound more tightly than T_3 so that, although the concentration of total T_4 in the blood is about fifty times greater than that of T_3, the free T_4 concentration is only three times that of T_3. It is likely that only the free hormone is available to the tissues.

LABORATORY ASSESSMENT OF THYROID DISEASE

The thyroid gland may produce an adequate amount of thyroid hormones (euthyroid state), an increased amount (hyperthyroid state) or a decreased amount (hypothyroid state). The functional state of the thyroid gland can be assessed by clinical examination but major disturbances of the thyroid function may be present without being clinically apparent.

THYROXINE AND TRIIODOTHYRONINE

As clinical effects of thyroid hormones correlate better with the concentration of free hormone, estimation of free T_4 and T_3 is preferred, although estimation of total T_4 and T_3 are still used. The measurement of free hormone is more difficult than measurement of the total concentration. This is because there is much less free hormone than bound hormone present and also because any attempt to use up the free hormone to measure it will alter the equilibrium between bound and free hormone. A further disadvantage of total hormone measurement is that it is dependent on the level of TBG. The TBG level may be increased by such factors as pregnancy and the use of the oral contraceptive pill and this could potentially give rise to a false positive diagnosis of hyperthyroidism. The opposite situation occurs when TBG levels are lowered, for example by systemic illness, protein losing enteropathy, androgens and corticosteroid excess. Genetic factors may be responsible for higher or lower concentrations of TBG than normal.

THYROID STIMULATINE HORMONE

Estimation of TSH is a useful indicator of thyroid function. A raised level indicates hypothyroidism. An exception to this is the rare situation of hypothyroidism secondary to dysfunction of the pituitary gland, in which the level of thyroid hormones is low, but, as the pituitary is unable to compensate, the TSH is not elevated. TSH concentrations may also be raised transiently during recovery from illness or starvation and in the very few patients who have TSH secreting pituitary tumours. If the TSH concentration is suppressed this is usually due to hyperthyroidism or to excessive thyroxine replacement therapy given for the treatment of hypothyroidism. Many laboratories use the measurement of TSH as a first line test of thyroid function and augment this with subsequent tests as necessary as is shown in Figure 21.2.

In compensated, or borderline, hypothyroidism laboratory investigations show that an adequate T_4 level can just be achieved by increased secretion of TSH. This may progress to overt hypothyroidism.

Interpretation of thyroid function tests is difficult in

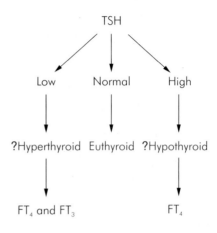

Figure 21.2 – Investigation of thyroid function using TSH as a first line test.

patients with systemic illness. The free T_3 concentration is often decreased as may be the free T_4 in the acute phase of an illness. This is termed sick euthyroidism and results from decreased peripheral deiodination of T_4, changes in the concentration of binding proteins and influences of non-thyroidal factors on the hypothalamic-pituitary thyroid axis. TSH levels may be decreased in the acute stages of an illness and increased during recovery.

The TRH test measures the TSH response to TRH. The TSH level is measured before and after an intravenous dose of TRH. With the advent of ultrasensitive assays for TSH its use has decreased, except in the assessment of TSH reserve in diseases of the pituitary or hypothalamus.

THYROID AUTOANTIBODIES

The detection of thyroid autoantibodies may be useful in the elucidation of the cause of a thyroid disorder. Thyroid microsomal antibodies, also known as antiperoxidase antibodies, are formed in most patients with autoimmune hypothyroidism. Some cases of hyperthyroidism are due to Graves' disease in which antibodies to the TSH receptor are produced and have stimulatory action.

THYROID SCANING

Thyroid scanning, involving the quantification of uptake of technetium by thyroid tissue, enables differentiation between Graves' disease and toxic multinodular goitre and between adenomas and carcinomas.

DISORDERS OF THYROID FUNCTION

An enlargement of the thyroid gland is termed a goitre. A goitre may occur in association with biochemically normal thyroid function or with both over and under production of thyroid hormones but does not invariably accompany either disorder.

HYPERTHYROIDISM

This is due to increased amounts of circulating thyroid hormones. Causes are shown in Table 21.1.

Graves' disease is an autoimmune disorder consisting of thyroid dysfunction together with involvement of the eyes and sometimes the skin. In addition to the clinical appearances a diagnosis can be made by the abnormal thyroid function tests and the presence of thyroid stimulatory antibodies. Toxic multinodular goitre causes hyperthyroidism because of autonomy of certain areas within a nodular thyroid gland. This is distinct from a single autonomously functioning toxic nodule. TSH secreting pituitary tumours are rare but laboratory tests show increased levels of thyroid hormones in the presence of detectable TSH.

Ingestion of thyroid hormone is usually due to self-administration by those with psychological disorders. Ingestion of excess iodine can induce hyperthyroidism particularly in patients with a pre-existing goitre due to iodine deficiency.

Thyroid tissue may occur in ovarian teratomas (struma ovarii) or, rarely, in cases of metastatic follicular carcinoma. Clinical features of hyperthyroidism are shown in Figure 21.3.

The cardiovascular effects of hyperthyroidism result from the stimulatory effect of thyroid hormones on the heart, increasing heart rate and stroke volume. There is a reduction in peripheral vascular resistance resulting in a rise in cardiac output. Weight loss commonly occurs, in spite of an increase in appetite. Effects on the nervous system lead to tremor and general agitation. Prolonged hyperthyroidism may cause osteoporosis as a result of increased bone turnover with a disproportionate amount of bone resorption. Hypercalcaemia may result. Occasionally patients with thyrotoxicosis may develop, or present with, thyroid storm – an acute emergency characterised by hyperpyrexia, dehydration and cardiac failure.

Hyperthyroidism can be treated by antithyroid drugs. These are normally prescribed for up to two years. If the patient then relapses a further course of drug treatment may be given. However surgical removal of thyroid tissue, or its destruction by radioactive iodine are alternative methods of treatment.

HYPOTHYROIDISM

Hypothyroidism results when circulating levels of thyroid hormones are low. Causes are shown in Table 21.2.

Hashimoto's thyroiditis is the result of autoimmune damage to the thyroid gland. In atrophic hypothyroidism there is atrophy of the gland, possibly as a late consequence of autoimmune disease. Iatrogenic hypothyroidism may occur after thyroid surgery or radioactive iodine treatment for thyrotoxicosis. It may also result as a side-effect of certain drugs for example

CAUSES OF HYPERTHYROIDISM
Graves' disease
toxic multinodular goitre
toxic nodule
ingestion of thyroid hormones, iodine or iodine containing drugs
TSH secreting pituitary tumour
ectopic thyroid tissue

Table 21.1

CAUSES OF HYPOTHYROIDISM
Hashimoto's thyroiditis
atrophic hypothyroidism
iatrogenic
iodine deficiency
congenital
secondary to pituitary or hypothalamic damage

Table 21.2

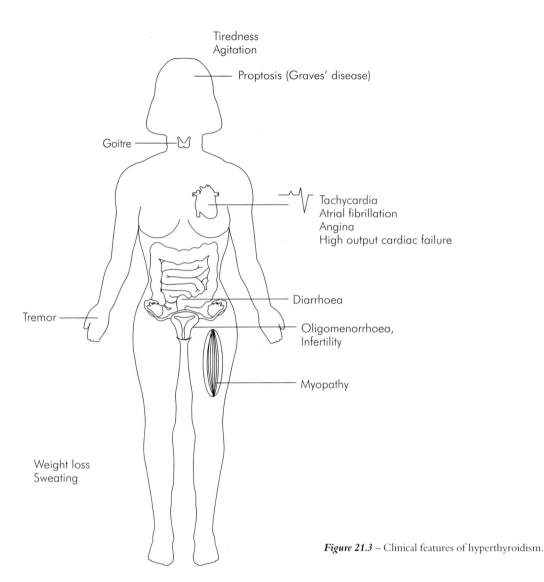

Tiredness
Agitation

Proptosis (Graves' disease)

Goitre

Tachycardia
Atrial fibrillation
Angina
High output cardiac failure

Diarrhoea

Tremor

Oligomenorrhoea,
Infertility

Myopathy

Weight loss
Sweating

Figure 21.3 – Clinical features of hyperthyroidism.

lithium. Pituitary or hypothalamic disorders may cause secondary hypothyroidism. In this situation TSH is not elevated in spite of a low T_4 Iodine deficiency leads to hypothyroidism together with enlargement of the thyroid gland (goitre). Whilst not a problem in the UK, it remains a major public health problem in areas where the iodine content of the soil is naturally low, although the incidence has decreased with the introduction of artificially iodised salt. Congenital hypothyroidism has an incidence of about 1/4000 live births. It may result from either a structural abnormality of the gland or, more rarely, from a defect in one of the enzymes involved in the production of thyroid hormones. If untreated it leads to severe developmental delay, short stature and delayed puberty. In many coun-

tries all neonates are screened for congenital hypothyroidism at the age of 5–7 days by the estimation of TSH concentrations on capillary blood samples. The sooner treatment with T_4 is instituted the better the prognosis, most treated children having near normal intellectual and skeletal development.

Clinical effects of hypothyroidism may occur slowly and pass unnoticed by the patient. They are shown in Figure 21.4.

Effects on the cardiovascular system are secondary to a decrease in cardiac output. There is a decrease in cutaneous blood flow leading to cold intolerance. Cardiac dilatation may occur together with pericardial effusion.

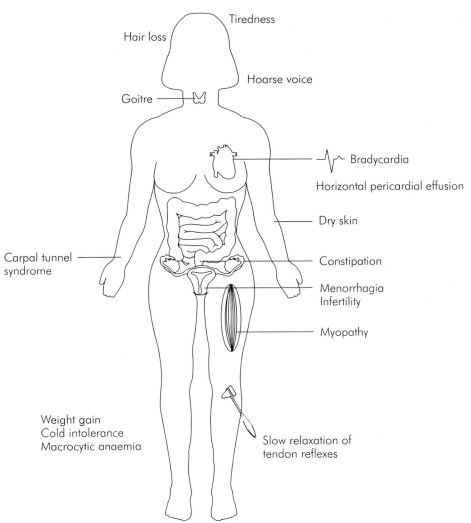

Figure 21.4 – Clinical features of hypothyroidism

Hoarseness of the voice may occur due to laryngeal oedema. There may be weight gain in the face of decreased appetite. In adults there is a dulling of intellectual function reversible with treatment, but in untreated children with congenital hypothyroidism permanent neurological damage occurs. Effects on the peripheral nervous system include delayed relaxation of tendon reflexes and there is often compression of the median nerve as it passes through the carpal tunnel at the wrist. Patients with hypothyroidism may occasionally present with myxoedema coma characterised by hypothermia and stupor. This presentation carries a high mortality.

Treatment of hypothyroidism involves the administration of thyroxine.

SELECTED READING

Braverman, L.E. and Utiger, R.D. *Werner & Inbar's The Thyroid*, 7th Edition. Lippincott–Raven, N.Y. 1997.

Reference ranges	
TSH	*0.3–5.0 mU/L*
Thyroxine	*10–26 pmol/L (free)*
	60–150 nmol/L (total)
Triiodothyronine	*3.0–10 pmol/L (free)*
	1.2–3.0 nmol/L (total)

22

THE ADRENAL GLANDS

Objective
To understand:

- The function of adrenocortical hormones – glucocorticoids, mineralocorticoids and androgens

- Disorders of the adrenal cortex – adrenal failure, Cushing's syndrome, Conn's syndrome, congenital adrenal hyperplasia

- Disorders of the adrenal medulla – phaeochromocytoma

- Investigation of abnormalities of the adrenal gland

The adrenal glands are situated on the superior poles of the kidneys. Each gland has two parts, a cortex and a medulla, which are functionally distinct. The adrenal cortex is essential to life and produces three types of steroid hormone – glucocorticoids, mineralocorticoids and androgens. The adrenal medulla is part of the sympathetic nervous system and produces catecholamines. It is not essential for life.

THE PHYSIOLOGY OF ADRENAL STEROID HORMONES

There are three types of steroid hormone synthesised from common precursors. However, there are different mechanisms for control of synthesis between the three types.

Glucocorticoids

Glucocorticoids are secreted in response to adrenocorticotrophic hormone (ACTH) from the anterior pituitary. ACTH is secreted in response to corticotrophin releasing hormone (CRH) from the hypothalamus. The most important glucocorticoid is cortisol which exerts feedback control on ACTH secretion. The functions of glucocorticoids are shown in Table 22.1.

In the blood about 95% of cortisol is bound to cortisol-binding globulin which is almost saturated under normal conditions. The plasma concentration of cortisol shows diurnal variation, reaching a peak in the morning and a nadir around midnight.

Mineralocorticoids

The most important mineralocorticoid is aldosterone which acts to stimulate the reabsorption of sodium ions in the kidneys.

FUNCTIONS OF GLUCOCORTICOIDS
Inhibition of ACTH secretion via negative feedback
Stimulation of protein catabolism
Stimulation of hepatic glycogen synthesis and gluconeogenesis
Sensitisation of blood vessels to noradrenaline
Enhancement of water excretion

Table 22.1

Androgens

The principal androgens produced by the adrenal gland are dehydroepiandrosterone and its sulphate, and androstenedione. They promote protein synthesis but are only mildly androgenic at physiological concentrations. In the circulation these hormones are protein bound to sex hormone binding globulin (SHBG) and to albumin.

DISORDERS OF THE ADRENAL CORTEX

Disorders of the adrenal cortex may result in under- or over-secretion of its hormones. In the inherited disorder congenital adrenal hyperplasia (CAH) there is hypersecretion of some hormones at the same time as undersecretion of others.

Adrenal hypofunction (Addison's disease)

Adrenal hypofunction is a rare occurrence of great importance. Causes of adrenal hypofunction are shown in Table 22.2.

Adrenal hypofunction most commonly occurs in patients in whom the pituitary-adrenal axis is suppressed secondary to the therapeutic use of glucocorticoids. In these patients the sudden withdrawal of steroids, or failure to increase the dose in inter-current

CAUSES OF ADRENAL HYPOFUNCTION
Autoimmune
Infection – e.g. tuberculosis, histoplasmosis
Infiltration – e.g. sarcoid, amyloid, malignancy
Adrenal haemorrhage (Waterhouse-Friedrickson syndrome)

Table 22.2

illness, may result in acute adrenal failure. Clinical features of adrenal hypofunction are shown in Figure 22.1.

The pigmentation that occurs in adrenal hypofunction is due to the melanocyte stimulating properties from the ACTH precursor pro-opiomelanocortin, secretion of which is increased due to loss of feedback control as a result of the lowered cortisol concentration. In cases of adrenal hypofunction secondary to disorders of the hypothalamus or pituitary, ACTH is not raised and no pigmentation occurs. Loss of body hair only occurs in adrenal failure in women, as in males the testes are the major source of androgens. Hyponatraemia and hyperkalaemia frequently occur in adrenal hypofunction. Aldosterone acts to enhance the reabsorption of sodium ions in exchange for potassium and hydrogen ions. Decreased aldosterone secretion therefore tends to result in hyponatraemia and hyperkalaemia. Cortisol has a permissive effect on water excretion, thus its lack may exacerbate hyponatraemia due to a dilutional effect.

Treatment of adrenal hypofunction is replacement therapy with the glucocorticoid hydrocortisone and the synthetic mineralocorticoid fludrocortisone.

Adrenal hyperfunction

Adrenal hyperfunction may manifest primarily as a disorder of glucocorticoid production (Cushing's syndrome) or of mineralocorticoid production (Conn's

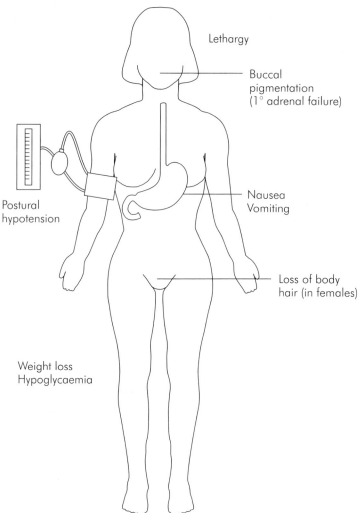

Lethargy

Buccal
pigmentation
(1° adrenal failure)

Postural
hypotension

Nausea
Vomiting

Loss of body
hair (in females)

Weight loss
Hypoglycaemia

Figure 22.1 – Clinical features of adrenal hypofunction.

syndrome). Causes of Cushing's syndrome are shown in Table 22.3.

The most common cause of Cushing's syndrome is the therapeutic administration of high doses of glucocorticoids, for example in the treatment of severe asthma. It is important to distinguish Cushing's syndrome from Cushing's disease. The latter term is used to describe adrenal hyperfunction secondary to pituitary over-secretion of ACTH. Clinical features of Cushing's syndrome are shown in Figure 22.2.

The majority of the clinical features are secondary to excess glucocorticoid secretion but, as glucocorticoids have inherent mineralocorticoid activity, sodium retention and potassium loss may occur. Over-

CAUSES OF CUSHING'S SYNDROME		
Treatment with corticosteroids		
Cushing's disease	increased pituitary secretion of ACTH	
Adrenal tumours	adenoma carcinoma	
Ectopic ACTH e.g. from carcinoma of the lung		

Table 22.3

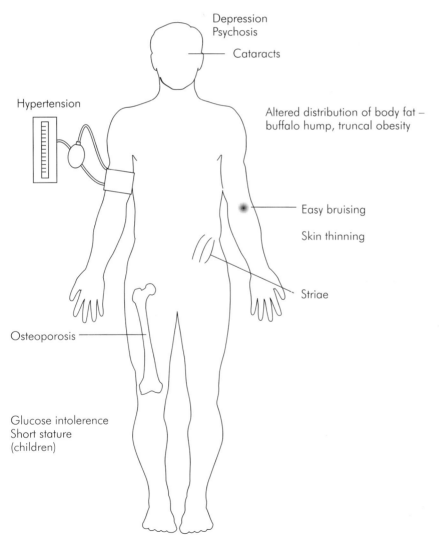

Figure 22.2 – Clinical features of Cushing's syndrome.

production of adrenal androgens may also be evident clinically, more so in women than in men.

In alcohol addiction and severe depression, pseudo-Cushing's syndrome may occur in which some of the biochemical features of true Cushing's syndrome may be present.

HYPERALDOSTERONISM

Hyperaldosteronism may be primary (Conn's syndrome) or secondary, the latter being more common. Causes of Conn's syndrome are shown in Table 22.4.

The most common cause of Conn's syndrome is an adrenal adenoma, although occasionally adrenal carcinoma occurs. Bilateral hyperplasia of the zona glomerulosa occurs in a small number of cases.

Clinical features of Conn's syndrome include hypokalaemia secondary to renal potassium wasting which can result in muscle weakness. Aldosterone excess results in sodium retention which may lead to hypertension. The drug carbenoxolone and liquorice confectionary have metabolites with mineralocorticoid activity and their ingestion may produce a biochemical picture similar to that of primary hyperaldosteronism.

Secondary hyperaldosteronism occurs in conditions in which there is long-standing hyperaldosteronism due to stimulation of the renin/angiotensin system by a low renal blood flow. This may occur due to a reduced circulating blood volume or to local abnormalities in the renal vessels. Very rarely, secondary hyperaldosteronism may occur due to a renin secreting tumour. Causes of secondary hyperaldosteronism are shown in Table 22.5.

In conditions in which there is a redistribution of extracellular fluid with a decreased plasma volume but a normal or high extracellular fluid volume, oedema may be present. In congestive cardiac failure the high venous hydrostatic pressure contributes to oedema.

CONGENITAL ADRENAL HYPERPLASIA

Congenital adrenal hyperplasia (CAH) comprises a

CAUSES OF CONN'S SYNDROME
Adrenal tumour –   adenoma
carcinoma
Bilateral adrenal hyperplasia

Table 22.4

CAUSES OF SECONDARY HYPOALDOSTERONISM
Congestive cardiac failure
Liver disease with ascites
Nephrotic syndrome
Renal artery stenosis
Renin-secreting tumours

Table 22.5

group of inherited disorders of the enzymes of adrenal steroid hormone biosynthesis. Symptoms and signs are related to overproduction of some hormones and underproduction of others. The biochemical basis of the disorders is shown in Figure 22.3.

The enzyme defects result in decreased synthesis of both glucocorticoids and mineralocorticoids. There is lack of feedback control of ACTH secretion by cortisol. The resulting increase in ACTH secretion results in adrenal hyperplasia and overproduction of androgens.

The most common disorder is deficiency of the 21-hydroxylase enzyme which has an incidence of 1 in 12,000 live births and accounts for about 95% of cases of CAH. Affected female infants may present at birth with ambiguous genitalia but individuals with a less severe defect may come to medical attention after puberty with hirsutism or oligoamenorrhoea. Affected males may present soon after birth with a life-threatening crisis characterised by hypotension with hyponatraemia and hypoglycaemia, precipitated by decreased concentrations of both cortisol and aldosterone. Boys may also present with pseudoprecocious puberty.

THE ADRENAL MEDULLA

The adrenal medulla, together with sympathetic ganglia, synthesise the catecholamines adrenaline and noradrenaline. Adrenaline is produced almost exclusively by the adrenal medulla and noradrenaline mainly at sympathetic nerve endings.

Adrenaline and noradrenaline are formed from the amine precursor tyrosine and metabolised to the inactive metabolite 4-hydroxy-3-methoxymandelic acid (HMMA), also called vanillylmandelic acid (VMA). Dopamine, adrenaline and noradrenaline are all catecholamines. Adrenaline, noradrenaline, the

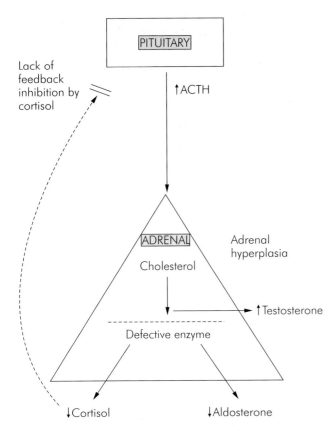

Figure 22.3 – Biochemical basis of congenital adrenal hyperplasia.

metabolites and their conjugates and HMMA can all be measured in urine. Adrenaline and noradrenaline act on the cardiovascular system, noradrenaline causing generalised vasoconstriction and hypertension and adrenaline causing vasodilatation in muscles with varying effect on blood pressure. Adrenaline may also increase the blood glucose concentration secondary to stimulation of glycogenolysis together with other anti-insulin effects.

DISORDERS OF THE ADRENAL MEDULLA

Phaeochromocytomas are tumours, usually benign, arising from the adrenal medulla in 90% of cases and occurring almost exclusively in adults. The symptoms and signs are secondary to increased levels of cate-cholamines and include hypertension, anxiety, sweat-ing and either pallor or flushing. Hyperglycaemia may also occur. These features are usually episodic although hypertension is often persistent. Whilst phaeochromo-cytomas account for only a very small minority of cases of hypertension the diagnosis should be considered,

particularly in young adults with hypertension, as there is a surgical cure. In 10% of patients phaeochromocy-tomas are associated with medullary carcinoma of the thyroid or tumours of the parathyroid glands (Multiple endocrine neoplasia type II).

Neuroblastomas are highly malignant tumours of sympathetic nervous tissue occurring in children. Approximately 40% of neuroblastomas are found in the adrenal gland. The presentation is usually with a rapidly enlarging abdominal mass.

LABORATORY INVESTIGATION OF DISORDERS OF THE ADRENAL GLAND

The diagnosis of adrenal hypofunction

As the plasma cortisol concentration is maximal at 9 am, blood samples for the investigation of adrenal hypofunction should be taken at 9 am. A 9 am cortisol concentration < 50 nmol/L confirms and a concentra-tion > 500 nmol/L excludes the diagnosis of adrenal hypofunction. In those patients in whom the diagnosis is unsure a Synacthen test is performed. This measures the response of the adrenals to a single dose of the ACTH analogue Synacthen. Adrenal hypofunction may be the result of adrenal atrophy secondary to decreased secretion of ACTH from the anterior pituitary. Measurement of ACTH concentration aids the distinction of primary from secondary adrenal hypofunction.

The diagnosis of adrenal hyperfunction

In the investigation of suspected Cushing's syndrome the presence of an increased plasma cortisol concentration must first be demonstrated and then its cause established. Demonstration of the loss of diurnal variation in cortisol secretion is a useful test but requires admission to hospital as the midnight sample should be taken whilst the patient is asleep. Cortisol is usually extensively protein bound within the circulation and its normal 24 hour urinary excretion is < 300 nmol. Increased 24 hour urinary cortisol excretion is highly suggestive of Cushing's syndrome, although it may also occur in pseudo-Cushing's and in obesity. Dexamethasone, a synthetic glucocorticoid, suppresses ACTH secretion by binding to cortisol receptors in the pituitary. Failure of suppression to a cortisol concentration < 50 nmol/L is characteristic of Cushing's syndrome. The CRH test may be helpful to differentiate between Cushing's disease and ectopic ACTH secretion. In normal individuals an iv bolus of CRH causes a rise in the plasma cortisol concentration. In Cushing's disease the usual occurrence is an exaggerated response, whereas in ectopic ACTH secretion the response is usually abolished.

The diagnosis of hyperaldosteronism

Primary hyperaldosteronism should be considered as a diagnosis in all patients with hypertension and hypokalaemia (plasma potassium concentration < 3.5 mmol/L). In most cases of hypokalaemia urinary potassium excretion should be minimal. However the finding of a urinary potassium concentration > 30 mmol/24 hours in the presence of hypokalaemia is suggestive, but not diagnostic of Conn's syndrome. These measurements are not valid if performed whilst the patient is receiving diuretics. To increase the sensitivity of these screening tests a high salt diet may be given. Secondary hyperaldosteronism can often be distinguished from primary by clinical observation. The sodium concentration may help to differentiate the two situations, often being high, or high normal, in primary and low or low normal in secondary hyperaldosteronism. The best way in which to distinguish, however, is the simultaneous measurement of aldosterone and plasma renin activity. Plasma renin activity is decreased in primary and increased in secondary hyperaldosteronism.

Diagnosis of catecholamine secreting tumours

Investigation of catecholamine secreting tumours usually begins by measuring 24 hour urinary excretion of HMMA. Foods including walnuts, bananas and vanilla as well as some drugs, may cause a false positive result and should be avoided. As the secretion from phaeochromocytomas is usually intermittent it is helpful to perform the urine collection when symptoms are present. If urinary HMMA is increased, urine or plasma adrenaline and noradrenaline should be measured. If these are raised the tumour should be localized using isotope studies, MRI scanning or selective venous cannulation with catecholamine estimation.

SELECTED READING

James, V.H.T. *The Human Adrenal Cortex*, 2nd Edition. Raven Press, N.Y. 1992.

23

THE GONADS

Objectives

To understand:

- Physiology of the hypothalamic-pituitary gonadal axis and the functions of the sex hormones

- Monitoring of pregnancy and principles of antenatal diagnosis

- Disorders of gonadal function – male hypogonadism, gynaecomastia, oligo-amenorrhoea, hirsuitism and virilism

The gonads are responsible for the production of hormones and of spermatazoa in males and ova in females. The most important hormone produced by the ovary is the oestrogen oestradiol and that of the testis is the androgen testosterone.

THE PHYSIOLOGY OF THE REPRODUCTIVE SYSTEM

The functions of the gonads are regulated by hormones secreted from the hypothalamus and pituitary. Pituitary gonadotrophins stimulate the gonads to produce sex hormones.

THE HYPOTHALAMIC-PITUITARY-GONADAL AXIS

Gonadotrophin releasing hormone (GnRH) is a decapeptide secreted, in pulsatile fashion, by the hypothalamus. This results in pulsatile secretion of the pituitary gonadotrophins follicle stimulating hormone (FSH) and luteinizing hormone (LH). The gonadotrophins are glycoproteins made up of two subunits. The β subunit of each hormone is unique whilst the α subunit is common to the gonadotrophins, thyroid stimulating hormone and human chorionic gonadotrophin (hCG). Secretion of FSH and LH can occur independently probably due to differences in the amplitude and frequency of pulses of GnRH. The gonadotrophins have some actions in common but FSH is more involved in germ cell maturation and LH in hormone production. In children, secretion of gonadotrophins is low. At puberty gonadotrophin pulses increase in both frequency and amplitude stimulating the production of sex hormones.

In the male, LH acts on the Leydig cells of the testis to increase production of testosterone. Testosterone then exerts feedback control on LH production. In the presence of high concentrations of testosterone, FSH acts on Sertoli cells to aid spermatogenesis. In both sexes FSH stimulates gonadal production of the hormone inhibin which exerts some feedback control on FSH production.

In the female, hormonal relationships are more complex, events occurring in a monthly menstrual cycle as shown in Figure 23.1

In the first part of the cycle, the follicular phase, FSH stimulates the secretion of oestrogen from the ovary. FSH and LH together bring about growth and maturation of follicular cells within the ovary. By about day seven of the cycle one follicle has become dominant and the remainder atrophy. The oestrogen concentration rises and FSH concentration falls, but at midcycle oestrogen causes a surge of LH production, together with production of a lesser amount of FSH. This brings about ovulation with the development of the corpus luteum. Concentrations of oestrogen and progesterone increase, inhibiting secretion of both FSH and LH. FSH is also inhibited by inhibin from the ovary. In the absence of conception the corpus luteum regresses and concentrations of oestrogen and progesterone fall resulting in FSH and LH release and the onset of a new cycle. In the biochemical evaluation of disorders of the menstrual cycle FSH and LH concentrations are measured in the early follicular phase. Progesterone concentration on day 21 can be used as an indicator of ovulation.

Androgens

Testosterone is the most biologically important androgen secreted by the testis. *In utero* testosterone is essential for the development of male internal genitalia. For development of male external genitalia testosterone must be converted to dihydrotestosterone by the enzyme 5α-reductase. Deficiency of this enzyme is a cause of male pseudohermaphroditism. Testosterone is necessary for the development of male secondary sexual characteristics and for spermatogenesis and also has anabolic actions. In early childhood plasma testosterone is barely detectable but the concentration rises rapidly at puberty. Testosterone is present in the female being both secreted from the ovaries and arising from the metabolism of androgens from the adrenal. Its concentration in the female is about one tenth of that in the male.

Oestrogens

The major ovarian oestrogen is 17β-oestradiol. Oestrone is secreted from the ovary and is also

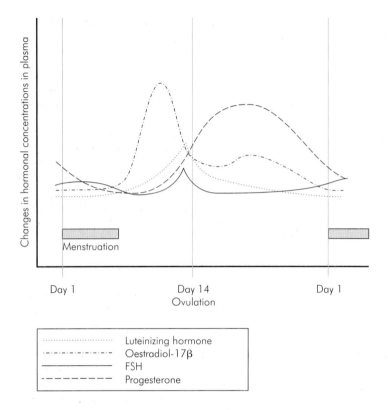

Figure 23.1 – Hormonal events during the menstrual cycle.

produced by conversion of ovarian and adrenal androgens in liver and adipose tissue. Oestrogens are necessary for the development of female secondary sexual characteristics and for maintenance of normal menstrual cycles. In the male oestradiol is secreted by the testes and produced by metabolism of testosterone, principally in adipose tissue.

Sex hormone binding globulin (SHBG) binds both testosterone and oestradiol within the circulation. About 97% of testosterone and 40% of oestradiol are bound to SHBG. The remainder is bound principally to albumin. SHBG has a greater affinity for testosterone than for oestradiol; SHBG concentrations in females are about twice those in males.

Progesterone arises from the corpus luteum and prepares the endometrium for implantation of a fertilised ovum. If a pregnancy arises progesterone is necessary for its maintenance.

PREGNANCY

If conception occurs, the fertilised ovum implants in the endometrium. The chorion and developing placenta produce hCG which has actions similar to LH. hCG prevents involution of the corpus luteum with the result that oestrogen and progesterone concentrations continue to increase and the endometrium is preserved. Prolactin secretion increases throughout the second and third trimesters of pregnancy secondary to the high circulating concentration of oestrogens. Together with oestrogen, progesterone and human placental lactogen (hPL), a peptide hormone synthesised by the placenta, prolactin prepares the breast for lactation. The presence of oestrogen inhibits milk secretion so that lactation does not occur until oestrogen concentrations fall at delivery. Oxytocin, from the posterior pituitary, is thought to have a role in the ejection of milk from the breast. Prolactin secretion is stimulated by suckling and high concentrations inhibit gonadotrophin secretion resulting in decreased fertility immediately following childbirth. Prolactin concentrations decrease to reach non-pregnant levels by about three months post-partum, even if lactation is continued.

MONITORING OF PREGNANCY

The presence of hCG can be used as a test for pregnancy. Most assays measure the β-subunit of hCG which can be detected in maternal blood at about one week after conception and in urine by about 10 days.

Monitoring of pregnancy includes that of both mother and fetus. Screening for maternal glycosuria and proteinuria is mandatory during pregnancy. It is usual to test for glycosuria at every ante-natal clinic visit and to measure the maternal random plasma glucose concentration at about 26 weeks of gestation. Whilst trace glycosuria is a relatively common event during pregnancy due to a decrease in the renal threshold for glucose, significant glycosuria or a random plasma glucose concentration > 6.6 mmol/L are indications for a glucose tolerance test to demonstrate or exclude the presence of gestational diabetes mellitus. Proteinuria may indicate the development of pre-eclampsia. Pre-eclampsia is a condition unique to pregnancy, in which there is a triad of proteinuria, oedema and hypertension. Elevation of plasma aspartate-transaminase activity and urate concentration can be used as early indicators of the development of liver and renal damage in pre-eclampsia. Careful maternal monitoring is also required in pregnancies in women with pre-existing medical conditions such as diabetes and phenylketonuria.

Formerly, fetal monitoring included measurement of substances such as hPL, hCG and oestriol in maternal serum or urine. Recent advances in ultrasound technology have meant that this is the method of choice for the monitoring of fetal wellbeing in most cases. The role of biochemistry in fetal monitoring is in the detection of fetal abnormalities.

Alphafetoprotein (AFP) is a glycoprotein synthesised by fetal liver and yolk sac. In abnormalities such as neural tube defects and exomphalos, maternal AFP concentrations are raised, reflecting leakage from exposed fetal blood vessels. Maternal AFP concentrations are decreased in Downs syndrome pregnancies as is the concentration of unconjugated oestriol. Maternal βhCG concentration is increased in Downs syndrome and these three measurements form the basis of the 'triple test' used as a screening test for Downs syndrome. However, this is being supplemented by the ultrasonic measurement of nuchal translucency thickness. A positive screening test for Downs can be confirmed by chromosome analysis performed on fetal material obtained by chorionic villus sampling or at amniocentesis. DNA analysis of chorionic villus samples enables rapid ante-natal diagnosis of a number of inherited disorders at an early stage of pregnancy.

ORAL CONTRACEPTIVES AND HORMONE REPLACEMENT THERAPY (HRT)

Gonadal steroids are used as oral contraceptives and as sex hormone replacement therapy. Oral contraceptives consist of a combination of oestrogen and progestogen or of a progestogen alone (the 'mini-pill'). Side-effects of oral contraceptives include adverse effects on glucose tolerance and on blood clotting. HRT is used after the natural menopause and in women with premature ovarian failure. HRT alleviates many of the symptoms of menopause and aids maintenance of bone mass, thus decreasing the tendency to osteoporosis. HRT also helps to protect against cardio-vascular disease. In males testosterone may be used in conditions where endogenous production is decreased.

DISORDERS OF GONADAL FUNCTION

Gonadal dysfunction may present with features of sex hormone deficiency or with infertility. In children it may present as pubertal delay. Hypogonadism may be primary, due to disease of the gonads themselves and this is characterised by raised levels of gonadotrophins and low levels of sex hormones. In secondary hypogonadism, due to hypothalamic or pituitary disturbance concentrations of both gonadotrophins and sex hormones are low.

Male hypogonadism

Gonadal failure occurring before puberty results in lack of development of secondary sexual characteristics and male musculature. There is delayed closure of the epiphyses which leads to a 'eunuchoid' habitus characterised by increased arm span and leg length. When gonadal failure occurs after puberty it can present as impotence or infertility and there may also be a decrease in body hair. Causes of male hypogonadism are shown in Table 23.1.

In Klinefelter's syndrome there is primary hypogonadism associated with the presence of one or more additional X chromosomes, the most common karyotype being 47XXY. Clinically these patients are found to have a eunuchoid habitus and small testes. Gynaecomastia is common due to an increase in the normal oestradiol-testosterone ratio.

Hypogonadotrophic hypogonadism may result from abnormalities affecting the hypothalamus or pituitary for example tumours or surgery and may also be congenital. In Kallman's syndrome hypogonadotrophic hypogonadism is associated with anosmia. Testosterone replacement therapy is used in the treatment of

CAUSES OF MALE HYPOGONADISM
Primary
structural abnormalities of testes
Klinefelter's syndrome
drugs (e.g. cytotoxics)
irradiation
Secondary
Disorders of pituitary gland
tumours
hypopituitarism
isolated gonadotrophin deficiency
Disorders of hypothalamus
Kallman's syndrome

Table 23.1

male hypogonadism and in hypogonadotrophic hypogonadism fertility may sometimes be successfully treated with GnRH.

Gynaecomastia

Gynaecomastia is the development of breast tissue in males and is usually due to perturbation of the oestrogen to androgen ratio. Causes of gynaecomastia are shown in Table 23.2.

In the neonatal period and during puberty gynaecomastia is due to temporary increase in circulating oestrogen. Decreased testosterone secretion in later life may also lead to gynaecomastia. Other causes include hepatic disorders in which oestrogens are increased and Klinefelter's syndrome in which androgen concentrations are low. Drugs causing gynaecomastia do so via a number of different mechanisms.

Oligo-amenorrhoea and amenorrhoea

The most common abnormalities of gonadal function in women are oligo-amenorrhoea and amenorrhoea. Oligo-amenorrhoea is infrequent menstruation and amenorrhoea is the complete absence of menstruation. Amenorrhoea may be primary, when menstruation has never occurred, or secondary. Causes of oligo-amenorrhoea are shown in Table 23.3.

Pregnancy is the most common cause of amenorrhoea and needs to be excluded from the differential diagnosis. Weight loss, emotional stress and excessive exercise are thought to cause oligo-amenorrhoea via hypothalamic mechanisms. Turner's syndrome is due to the

CAUSES OF GYNAECOMASTIA	
Physiological	neonatal
	pubertal
Increased oestrogens	liver disease
Decreased androgens	Klinfelter's syndrome
	androgen insensitivity
Drugs	digoxin
	spironolocatone
	cimetidine

Table 23.2

CAUSES OF OLIGO-AMENORRHOEA	
Primary	
Congenital	Turner's syndrome
Premature menopause	autoimmune
	idiopathic
Secondary	
Pituitary dysfunction	tumours
	hypopituitarism
	isolated gonadotrophin deficency
Hypothalamic dysfunction	stress
	weight loss
Polycycstic ovary syndrome	
Thyroid dysfunction	

Table 23.3

presence of an XO karyotype and is characterised by short stature, dysmorphic features and gonadal dysgenesis. In the polycystic ovary syndrome (PCOS) cystic ovaries are associated with oligo- or amenorrhoea and sometimes with hirsutism, insulin-resistance and obesity. Biochemical investigation usually shows normal FSH but elevated LH concentrations.

Replacement of female gonadal hormones can be achieved by the use of oestrogens and progestogen given in a cyclic way, usually in the form of an oral contraceptive pill. To aid fertility in hypothalamic or pituitary disorders FSH and LH can be given, with hCG used to simulate a mid-cycle LH surge. Whilst sex hormone replacement should be given in primary ovarian failure, fertility cannot be restored. Clomiphene is an oestrogen receptor blocker which brings about increased GnRH and thus FSH and LH secretion. It can be used to promote ovulation in PCOS.

Hirsutism

Hirsutism is an increase in a woman's body hair with a male pattern distribution. It can be due to increased tissue sensitivity to androgens, increased androgen secretion or a decreased concentration of SHBG. PCOS is the commonest cause of hirsutism. Other endocrine causes include Cushing's syndrome, congenital adrenal hyperplasia and androgen secreting tumours. Biochemical evaluation should include measurement of FSH, LH testosterone, SHBG and 17-hydroxyprogesterone. Cyproterone is an anti-androgenic agent which can be effective in the treatment of hirsutism. Hirsutism may be associated with other androgenic effects such as temporal balding and cliteromegaly. This is termed virilisation and is often a manifestation of a serious underlying cause, such as an androgen secreting tumour.

SELECTED READING

Brook, C.G.D. and Marshall, W.J. *Essential Endocrinology*, 3rd Edition. Blackwell Science, 1996.

Reference ranges		
		Serum
FSH	adult females:	2–8 U/l (follicular phase)
		>15U/l (post-menopausal)
	adult males:	2–10 U/l
LH	adult females:	2–10 U/l (follicular phase)
		>20 U/l (post-menopausal)
	adult males:	2–10 U/l
Progesterone		>30 nmol/l (day 21 sample)
		indicative of ovulation
Testosterone		
	adult males:	10–30 nmol/l
	adult females:	0.5–2.5 nmol/l

24

METABOLIC ASPECTS
OF MALIGNANCY

Objectives
To understand:

- The mechanisms of neoplastic change
- The metabolic consequences of malignancy
- The use of tumour markers

FACTORS INVOLVED IN TUMOUR FORMATION	
Factor	Example
Biological	Tumour viruses Genetic factors Diet Immune deficiency
Chemical	Carcinogens
Physical	Radiation

Table 24.1

In the UK malignant tumours are the second most frequent cause of death. The most common tumours in males are those of the lung, stomach, prostate, colon and rectum. In females carcinoma of the breast is the most common. Cancer cells are not under the control of the normal regulatory mechanisms governing cell growth. They are able to invade adjacent tissue and they metastasise to distant tissues via the blood or lymph. Changes in adhesion properties, proteolytic enzymes and factors involved in angiogenesis are known to be important in the metastatic process. Disturbance of cell growth results from a decrease in its control resulting in uncontrolled proliferation. This process is due to a mutation in some part of the DNA of the cell either directly or in the genes regulating proteins involved in cell division.

MECHANISMS OF NEOPLASTIC CHANGE

Carcinogenesis results from a varying interaction between inherited and acquired genetic change. The exact mechanisms of this change are not clear for most cancers but a number of factors have been found to be important as shown in Table 24.1.

Certain viruses are known to be important in tumour formation – one of the best known associations is that of the papilloma virus and carcinoma of the cervix. A number of carcinogens have been described, for example N-nitroso compounds in cigarette smoke have been implicated in the aetiology of carcinoma of the lung. A low level of dietary fibre is associated with colonic and rectal tumours and immune deficiency is a known aetiological factor in the development of lymphoid malignancies. Irradiation by ultraviolet, gamma and X-rays is also known to be associated with tumour formation.

At a molecular level, changes in oncogenes and in tumour suppressor genes are important in neoplastic transformations.

ONCOGENES

These are closely related to proto-oncogenes which are normal cellular genes. If these proto-oncogenes become altered or activated in normal cells they are converted to oncogenes and transformation of normal cells to malignant cells takes place. Oncogenes may therefore form increased amounts of growth factors, growth factor receptors or DNA-binding proteins influencing gene expression or control of the cell cycle. A number of mechanisms are known to account for the transformation of proto-oncogenes to oncogenes. These include point mutations leading to the potentiation of the function of a gene product, amplification of the region of DNA containing the oncogene, translocation of a regulatory gene to the vicinity of the proto-oncogene or insertion of a viral gene. An example of an oncogene is *erb* B which codes for a truncated form of the epidermal growth factor.

TUMOUR SUPPRESSOR GENES

Cancer may also be the result of abnormal function of tumour suppressor genes which are important in the regulation of cellular proliferation. Failure of the action of tumour suppressor genes may result in an increase in cell proliferation or abnormal cell differentiation. An example of a suppressor is p53 which is involved in apoptosis. An abnormality of the p53 gene is therefore likely to predispose to increased cell proliferation and tumour formation. Defects of p53 have been found to be important in some tumours of the colon, rectum and breast.

METABOLIC CONSEQUENCES OF MALIGNANCY

Metabolic consequences may be the first signs of malignancy and contribute greatly to the associated morbidity and mortality. Amongst the most frequent effects are weight loss, fever, anaemia and hypercalcaemia. These changes may occur secondary to the secretion of substances by the tumour or be due to metabolism by the tumour itself.

Weight loss

Weight loss is extremely common and is usually multifactorial in origin, causes including anorexia, vomiting, secondary infections and the effects of treatment. There may be an increase in metabolic rate which may in part be due to release of cytokines, such as TNF-α, by tumours.

Anaemia

Anaemia in malignancy is also multifactorial – causes include chronic blood loss, bone marrow infiltration by malignant cells and defects in iron utilisation.

Fever

Fever may result from effects of the tumour itself or from associated problems such as infection. Tumour-induced fever is thought to be caused mainly by the action of cytokines and prostaglandins. It is particularly common in lymphomas and leukaemias.

Hypercalcaemia

Hypercalcaemia associated with malignancy is usually of sudden onset and is rapidly progressive. Mechanisms include the production of PTH-related peptide (PTH-rP) and the effects of cytokines on osteoclasts. PTH-rP is similar in structure to PTH with which it shares a receptor. Osteoclast activating factors include TNF-α and interleukins.

Paraneoplastic syndromes

Paraneoplastic syndromes occur examples including digital clubbing and acquired ichthyosis. Clubbing of the fingers comprises increased curvature of the nail bed together with swelling and thickening of the digits and may occur in non-malignant conditions but is particularly common in squamous carcinoma of the lung. In acquired icthyosis, thickening and scaling of the skin in a characteristic manner is associated particularly with lymphoid malignancies. Neurological syndromes include dermatomyositis and polymyositis, most commonly associated with carcinoma of the bronchus, breast and ovary, and peripheral neuropathy in lung tumours.

ECTOPIC HORMONE SECRETION

Tumours composed of cells that do not in health have an endocrine function may sometimes secrete hormones. The genes involved in hormone production are present in all cell types but are usually suppressed in non-endocrine tissues.

In some malignant tumours this suppression is altered and the genes are able to bring about hormone production. The products of these ectopic hormone-secreting tumours are most commonly ADH, ACTH and PTH – all peptide hormones. Ectopic secretion of ADH is most commonly due to small cell carcinoma of the bronchus but may also be found associated with pancreatic or carcinoid tumours. The secretion of ADH is not subject to normal physiological control and water retention occurs leading to dilutional hyponatraemia. ACTH production from tumours, particularly of the bronchus, may be sufficient to give rise to Cushing's syndrome.

CARCINOID TUMOURS

Carcinoid tumours arise from argentaffin cells of the APUD system. They usually occur within the small intestine, particularly the appendix, but may also arise from the bronchi, pancreas, thymus and ovary. They are reasonably common but rarely metastasise. The carcinoid syndrome occurs when products of the tumour are released into the circulation causing characteristic symptoms. This syndrome is seen most often in association with bronchial tumours as their secretions pass directly into the systemic circulation. It may occur due to the presence of hepatic metastases from a gastrointestinal tumour. The main presenting symptoms are flushing and diarrhoea. Wheezing may also occur as may fibrosis of the right side of the heart. The tumour products responsible are serotonin and various peptides.

MULTIPLE ENDOCRINE NEOPLASIA (MEN)

MEN are rare disorders inherited in an autosomal dominant manner characterised by tumours, which may be benign or malignant, of two or more endocrine glands. Once an affected patient is found screening of family members is essential. MEN can be divided into two types according to the site of the tumours as shown in Table 24.2.

CLASSIFICATION OF MEN

Type 1 (Wemer syndrome):
    Pituitary
    Pancreas
    Parathyroids

Type 2 (Sipple syndrome):
    Medullary carcinoma of the thyroid
    Phaeochromocytoma
    Parathyroids

Table 24.2

TUMOUR MARKERS

A tumour marker is a substance which can be related to either the existence or progression of a tumour. It may be secreted by a tumour or be present on its surface. Ideally a tumour marker could be used for screening and diagnosis, to predict prognosis, to monitor response to therapy and to detect residual disease or recurrence. As yet there is no tumour marker which completely fulfils all these functions but a number of markers have become established in clinical practice.

Alpha-fetoprotein (AFP) and human chorionic gonadotrophin (hCG)

Alpha-fetoprotein (AFP) and human chorionic gonadotrophin (hCG) are glycoproteins useful in the management of germ cell tumours. The measurement of AFP alone is useful in the management of primary hepatocellular carcinoma and is useful in screening patients at high risk, for example those with hepatitis B infection or known cirrhosis. βhCG measurement can be used in screening for choriocarcinoma in at risk women who have had a previous pregnancy associated with a hydatidiform mole.

Prostate specific antigen (PSA)

Prostate specific antigen (PSA) is used as a tumour marker in carcinoma of the prostate. However a raised concentration may be present in benign prostatic hypertrophy which means its measurement is not of use as a screening test. Measurement of PSA is of value in the diagnosis and follow up of carcinoma of the prostate.

Calcitonin

Calcitonin is a tumour marker for medullary carcinoma of the thyroid. This condition may be hereditary and measurement of calcitonin is useful for screening family members. Affected family members may have normal basal calcitonin concentrations but show an exaggerated rise after stimulation with alcohol or pentagastrin.

Carcinoembryonic antigen (CEA)

Carcinoembryonic antigen (CEA) is elevated in colorectal carcinoma but may be elevated in normal subjects, especially those who smoke and in non-malignant disorders such as liver disease and pancreatitis. The measurement of CEA is not of use in screening or to make a diagnosis of colorectal cancer but may be useful in monitoring response to treatment.

Paraproteins

Paraproteins are immunoglobulins produced by a single clone of B cells and are detectable in the serum and urine of almost all patients with myeloma. The presence of a paraprotein is useful in the diagnosis of myeloma and serial measurements can be used to monitor response to treatment.

Carbohydrate antigen (CA)

Carbohydrate antigen (CA) markers are glycoproteins recognised by monoclonal antibodies to tumour cells. A number have been identified but none, as yet, is specific for a particular tumour. Their use therefore is mainly in monitoring and follow up rather than for diagnosis. Examples include CA 125 for ovarian carcinoma and CA19–9 for pancreatic tumours.

SELECTED READING

Marshall, W.J. and Bangert, S.K. (eds). *Clinical Biochemistry: Metabolic and Clinical Aspects*. Churchill Livingstone, Edinburgh. 1995.

25

NUTRITION AND NUTRITIONAL DISORDERS

Objectives

To understand:

- The assessment of nutitional status

- Dietary components - carbohydrate, fat, protein vitamins and trace elements

- The principles of artificial nutritional support

Food is a requirement for life. The quality and quantity of the diet taken are important — overnutrition leading to obesity with increased morbidity and mortality, undernutrition leading to weight loss and eventual starvation. Poor quality diets have significant effects on health — for example a high fat intake predisposes to cardiovascular disease.

ASSESSMENT OF NUTRITIONAL STATUS

This can be performed by clinical examination, anthropometric measurements or laboratory investigations. Whilst carefully performed clinical examination is informative, anthropometry — measurement of the body — may provide a more accurate indication of nutritional status. In children growth is an important indicator, in adults the usefulness of height is in assessing the significance of weight as can be seen from Table 25.1. Measurement of the mid-arm circumference gives an indication of tissue bulk. Measurement of skinfold thickness, most usually in the triceps or subscapular regions, measured with specially designed callipers, gives an indication of body fat stores. Unless carefully performed skinfold measurements can be

THE USE OF BODY WEIGHT IN THE ASSESSMENT OF NUTRITIONAL STATUS	
Body mass index (BMI) = $\dfrac{\text{weight (kg)}}{(\text{height in metres})^2}$	
BMI Description	
<20	Underweight
>20-25	Desirable
>25-30	Overweight
>30	Obese

Table 25.1

subject to errors, both inter-and intra-observer. The triceps skin fold and mid-arm circumference may be used to calculate the mid-arm muscle circumference, which reflects muscle mass, as a further nutitionl indicaor. All these indices are particularly useful as serial measurements of nutritional status.

Laboratory investigation of specific nutritional deficiencies, for example those of folate and iron can be easily performed. The quantification of general malnutrition by laboratory indices is more difficult. Albumin is frequently measured and, whilst low plasma concentrations can reflect poor dietary protein intake albumin concentration is affected by liver disease, fluid balance and the acute phase response. The half-life of albumin is about a month. Proteins with a shorter half-life sometimes used as nutritional indicators include pre-albumin, transferrin and retinol binding protein.

ENERGY

Dietary energy is obtained from a combination of carbohydrate and fat. Energy requirement is dependent upon basal metabolic rate (BMR), which can be measured accurately using isotopic methods or direct or indirect calorimetry. More practically, BMR is calculated using the Harris-Benedict or Schofield equations with adjustments made for factors such as activity levels or severe illness.

CARBOHYDRATE

Dietary carbohydrate include sugars, oligosaccharides and starches and provides 4kcal/g. Some tissues require carbohydrate as an obligatory energy substrate, for example brain and erythrocytes.

FAT

The majority of dietary fat is in the form of triacylglycerols but also includes phospholipids and sterols, for example cholesterol. Fat has a higher energy content than carbohydrate, providing 10kcal/g.

PROTEIN

Protein provides about 12% of total calories of the Western diet and contains 4kcal/g. Human protein contains twenty amino acids, nine of which are "essential" and must be provided in the diet. Essential amino acids are shown in Table 25.2.

ESSENTIAL AMINO ACIDS
Histidine
Isoleucine
Leucine
Lysine
Methionine
Phenylalanine
Threonine
Tryptophan
Valine

Table 25.2

Protein energy malnutrition (PEM) is prevalent in the developing world, particularly in children, secondary to their high energy requirements for growth. Two syndromes of PEM are recognised — marasmus and kwashiorkor. Marasmus tends to occur within the first year of life and is associated with severe energy deficit. The presentation of kwashiorkor is normally more acute in a young child whose diet contains very little protein. Classically there is associated oedema, skin rash and hepatomegaly. The relatively increased carbohydrate content of the diet in kwashiorkor may result in the maintenance of insulin secretion. Whilst this spares muscle protein it limits the amino acids available for hepatic protein synthesis — particularly of albumin, which may explain the oedema.

TRACE ELEMENTS

Trace elements are those present in tissues at a concentration of less than 50mg/kg. At least eight are known to be essential, deficiency being associated with specific disorder, usually occurring in association with protein-energy malnutrition, severe systemic disease — particularly of the gastrointestinal tract, or inappropriate artificial feeding. Due to changes in protein binding, plasma concentrations do not necessarily reflect tissue stores, which may make assessment of trace element stores difficult. Recommended daily intakes have been established for enteral but not for intravenous intake.

ZINC

Zinc is important for many enzymes including those involved in DNA synthesis. In the inherited disorder acrodermatitis enteropathica there is a defect in zinc absorption. Severe deficiency results, characterised by a symmetrical skin rash and diarrhoea. Lesser degrees of deficiency have been associated with delayed wound healing and increased susceptibility to infection.

COPPER

Copper-containing proteins include dopamine hydroxylase and cytochrome C oxidase. Features of deficiency, described in infants with poor nutrition, and with the inherited disorder of copper metabolism Menke's disease, include hypochromic, microcytic anaemia, neutropenia and fractures.

SELENIUM

Selenium is part of the glutathione peroxidase complex and is also important for the conversion of thyroxine to triiodothyronine. Deficiency has been linked to the cardiomyopathy Keshan disease and the osteo-arthropathy Kashin-Beck disease, endemic to parts of China. Very low plasma levels are usually only seen in patients on parenteral nutrition or very severely restricted diets for the treatment of inherited metabolic disease.

MOLYBDENUM

Molybdenum is required as a cofactor for activity of certain oxidase enzymes. Deficiency has been described in a patient receiving parenteral nutrition and an inherited abnormality of the cofactor exists associated with neurological abnormalities, lens dislocations and xanthinuria.

MANAGANESE

Manganese is a component and activator of enzymes. Deficiency has been described in animals and in association with PN. Toxicity has been described in patients receiving long term PN and in manganese miners and is clinically similar to Parkinson's disease.

CHROMIUM

The exact role of chromium is unsure but deficiency is known to affect glucose tolerance and peripheral nerve function.

COBALT AND IODINE

Cobalt is necessary as a constituent of Vitamin B_{12} (Chapter 21) and iodine for the formation of thyroid hormones (Chapter 21)

VITAMINS

Vitamins are divided into water-soluble and fat-soluble (vitamins A, D, E and K). Distinction is useful as, in those disorders where fat absorption is particularly compromised, it predicts which deficiencies are likely to occur. Plasma concentrations of Vitamin B_{12} and folate are measured in the assessment of anaemia and vitamin D in the evaluation of metabolic bone diseases. Measurement of some vitamins is not made by assay of plasma concentrations — for example assessment of riboflavin status involves measurement of red cell glutathione reductase. However toxicity of most vitamins is rare and the response to a trial of therapy is often taken as proof of deficiency so measurement is rarely required.

VITAMIN A

Vitamin A is ingested as carotene or retinol, found in large quantities in liver, vegetables and fruit. Its active form 11-cis retinal is required by the rods of the eye and, as retinoic acid, it is important for epithelial cell differentiation. Vitamin A deficiency leads to night blindness and corneal ulceration and keratinisation. Deficiency also predisposes to infection of the gastrointestinal and respiratory tracts.

VITAMIN D

Vitamin D is discussed in Chapter 19.

VITAMIN E

Eight structurally similar compounds with anti-oxidant effects have vitamin E activity. Dietary sources include those rich in polyunsaturated fatty acids, particularly vegetable oils. Deficiency can occur in steatorrhoea and in the inherited disorder abetalipoproteinaemia — haemolytic anaemia and neurological features result.

VITAMIN K

Vitamin K is found in liver and leafy vegetables but is also synthesised by colonic bacteria. It is necessary for the γ-carboxylation of clotting factors and bone matrix proteins. Deficiency leads to bleeding and can be monitored by assessing clotting times.

THIAMIN (VITAMIN B_1)

Thiamine is important as a coenzyme in carbohydrate metabolism dietary sources including yeasts, vegetables and some meats. It is the vitamin with the smallest body store and deficiency may be unmasked by refeeding a carbohydrate-rich diet. The clinical features of beri-beri respond to thiamine treatment suggesting it is caused by deficiency. Deficiency may also present as Wernicke's encephalopathy or Korsakoff's psychosis. Measurement of erythrocyte transketolase activity may be used for confirmation of deficiency.

RIBOFLAVIN (VITAMIN B_2)

Riboflavin is found in offal and dairy products and is essential for oxidative metabolism. Deficiency leads to skin lesions, cheilosis and stomatitis.

NIACIN

The term niacin refers to nicotinic acid and its amide, a component of NAD and NADP. The daily requirement can be met from the diet and from metabolism of tryptophan. Dietary deficiency leads to pellagra, characterised by dermatitis in sun-exposed areas, diarrhoea and dementia. Pellagra can also rise in the inherited disorder of tryptophan absorption Hartnup disease and in carcinoid syndrome, in which tryptophan is used for the metabolism for large quantities of 5-hydroxytryptamine.

VITAMIN B_6

Vitamin B_6 activity is possessed by pyridoxine and related compounds which catalyse reactions of amino acids. Vitamin B_6 is obtained from many dietary components and synthesised by gut bacteria thus isolated deficiency is rare but has been described and results in neuropathy. Drugs, for example isoniazid, can interfere with the vitamin's metabolism causing a relative deficiency.

VITAMIN C

Vitamin C in the tissues is mostly in the form of L-ascorbic acid. It functions as an anti-oxidant and is important in collagen formation and in the intestinal absorption of non-haem iron. Main dietary sources are fruits and vegetables and deficiency causes scurvy characterised by bleeding gums, poor wound healing and impaired iron absorption.

NUTRITION SUPPORT

The incidence of malnutrition in hospitalised patients has been shown to be as high as 50%. However, the degree of nutrition support required varies from simple encouragement to eat the food provided through to the administration of all nutrients by an intravenous route. The usefulness of simple, practical measures should not be overlooked, for example providing a liquid diet for a patient with chewing or swallowing difficulties or a carer for a patient who needs to be fed.

ENTERAL FEEDING

Nutritional support via the gut (enteral feeding) should be used if possible. Integrity of the gastro-intestinal mucosa requires nutrients from the lumen, some of the substrates required such as glutamine and short chain fatty acids not being routinely provided in intravenous feeding solutions. Compared with intravenous feeding enteral feeding stimulates gall bladder contractility, therefore decreasing the likelihood of gallstones, results in fewer metabolic complications and is cheaper.

Supplements and sip feeds

A range of supplements and sip feeds exist in many flavours, some of which can be used as an adjunct to a normal diet and others, which are nutritionally complete, as its replacement.

Tube feeds

Tube feeds are of two basic types — polymeric and elemental. Polymeric feeds are the most widely used and contain whole protein, carbohydrate and hydrolysed fat. They can be provided with a composition adjusted in a particular disease state — for example low sodium content in a patient with liver disease and ascites. Elemental formulae contain protein in the form of short chain peptides or amino acids, monosaccharides and an increased proportion of medium chain triglycerides. The feed is usually administered through a fine-bore nasogastric tube. Alternatives include a gastrostomy tube, placed directly though the abdominal wall into the stomach, or via a jejunostomy. Complications of enteral feeding include regurgitation, pulmonary aspiration, tube malposition, displacement and occlusion, abdominal pain, bloating and diarrhoea. Drug interactions may occur with the feed and less commonly, metabolic abnormalities such as hypergly-

caemia, hyperkalaemia and hypophosphataemia can occur.

PARENTERAL NUTRITION

The absolute indication for parenteral nutrition (PN) is a non-functioning gut, for example secondary to the short bowel syndrome or radiation enteritis. Other indications include paralytic ileus and complex fluid balance problems due to sequestration of fluid within the gut lumen.

Parenteral feeds usually consist of lipid emulsions, amino acids and hypertonic glucose with vitamins and trace elements supplied in one "big bag" ready for intravenous infusion. Energy requirement is the same as for enteral nutrition. Whilst trace elements and vitamins are given according to recommended daily intakes, these values are for a normal diet. As much of the control of absorption of these substances takes place at gut level it is less certain how much should be given intravenously. Meeting up to 50% of energy requirements with lipid decreases the osmolality of the mixture and the incidence of hyperglycaemia and has the benefit of limiting the formation of carbon dioxide, which can be of benefit in patients with respiratory problems.

Monitoring of patients receiving PN should include careful recording of fluid balance and regular measurement of body weight. Biochemical measurement should be performed to ensure that the potential complications of hyper- or hypo-natraemia, kalaemia, phosphataemia and magnesaemia can be detected and corrected before becoming severe. Regular blood glucose monitoring should be performed because hyperglycaemia may occur, particularly in patients with intercurrent sepsis or pre-existing diabetes mellitus, and requires insulin for its control. Hepatobiliary dysfunction may occur, initially obvious as increased activity of enzymes that indicate cholestasis, for example alkaline phosphatase and γ-glutamyl transferase. If PN continues impaired hepatic function can occur and, in children may progress to irreversible liver failure requiring transplantation.

SELECTED READING

Truswell, A.S. (ed). *ABC of Human Nutrition*, 3rd ed. London: BMJ Books, 1999.

Garrow, J.S. and James, W.P.T. (eds). *Human Nutrition and Dietetics*, 9th Ed. Edinburgh: Churchill Livingstone, 1993.

Index

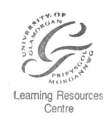